Microdosing

WITH

Amanita Muscaria

Microdosing
WITH
Amanita Muscaria

Creativity, Healing, and Recovery
with the Sacred Mushroom

Baba Masha, M.D.

Park Street Press
Rochester, Vermont

Park Street Press
One Park Street
Rochester, Vermont 05767
www.ParkStPress.com

Park Street Press is a division of Inner Traditions International

Cataloging-in-Publication Data for this title is available from the Library of Congress

ISBN 978-1-64411-505-3 (print)
ISBN 978-1-64411-506-0 (ebook)

Printed and bound in China by Reliance Printing Co., Ltd.

10 9 8 7 6 5 4 3 2

Text design by Priscilla H. Baker and layout by Virginia Scott Bowman
This book was typeset in Garamond Premier Pro and Futura with Bigola Display
and Gill Sans used as display typefaces

To send correspondence to the author of this book, mail a first-class letter
to the author c/o Inner Traditions • Bear & Company, One Park Street,
Rochester, VT 05767, and we will forward the communication, contact the
author via comments on her YouTube channel **https://www.youtube.com/c
/AMANITAMicroDosingbabaMasha** (in Russian with English closed captioning),
or contact her on Telegram at @ **babMaiiia**.

❖❖❖

Dedicated to James Fadiman

Contents

Foreword

James Fadiman

Most people stop at the Z, but not me . . .
You'll be sort of surprised what there is to be found
Once you go beyond Z and start poking around!
DR. SUESS, *ON BEYOND ZEBRA* (1955)

Baba Masha, the name the author of this book goes by, says its contents came about through a series of "mystical accidents." While there is a certain honest humility in that description, she does not give herself nearly enough credit. This is not only a book of discovery, but a wonderful example of how actual discovery happens, how much work there is to bring it about, and what it is in a life that makes a person sensitive or able to appreciate the import of the new knowledge when it appears. As important as being able to recognize what you have found, is to have the capacity to follow up on the initial discovery, and to keep opening other unanticipated doors. Baba Masha has done all that and more.

The book details thousands of healings that are not only unusual, but, as you will see, invaluable. To recognize them Masha had to overcome the most difficult of all obstacles—a strong, well-educated, and substantiated disbelief in what you are being told.

Science, in spite of its own opinion of itself, is often dead wrong. For example, there was a period in relatively modern European history when a number of natural history museums disposed of their collections of meteorites since the scientists of the day agreed, "Meteorites cannot exist, because there are no stones in the sky to fall." Before you smile at their folly, reflect first on the accuracy of their statement. While we know that meteorites originate beyond the sky, that reality was not the obvious wisdom it is today. Right logic, wrong assumptions.

What is the science of today as it pertains to *Amanita muscaria*? Right now, if you open any mushroom identification book to *Amanita muscaria,* after it describes its shape, color, varieties, where found and so forth, it will add that it is toxic. In some books the toxic descriptions can be quite extensive, but even this brief one from Wikipedia should cool most anyone's interest in trying any:

> Fly agarics [*Amanita muscaria*] are known for the unpredictability of their effects. Depending on habitat and the amount ingested per body weight, effects can range from mild nausea and twitching to drowsiness, cholinergic crisis-like effects (low blood pressure, sweating, and salivation), auditory and visual distortions, mood changes, euphoria, relaxation, ataxia, and loss of equilibrium like with tetanus.

What these reference books usually leave out is that *Amanita muscaria* has centuries of good press. It is probably the best-known mushroom by sight to children and adults alike, appearing as the Christmas mushroom on everything from those Victorian lithographs with Santa, elves, and reindeer, to contemporary holiday cards and animations.

It is the mushroom credited by the mycological scholar R. Gordon Wasson and later by John Brough as "Soma" a substance described in detail in the *Rig-Veda* (ca. 1500 BCE) that, when ingested, makes one aware of one's relationship to Divinity. As Soma was not described as having seeds, flowers, leaves, or roots, the scholars reasoned that Soma was likely a mushroom and most likely *Amanita muscaria.*

As is always the case, other scholars disagreed.

More controversial was a theory proposed by John Allegro, a philologist, archaeologist, and Dead Sea scrolls scholar, that Christianity itself was a religion centered on the ritual use of this mushroom and that perhaps Christ was not a living person, but the essential nature of *Amanita muscaria.*

Even more scholars disagreed with this possibility. Among the arguments put forth by those who have a very different idea of the origins of Christianity is that *Amanita muscaria* grows predominantly in Northern Hemisphere forests and the necessary trees the mushroom needs to propagate were unlikely to have even been in the Holy Land in that era. More recent scholarship has found paintings in a number of medieval churches clearly linking Jesus and saints with this specific mushroom.[1]

Fairly impressive credentials for a "toxic" mushroom.

As positive as all these possibilities are, contemporary descriptions and cases like the following are what gives *Amanita muscaria* its toxic designation.

On March 3, 1897, Count Achilles de Vecchj, an Italian diplomat being hosted by people in Virginia, requested a breakfast of *Amanita muscaria,* sadly confusing it with *Amanita caesarea,* an edible Italian mushroom that looks much the same. He ate between one and two dozen mushrooms and died several hours later. His convulsions were so severe that he broke the bed he was lying on. "Out of his death and its ensuing lurid and widespread publicity, sprang a renewed North American interest in mushroom societies, especially in the Northeast, to provide much needed public education about edible and poisonous wild mushrooms."[2] Yet, in 2008, a paper was published in the highly respected journal *Economic Botany* that proposed that *Amanita muscaria* be considered as a "safe" and broadly accepted "edible" species.[3]

Dismayed, perhaps even horrified, by the suggestion, the distinguished botanist, naturalist, and *Amanita* expert, Debbie Viess wrote an extensive scholarly article savaging almost every assertion and reexamining every reference in the earlier article to make it clear that to describe *Amanita muscaria* as anything other than toxic was a disservice to science and a danger to mushroom finders, professional or amateur.[4]

What then happens when Masha, a well-trained researcher and physician in her own right, hosting an extremely popular nationwide program in Russia discussing people's experiences using all kinds of psychedelics, gets a single report from someone who has been taking low doses of *Amanita muscaria* for his "health"? Her initial reaction: In his ignorance he might be killing himself.

If I were reporting about a video drama series, this would be a moment of dramatic tension. We, the viewers, would be left to wonder, is this doctor going be able to intervene and save this person? (And will it take several more episodes in the series before we find out?)

Reality, of course, is far stranger. Masha pushed past her training, past her own belief system, and thus began a counter-intuitive adventure where the looming edifice of prior science gets replaced with stacks and stacks of real-world evidence. What unfolds is a groundbreaking, paradigm-busting, citizen-science driven, alternative finding that the experts had never noticed, maybe never considered looking for.

There is a Sufi story about a person who passes by opportunity after opportunity for his own enlightenment. The story ends with the teacher saying, "That's why there are so many seekers and so few finders." Masha is one of those rare individuals, more enticed by an unmarked trail than what's already on the map. This was not her first encounter acting against conventional culture and likely not her last.

She was trained not only to be a physician, but to be an observer, paying more attention to the whole patient than to symptoms. That she had become adept in the use of contemporary media also aided her when the first reports about using *Amanita muscaria* came to her. Perhaps no one else had had the background or the opportunities. If they had, they walked by them out of ignorance or, perhaps, lacked sufficient curiosity.

I've been working with microdoses of conventional psychedelics like LSD and psilocybin mushrooms for ten years. Early on, I felt I was discovering a secret that everyone else had overlooked. Fairly inflated with myself, I spoke to a friend with a background in anthropology and a knowledge of substances. He said, "Has it occurred to you that indigenous people might have tried smaller doses of these substances over the few thousand years they have been using them?" It had not.

I was almost convinced that, like Masha, a series of mystical accidents and years of preparation had favored me. However, I recently got back in touch with my friend to ask about using microdoses for better sleeping, since all of the reports I had were from people taking them early in the day. He told me how to use them for sleep, but then told me the following account, about his 1976 visit to the village where Maria Sabina lived. She was the curandero who first shared the existence of, and the rituals associated with, psilocybin mushrooms for healing and divination. As related to me by my friend:

> Back to the trail and our foray . . . on the climb up—and the 600-meter ascent (1,969 feet) really is a climb even for a mule—we encountered people backpacking up loads of firewood and tried to keep up with two guys who were quite open to sharing information and had some (mushroom) fruitings at their home, but they outpaced us even with their heavier loads. I told them we couldn't keep up. We rested a bit and the conversation turned to their fitness. They divulged that they microdosed so they would be able to walk right up the mountain under a heavy load without feeling tired. That was my first exposure to the idea, two informants actually microdosing, when they told us. I thereafter used the technique myself to backpack up mountains and can attest to how well it works.

In short, although the village had been overrun for years with gringos looking for mushrooms for everything from an exotic high to a profound encounter with God as well as researchers from all over the world, common microdose use had gone unnoticed or been ignored. In 1976 my friend had encountered a society that used microdoses, cultivating the mushroom in their own gardens, and had fully integrated them into their lives. Perhaps he was not the person, perhaps it was not the time, and perhaps it was just as well that it stayed unknown.

Thirty-five years later, when I first started to explore microdoses, having been told about them by Robert Forte, who had heard about them from Albert Hoffman, times had changed. Perhaps I was the person with enough curiosity and more than enough ignorance to start asking other people to microdose and tell me what their experience was like.

Masha's discoveries are a different order of magnitude. In this fore-word I have this opportunity to thank her. People who work in altered states of consciousness like opportunities to support one another, shar-ing data, opportunities, and in this case, congratulations. Just because Masha's interest is in presenting what the thousands of people who con-tributed their own stories told one another, you are reading what a dif-ference citizen science can make.

It could have gone another way. Masha could have counseled that first person to stop using the *Amanita*. She could have not told her audience about it. If she had done that, we would still not know of its healing properties.

As I was completing this foreword, I asked Masha a question. Along with her answer, she told me that she's looking at some new conditions. "More data is coming in," she said.

An explorer who, after a long voyage, comes back into port to unload treasure found where no one else had been, delivers a long report to those who sponsored the voyage. While in port she is honored by dignitaries, interviewed by academics, given awards, and asked to make speeches. However, after a while she is back down at the port, hiring on a new crew, and testing the new sails and ropes. A few days later she is gone, taking advantage of a strong breeze and a rising tide.

Good sailing, Masha!

When you return there will be a lot of us welcoming you at the dock.

Thank you for what you've done. Thank you for what you're doing. Thank you.

JAMES FADIMAN, PH.D., has been researching psychedelics since 1961 and the effect of microdosing since 2010. As well as holding consulting, training, counseling, and editorial jobs, he has taught psychology and design engineering at San Francisco State, Brandeis, and Stanford and, for three decades, taught Sufism and other classes at Sophia University, which he cofounded. He has published textbooks, professional books, a self-help book, a novel, a produced play, and videos, including *Drugs: The Children Are Choosing* for National Public Television. He was featured in a National Geographic documentary and had three solo shows of his nature photography. His most recent books are *The Psychedelic Explorer's Guide: Safe, Therapeutic, and Sacred Journeys* and *Your Symphony of Selves: Discover and Understand More of Who We Are* (coauthored with Jordan Gruber).

Opening Remarks

The important thing is not to stop questioning. Curiosity has its own reason for existing.

ALBERT EINSTEIN

This book is the result of an international study of the medicinal effects of *Amanita muscaria* microdosing with more than 3,000 volunteer trials. This endeavor was inspired by a series of mystical accidents, the so-called synchronicity. The project was created and supported by public efforts, gaining strength and unfolding before the participants' eyes. The information captured in this book is a reflection of inexhaustible curiosity, incredible activity, and the enthusiasm of the contributors to this research. It was a prodigious community effort.

I am incredibly grateful to my YouTube followers, Telegram subscribers, community members, my associate Thomas, and administrators in my chat rooms who generously engaged with me during this research. I am also indebted to J. Fadiman for guiding and motivating me to write this book. Finally, my deepest love and gratitude go out to my family. Their encouragement and support enabled me to finish my research. Thank you very much.

The primary goal of this book is to share with the readers the data I compiled on *Amanita muscaria* microdosing. The information is based on accumulated and publicly well-documented data in progress. It presents the experiential material of *Amanita muscaria* microdosing reception on a large, international scale.

The information provided in this book is for educational purposes only and should not be taken as advocacy for *Amanita muscaria* use.

All men by nature desire to know.

ARISTOTLE, *METAPHYSICS*

PART ONE

Meeting
Amanita muscaria

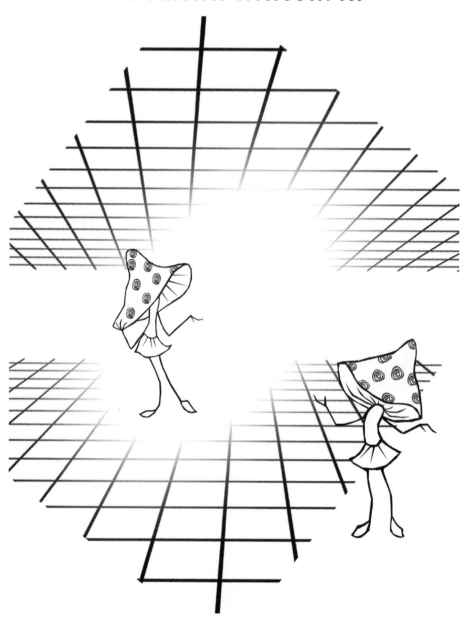

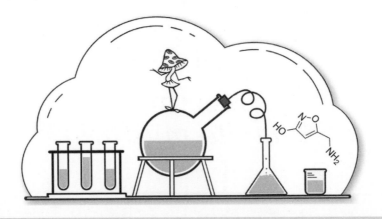

CHAPTER 1

Introduction to *Amanita muscaria*

Whenever you find yourself on the side of the majority, it is time to pause and reflect.

MARK TWAIN

Amanita muscaria in History

The original name *Amanita muscaria* comes from the ancient Greek αμανίτης (amanítis), modern amānītai—*Amanita* (a fungus) + Latin *musca* ("fly"). The *Amanita muscaria* (AM)* has a surprising equivalent all over the world and is connected to the "flykiller": fly agaric (English); *Haetorimodashi* (Japanese); *Hongomosquero, Ho Hongomosquero,* and *Hongo Matamoscas* (Spanish); *Amanite Tue-mouches* (French); *Fliegenpilz* (German); *Mukhomor* (Russian); and *Moscario* (Italian).

Amanita muscaria is widespread throughout the Earth and is present on all continents from far north to south, occurring in Europe, Asia,

---

*Amanita muscaria is often abbreviated as AM throughout this book.

Africa, Australia, New Zealand, North America, Central America, and South America.

A growing number of molecular studies show that *Amanita muscaria* has phylogeographic structures and that its distinct lineages are usually limited to different continents.[1] Phylogenetic work indicates three geographic clades (Eurasian, Eurasian-alpine, and North American groups) within *Amanita muscaria*. Nested clade analyses (NCA) confirmed that the ancestral population of *Amanita muscaria* likely evolved in the Siberian-Beringian region and expanded their range in North America and Eurasia. In addition to range expansions, populations of all three species remained in Beringia and adapted to the cooling climate.[2]

Amanita muscaria is the oldest entheogen mushroom known to humans. The fungus was used before the Common Era (BCE) by distant ancestors, confirmed by a caveman's text carved in stone for descendants and the folklore world.

Use of the *Amanita muscaria* mushroom started in ancient times and is connected with mysticism.[3] *Amanita* goes back 50,000 years, painted by Aboriginals in Australian caves. Mushrooms and toadstools were believed to be fallen stars endowed with magic. As such, they were considered taboo, and their consumption was forbidden.[4] Representations of *Amanita* mushrooms, most prominently *Amanita muscaria,* have been reported in polychromatic rock paintings in the Sahara,[5] dating from the Paleolithic era from 9000–7000 BCE.[6] *Amanita muscaria* has had a reputation for killing flies at least as far back as the *De vegetabilibus* of Albertus Magnus in the thirteenth century. The psychoactive *Amanita* mushrooms have a well-attested entheogenic use among Siberian, European, and Pan-American shamanic peoples and are specifically implicated in the mysteries of ancient Greece (the Mysteries of Dionysus) and Rome (Mithraic Mysteries),[7] and as the original Vedic plant-god Soma,[8] and the Avestan haoma among the gnostic Manicheans and early and mystically inclined Christians of later periods.[9]

Besides various symbols that might correspond to *Amanita muscaria* and originate from northern and southern Asian traditions, some may also be discerned in Buddhist myths. In the legendary biographies of some Buddhist adepts from the second and ninth centuries, there are some clues that can be interpreted to reveal that the adepts were consuming psychedelic *Amanita muscaria*—fly agaric—mushrooms to achieve enlightenment. They appear to be echoed in Germanic tradition, possibly in some characteristics related to the god Odin.[10]

A few publications argue that Christianity originates from a cult of *Amanita muscaria*. Jesus was supposedly being invested with the energy of the mushroom,[11] but other religious and secular biblical scholars discredit this.[12]

P. J. von Strahlenberg, a Swedish colonel who was in a Siberian prisoner of war camp for twelve years, wrote the first published documentation of the effects of *Amanita muscaria* on humans. In written observations von Strahlenberg noted this:

> The Russians who trade with them (Koryak), carry thither a Kind of Mushrooms, called in the Russian tongue, Muchumur, which they exchange for Squirrels, Fox, Hermin, Sable and other Furs: Those who are rich among them lay up large Provisions of these Mushrooms, for the Winter. When they make a Feast, they pour Water upon some of these Mushrooms and boil them. They then drink the Liquor, which intoxicates them: The poorer Sort, on these Occasions, post themselves round the Huts of the Rich, and watch the Opportunity of the Guests coming down to make Water; And then hold a Wooden Bowl to receive the Urine, which they drink off greedily, as having still some Virtue of the Mushroom in it, and by this Way they also get Drunk.[13]

Known as mukhomor in Russian, the *Amanita muscaria* toadstool is the center of iconic myths and legends of the indigenous peoples of Siberian tribes—Chukchi, Koryaks, Kamchadals, Yakuts, and Yukagirs. *Amanita muscaria* was used as medicine, an entheogen for rituals, a food source, and a ceremonial drink.[14] Detailed description of the use of *Amanita muscaria* by the peoples of the far Northeast in the middle of the eighteenth century was carried out by the Imperial Academy of Sciences in St. Petersburg where, in 1755, a two-volume work of Professor S. P. Krasheninnikov, a participant of the Great Northern Expedition of 1733–1743, was published. In his book *Description of the Land of Kamchatka*, Krasheninnikov described the mukhomor (*Amanita muscaria*) intoxication in entheogen ceremonies of the Koryaks and Kazaks:

> The first and usual sign by which one can recognize a man under the influence of the mukhomor is the shaking of the extremities which will follow after an hour or less, after which the persons thus intoxicated have hallucinations, . . . while some might deem a small crack to be as wide as a door, and a tub of water as deep as the sea. But this applies only to those who overindulge, while those who use a small quantity experience a feeling of extraordinary lightness, joy, courage, and a sense of energetic wellbeing.[15]

An ethnological study of mukhomor as food, medicine, and an intoxicating and hallucinogenic agent was documented by other participants of the previously mentioned expedition—G. Steller, *Description of the Land of Kamchatka, Its Inhabitants, Their Culture, Way of Life and Customs* (1793) and Y. Lindenau, *Description of the Peoples of Siberia in the First Half of the 18th Century* (first published in 1983)—in which historical and ethnographic materials about the peoples of Siberia and the Northeast were studied. K. Merck was also part of the Northeastern Geographical Expedition of Billings-Sarychev (*Ethnographic Materials of the Northeastern Geographical Expedition of 1785–1795*), and the materials he presented must be noted as well.

Oliver Goldsmith in *The Citizen of the World* (1762) elevates mushroom intoxication to the nobility in order to comment on a moral about excessive flattery, likened to making use of excreted material. However, the central effects he describes are those of mild alcohol intoxication.

In the late nineteenth century through the mid-twentieth century, mukhomor was studied by ethnographers V. G. Bogoraz-Tan (1904) and V. I. Iohelson (1900) on the Jesup Northern Pacific Expedition. In 1957, the monumental two-volume *Mushrooms, Russia and History* by R. G. Wasson and V. P. Wasson was published, which for the first time combined well-known research in the fields of mycology and ethnobotanics, including data on the red mukhomor.

Amanita muscaria Chemistry

The chemical constituents of *Amanita muscaria* have been thoroughly investigated. Ibotenic acid, muscimol, muscarine, and muscazone are the most studied compounds. These four chemicals are found in certain species of *Amanita muscaria* throughout the world. The website inchem.org explains that they are related and are all isoxazole derivatives. Detailed mycological data have already been published.[16]

Ibotenic acid (a-amino-3-hydroxy-5-isoxazoloacetic acid 1) is an analog of the neurotransmitter glutamate, which acts as a non-selective glutamate receptor agonist.[17] Ibotenic acid is water-soluble. Any attempt at dehydration leads to decarboxylation of ibotenic acid, turning it to muscimol. Ibotenic acid is decarboxylated to muscimol in the body.[18] The molecular formula is $C_5H_6N_2O_4$.

Muscimol (3-hydroxy-5-aminomethyl-isoxazole) is a GABA analog,[19] a specific agonist of the GABAA receptor.[20] Muscimol is also water-soluble.[21] The molecular formula is $C_4H_6N_2O_2$.

Muscarine (4-hydroxy-5-methyloxolan-2-ylmethyl-trimethylazanium) is the first parasympathomimetic substance ever studied. Muscarine mimics the function of the natural neurotransmitter acetylcholine in the muscarinic part of the cholinergic nervous system.[22] Muscarine is only a trace compound in the *Amanita muscaria*.[23] The molecular formula is $C_9H_2ONO_2$.

Muscazone (a-amino-2,3-dihydro-2-oxo-5-oxazoleoacetic acid 3) is a heterocyclic glycine derivative found only in *Amanita muscaria*.[24] The structure was confirmed by synthesis.[25] The molecular formula is $C_5H_6N_2O_4$.

Other active constituents detected in *Amanita muscaria* are only in trace amounts, and their contribution to the biological effects of *Amanita muscaria* is apparently negligible.[26] Constituents include acetylcholine, amavadin, betain, betalamic acid, choline, quaternary trimethylammonium salt of 6-amino-2,3-dihydroxy-hexan, hercynin, hypoxanthin, (x)-R-hydroxy-4 pyrrolidone, uracile, stizolobic acid, muscaridin, muscarufin, muscaflavin, xanthin, adenosin, a carbolinic derivative, and b-D-n-butylglycopyranoside, muscapurpurin, muscarubin.[27]

The caps and stems were studied separately, revealing different metabolic compositions. Compared to the stems, *Amanita muscaria* caps exhibited higher concentrations of isoleucine, leucine, valine, alanine, aspartate, asparagine, threonine, lipids (mainly free fatty acids), choline, glycerophosphocholine, acetate, adenosine, uridine, 4-aminobutyrate, 6-hydroxynicotinate, quinolinate, UDP-carbohydrate, and glycerol. Conversely, stems exhibited lower concentrations of formate, fumarate, trehalose, and α- and β-glucose. Six metabolites—malate, succinate, gluconate, N-acetylated compounds (NAC), tyrosine, and phenylalanine—were detected in whole *Amanita muscaria* fruiting bodies but did not show significant differences in their levels between caps and stems.[28]

Fresh *Amanita muscaria* contains 258–471 ppm of ibotenic acid with the entirety of the fungi.[29] Nearly all the ibotenic acid is concentrated in the caps. Typically, the ibotenic acid to muscimol ratio of fungal cap tissue would be 9:1 or greater in fresh samples.[30] A portion of the ibotenic acid converts to muscimol while drying *Amanita muscaria,* so the conversion is incomplete and highly variable depending on conditions. A relatively low conversion rate of only 30% after drying, leaving a concentration of ibotenic acid, is typically 180–1800 ppm.[31] A common ibotenic acid to muscimol ratio would be 3:2 in dried specimens, such that the neurotoxin amounts far exceed the GABA analog.[32]

Additionally, multivariate data analyses of the fungal basidiomata and the types of soil were performed. A biogeochemical study of *Amanita muscaria* confirmed that elemental distribution in different parts of fruiting bodies is variable for each element and may change during maturation. Soil properties, species specificity, and the pattern of fruitbody development may all contribute to the various types of elemental distribution and suggest that the results for one species in one location may have only limited potential for generalization.[33]

Amanita muscaria Toxicology

Amanita muscaria may concentrate vanadium to 200 ppm (30 times those reported in living organisms). Isolation, structure determination, and synthesis of the pale blue vanadium complex amavadin 18[34] were confirmed by crystallography.[35] Similarly, unusually high levels of selenium to 17.8 ppm[36] and heavy metals have been reported: cadmium 13.9, cobalt 2.6, chromium 1.7, lead 33.3, mercury 61.3, and nickel 7.5 ppm.[37] Arsenic compounds were identified and quantified in the mushroom *Amanita muscaria* collected close to a facility that had roasted arsenic ores.[38]

A prognosis of poisoning is generally minor, and very seldom are lethal cases mentioned. Subsequent gastrointestinal disorders with vomiting are inconsistently reported and not characteristic of the syndrome.[39] Central nervous system dysfunctions primarily characterize this poisoning.[40] No damage to organs has been reported, although the active components may induce in vivo brain lesions. Regular consumption of the mushroom would probably be harmful, even though most human poisoning cases do not report any aftereffects. Brain lesions in rodents treated with ibotenic acid and muscimol can occur.[41] A study of several poisoning cases in which *Amanita muscaria* was consumed to evoke hallucinations showed that the poisoning regressed with no organ complications. The remaining persons who had eaten the fly agaric were free of any complaints.[42]

The onset of symptoms of *Amanita muscaria* poisoning is rapid after significant exposure (0.5–1.5 hours). Gastrointestinal discomfort is uncommon, and neurologic and psychotropic effects dominate. Inebriation, euphoria alternating with anxiety, confusion, illusions, delusions, hallucinations, agitation, and violent behavior are also common. More uncommon symptoms are myoclonic jerks, muscle fasciculation, and convulsions. CNS depression and unconsciousness may follow heavy exposure, especially in *Amanita pantherina* cap poisoning.[43]

If *Amanita muscaria* is ingested for a psychoactive experience, manifestations occur within two hours and are characterized by the GABAergic effects of drowsiness, hallucinations, dysphoria, dizziness, delirium, glutaminergic effects of hyperactivity, ataxia, hallucinations, myoclonus, and seizures.[44] Since the mushrooms contain both muscimol and ibotenic acid, their ingestion may result in alternating excitatory and inhibitory symptoms. Other than tachycardia, which is nonspecific and may occur due to hypovolemia or hypoxia, adverse cardiac effects with these mushrooms are uncommon.[45]

There is a relationship between the psychochemical properties of the active components and the mode of consumption. For instance, Mexican people eat the carpophore of *Amanita muscaria* without the cuticle that has been peeled off and also discard the cooking water.[46] In Italy, after boiling and rejecting excess water, the mushroom is preserved in brine prior to consumption.[47] In North America the red cuticle is peeled off, and the remainder is dried and then smoked.[48] These procedures eliminate or destroy the greater part of the active water-soluble substances. The red skin of the cap and the yellow tissue beneath it contain the highest amounts of these substances, so that might explain the practice of removing it.[49] From my own experience, Russian people eat AM stems after boiling them twice and frying.

Amanita muscaria in Pharmaceutical Science

I was not able to find any methodical data, clinical research, or medical tests that relate to the effects on the human body of a regular intake of very small *Amanita muscaria* doses. However, I found several studies that show the medicinal properties of *Amanita muscaria*'s components.

It has been proved that muscimol microinjections in the subthalamic nucleus reverse Parkinsonian symptoms, and muscimol has suppressive effects on essential tremors without impairing speech and coordination.[50]

Possible neuroprotective effects of an extract from *Amanita muscaria* that contains high amounts of muscimol have been evaluated, revealing statistically significant neuroprotective effects on in vitro neurotoxicity models.[51]

In patients with Huntington's disease and chronic schizophrenia, oral doses of muscimol have been found to cause a rise of both prolactin and growth hormone. Muscimol is a GABA agonist therapy in schizophrenia. At dose levels below 5 milligrams, many patients experienced a tranquilizing effect from muscimol. These subjects, when receiving the active drug, reported feeling more relaxed and less anxious and claimed a positive drug experience despite their lack of relief from psychotic thinking.[52]

Improvement in tardive dyskinesia was found after muscimol therapy. At oral dose levels from 5–9 milligrams, involuntary movements were consistently attenuated, usually in the absence of sedation.[53] Another study says that ibotenic acid and muscimol both have beneficial effects on human epilepsy and perhaps Huntington's disease or other neurological disorders. Muscimol was involved in synthesis of anticonvulsants such as tiagabine (Gabatril). It was marketed as a therapeutic agent for the treatment of epilepsy.[54]

The chemically related hydroxypyrollidone derivative found in *Amanita muscaria* is a known antibiotic and antifungal. The hydroxypyrollidone chemical frame is common in some micromycetes, which generally exhibit a potent biological activity against bacteria and other fungi (e.g., aureothrycin, equisetin).[55]

Cycloserine is an antimicrobial tuberculostatic agent that exhibits a carbon backbone similar to muscimol. It is known to induce effects on the central nervous system but with a longer latency period. Somnolence, confusion, and nervousness distinguish untoward effects.[56]

Muscimol is widely used as a ligand to probe GABA receptors and was the lead compound in the development of a range of GABAergic agents, including nipecotic acid, tiagabine, 4,5,6,7-tetrahydroisoxazolo (5,4-c), pyridin-3-ol (gaboxadol), and 4-PIOL.[57] Gaboxadol is currently studied as a potential therapeutic agent in Angelman syndrome. Gaboxadol shows potent, non-opioid analgesic effects. Sedative effects did, however, prevent therapeutic use as an analgesic but were subsequently shown to reflect unique hypnotic properties. Gaboxadol was described as an agent "capable of restoring a normal sleep architecture."[58] Gaboxadol is a conformational analog of muscimol with analgesic and sleep-promoting properties. It was investigated for the treatment of insomnia[59] and has shown activity as an analgesic as well as a novel type of hypnotic that increases non-REM sleep and enhances delta activity.[60]

Transmeningeal muscimol can prevent focal EEG seizures in the rat neocortex without stopping multineural activity in the treated area.[61]

Ethanolic extract of *Amanita muscaria* shows anti-inflammatory activity and deserves a modern evaluation.[62] A, β, and β-d-glucan (AM-ASN) isolated from the alkaline extract of the fruiting bodies of *Amanita muscaria* exhibited significant antitumor activity against Sarcoma 180 in mice.[63] The chemical AM-ASN, a beta-glucan, is extremely interesting for its antitumor activity.[64]

Fucomannogalactan and glucan isolated from *Amanita muscaria* showed inflammatory pain inhibition. Both the homo- and hetero-polysaccharides were evaluated for their anti-inflammatory and antinociceptive potential, and they produced potent inhibition of inflammatory pain.[65]

Muscimol has been used to reduce conditioned fear expression in lateral amygdala,[66] to eliminate cortical cell response in ferrets,[67] and to inactivate the lateral magnocellular nucleus of the nidopallium in zebra finches.[68]

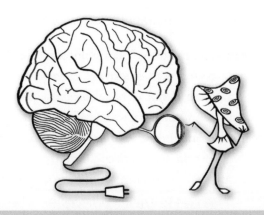

2 Project *Amanita muscaria* Microdoses Development

The problem is not to find the answer, it's to face the answer.

TERENCE McKENNA

At this time there is no documented comprehensive scale study on the medicinal effects of *Amanita muscaria* in modern international pharmacology or medicine, including reliable data on the systematic reception of this fungus in microdoses and their effect on nosological units in the transcontinental range.

This project does not offer theories or hypotheses and reflects only systematized material accumulated over two years. This study is also not a claim of scientific discovery and its proof. The data I demonstrate have many limitations that separate this book from scientific literature. The information that I collected and documented is based on various individual experiences with *Amanita muscaria* collected in different geographic zones from all continents of our planet. I present descriptive statistics to aggregate *Amanita muscaria* microdosers' experiences, and it should be regarded as a qualitative examination of individuals' experiences with *Amanita muscaria* microdosing. As a preliminary survey and the opinions of random *Amanita muscaria* microdosers, this study highlights only the facts and offers unique information from the first public *Amanita muscaria* microdose volunteer trial that included more than 3,000 participants from all continents.

Project Objectives

- Explore the range of diseases that might be corrected by AM microdosing
- Study the degree of influence of AM microdosing on nosological groups
- Determine the stability of AM microdosing effects
- Note the analgesic properties of AM
- Optimize the personal microdose size of AM based on the results of voluntary experiments
- Determine the optimal form of AM microdose reception
- Calculate the optimal duration of AM microdose reception
- Inquire into AM microdosing as a dependency antidote
- Learn the possible negative effects of taking AM
- Detect the optimal conditions for harvesting and storing AM

Project History

Psychedelic plants crossed my path at a later point in my life. My early adulthood was dedicated to the professional study of classical piano, chemical engineering, and medicine. My prefatory opinions and beliefs on psychedelics were based on erroneous observations made by my mentors and professors. During my fifth year of medical school, my professor, while suturing a patient's stoma, very casually said to "never try LSD since the option after the reception will be unambiguous. . . . You will grind iron rods of a cage for the rest of your life." Of course, I believed the professor. Why wouldn't I? After all, he was my teacher who could skillfully penetrate a patient's stomach and save his life. I did not seek further clarification. Life in Soviet Russia did not provide a rich palette for openly questioning authority or rank.

One day I decided to quit my warm, cozy position at the Science Research Institute of Obstetrics and Gynecology and follow my childhood dream to go around the world, which had already been blighted significantly due to my stealthy rebellious run-ins with the Soviet authoritarian system. Fate was on my side. The Soviet Union collapsed, and the wind of change brought me to the United States.

Significant life experiences followed. I discovered new culture, new thinking, new artists, and other personalities that were prohibited in Soviet Russia. By immersing myself in a new environment, I encountered culture shock, but I also had the chance to learn new skills and learn more about myself. My own culture has shaped my views, whether I realized it or not, and learning new points of view substantially enriched and refreshed my mind.

In three years I achieved my American dream—a house, two cars in the garage, chicken in the pot, and a corporate nest egg that generously paid for my expenses. But something was missing in that picture. Several years later I dropped all that, married my long-haired bohemian musician boyfriend, and moved to the foggy embrace of Big Sur, California.

The Pacific West graciously offered even more enlightening experiences—yoga and a chorus of Tibetan voices. Later, Timothy Leary, Robert Anton Wilson, Alan Watts, and Terrence McKenna joined these voices. Mysterious stories about the medicinal properties of some plants attracted my attention, and I devoted the next ten years of my life to the dense study of the therapeutic potential of plant psychedelics through my own self-induced experiences and in-depth study of all available material on this topic.

Growing up I learned to live in the material world and disregarded my ethereal relationship with the universe. The system had me believe that the transcendental world was irrelevant and did not exist. This perspective made the world around me empty, gloomy, and difficult. The world was a dangerous place, and enemies surrounded my motherland. Communism was my only hope. I had to subjugate myself to authoritarian rules in order to survive. My psychedelic experiences had a profound impact on my psyche and liberated me from this dazed and confused state. My first ayahuasca journey was a turning point in my life, so much so that I started going to the ceremony twice a year to experience a sense of calmness, divorced from such influencers as propaganda, ideologies, and politics. I felt a sense of spiritual awareness and tranquility, healing feelings I did not believe existed. During these self-induced journeys managed by trusted shamans, I could observe my psyche without age, gender, given name, culture, language, stereotypes, dogmas, and even knowledge of the species I belonged to. My conditioned view of myself and the universe blew up into a million pieces.

As I tried psychedelic and nonpsychedelic shamanic remedies, I gradually started noticing positive changes in my physical and psychological well-being. The results were far superior to what I had noticed during my years of study, research, and practice in the medical field. I cured serious conditions I could not correct with official medicine. When I tried to share with my former medical colleagues the knowledge I had gained through my study of and experience with plant psychedelics and nonpsychedelic shamanic remedies, they thought I had turned into a charlatan and a quack. They labeled me a substance abuser. I could not convince my fellow medical professionals that the medical training we had received, which was based on specialization and predefined disparate learning modules, overlooked the human body as a whole. Instead, I was met with skepticism, and I was ridiculed.

After studying psychedelic plants for a decade, I created a video podcast in Russian called *Radio Psychedelix*. It helped me organize my thoughts and provided me with an effective way to release the overwhelming burden I was carrying with all the knowledge I had gained.

Discussions on psychedelic plants, including discussions of medicinal properties, are considered propaganda for narcotic usage and are crimes in Russia. In order to produce my podcast, I had to be creative and hide my real identity. I created a character with a funny voice to convey the narrative and used a pseudonym—Baba Masha, my grandmother's name, and Some as my last name. The video format was simple: a psychedelic-colored mouth speaking out of blackness, constantly giggling and whispering the incredible adventures of the Psychedelix Kingdom.

Comments on the video podcast had to be shut down the first year. From the start I was declared a sneaky foreign agent working with a group of trained individuals to infuse insanity among the communities living in Russian-speaking territories. Podcast subscribers had all kinds of questions—had I had sex with aliens and in what positions, and so on. However, Baba Masha Some did not give up. Between giggles and stories about her visits to strange worlds and meetings with spirits, Baba Masha inserted translations of modern scientific articles, chemistry and medical research, book translations, podcasts, and lectures on psychedelics by world-renowned gurus. Camouflaged by jokes and equivocations, my podcast addressed the medicinal benefits of cannabis, ayahuasca, iboga, San Pedro and peyote cacti, magic mushrooms, sananga, rappe, and kambo, among others.

Even though some viewers demanded that I show my face to the public, accept charges for betraying the motherland in exchange for American sausages and drugs, and conduct and reveal the results of my sanity test, the brilliant minds that Baba Masha had translated into Russian had already captured part of the audience. Timothy Leary, Aldous Huxley, A. R. Wilson, T. K. McKenna, Ram Dass, S. Groff, James Fadiman, Rick Strassman, David Nutt, Paul Stamets, J. Rogan, B. Lipton, J. Peterson, G. Hancock, Rick Doblin, and others had already leaked into the consciousness of the crowd, and clearly the layer of "ours" had been marked.

Subscribers formed Masha's first secret group, Radio Psychedelic, on a social media outlet. Masha was admitted as a guest of honor to the underground Russian Central Committee of Psychedelics. She finally made her appearance to an audience in the form of a cartoon with a joint in her hand. She was flying through the universe on a tiny rock covered with magic cacti and mushrooms. Terence McKenna flew by, waving to Masha, from the window of the mushroom ship.

The ice had broken, and Masha had successfully made direct contact with subscribers who supported the work. The first contact had suffered from depression and panic attacks since early childhood. By the time he was twenty-seven, he had tried all possible conventional methods to address his issues, including going through psychotherapy and taking antidepressants, as well as following unconventional paths such as working with various gurus and practicing meditation and holotropic breathing. However, the outcome was not favorable. But after one year of our virtual communication and the use of microdoses of psychedelic mushrooms, this contact was cured of his long-term illness and became my first interviewee* for *Radio Psychedelix.*

After that first published interview, reports of other people's psychedelic experiences poured in like an avalanche. My audience was growing fast. On March 8, 2018, the government of the Russian Federation blocked *Radio Psychedelix.* By that time the number of views on the channel had reached a million.

It was a fatal mistake on the Russian Federation's part. The act of suppressing Baba Masha had the opposite result. Ironically, the government's blocking of the podcast earned me legitimacy and trust on the subject matter from the young population in Russian-speaking territories. My subscribers encouraged me to open a new channel. Soon, I was contacted with a multitude of reports from my listeners on the use and benefits of psychedelic plants on the mind and body.

A year later the number of subscribers and viewers on the new channel had tripled. The Baba Masha virus had spread to eighteen channels in the virtual subsoil with live chatrooms, support groups, channels with reports of the effects of psychedelic plants, and livestreams for Russian-speaking audiences on all continents. My second YouTube channel was blocked by the Russian Federation on September 1, 2020. By that time the number of views on the channel had reached 3 million.

Right before creating my *Psychedelic Plants* broadcast in 2014, my psychedelic search was crowned by iboga, the brain-smashing, seventy-two-hour experience with a blast of information, visions, and

---

*Reports were posted anonymously and/or compiled for this book with names removed.

insights. There was a recurring telepathic message in all the experiences I had with iboga. "Look for homeopathic doses," I thought. "Look for homeopathic doses." And synchronicity kicked in! A few weeks after an iboga trip, a random internet search exposed me to James Fadiman's book *The Psychedelic Explorer's Guide*. Bingo! A new word—*microdose*—entered my life. After reading Fadiman's work on psilocybin mushroom microdosing, I tried his method myself in two six-month sessions with a six-month break between. The results were astounding. I included this method in my Russian broadcast. Psychedelic microdosing quickly took over Russian-speaking territories, and there were hundreds of cases of depression recoveries among my podcast subscribers.

Soon after, a fifty-two-year-old subscriber mentioned that for several years he had regularly used small doses of dry *Amanita* for health benefits and was still in good health. My response was very dry and dismissive—"Are you crazy? Are you trying to kill yourself?"

Over the next couple months, I received more reports from *Amanita* microdosers. A forty-year-old woman was successfully using *Amanita muscaria* in microdoses to treat systemic lupus erythematosus. Two older people (eighty-two and eighty-seven years old) reported quick recoveries from stroke. Soon, I encountered more people taking *Amanita muscaria* in small doses with significant medical benefits. However, my obedient brain reacted to AM with the standard skepticism instilled in me—"stay away from this particular poisonous mushroom."

As soon as I shared my recent discoveries with *Amanita muscaria* microdosing on my broadcast, sixty-seven more people contacted me and shared similar positive outcomes. Depending on the time of consumption, *Amanita muscaria* microdosing showed great benefits in certain aspects of calming and energizing the mind and body, as a mood enhancer, and in relieving the symptoms of depression and asthenia. Subscribers also claimed pain-relief properties and that *Amanita muscaria* microdosing was an extremely potent sleep aid. Personal conversations with AM microdosers—unknown to each other—showed unbelievably consistent data.

I then found myself hunting in the Pacific Coast woods for fly agaric and preparing it with recipes the members of my online community gave me. Yes, I experienced mood elevation, blasts of energy, a prolific workday, and a perfect restful sleep. Then the most amazing thing happened. The *Amanita muscaria* alcohol extract completely took away the pain from my bulged L5 disk. I was able to go back to the gym and go for long hikes. Additionally, by using *Amanita muscaria* ointment, I got rid of most of the age spots on my skin.

My personal results combined with data I received from sixty-seven responders were amazing resources. I published this information on my podcast in February 2019. In a few months I received hundreds of reports that highlighted the health benefits of microdosing AM, the online price of AM skyrocketed in Russian-speaking territories, Baba Masha was declared the responsible party for the Golden Amanita Fever of 2019, and Russian vocabulary was enriched with a new phrase— *Amanita muscaria* microdose. Businesses selling *Amanita* products filled the internet.

CAUTION

Dealers were quick to register *Amanita* products as a brand trade, and new food supplements with *Amanita* grew like mushrooms. The quality of sold and purchased *Amanita* is critical and under question in general. Many sellers are irresponsible and pushing totally unknown powder in capsules, or the previous season's AM, or AM picked in an environment that is not chemically safe, or AM that has been stored incorrectly and so is moldy, and so on. I have letters from witnesses who work at such facilities detailing hygienic violations such as dirty conditions, AM eaten by worms, and other mushrooms in the powdered end product. I have pages of complaints on side effects and negative effects of *purchased* AM—pimples, allergic reaction, kidney and liver pain, and so on.

In addition, many of these businesses push *Amanita pantherina,* which has different chemical compounds and is not suitable for microdosing. The results of microdosing *Amanita pantherina* are 50/50, with many negative effects on mental and emotional health such as weird behavior, depression, and more.

Currently, all information is available on the online platform Telegram. Telegram channels include the following:

- Effects of rappe, sananga, ayahuasca, and iboga: User reports
- Effects of psilocybin mushrooms: User reports; Trips and microdosing
- Marijuana health benefits: User reports
- Marijuana addiction: Poll votes; Questionnaire
- Information and help for marijuana product addicts
- Live chat support room: Psychedelic plants
- Live chat support room: *Amanita muscaria* microdosing
- HPPD: Support for victims of designer drugs
- *Radio Psychodelix* channel, a duplicate of two YouTube channels
- Baba Masha: Q & A
- AM microdosing effects: Poll votes; Questionnaire
- *Amanita muscaria* effects report collection
- AM microdosing for sport fighters: Poll votes; Questionnaire
- Live stream with Baba Masha
- Grower's library
- Collection of books: Conciseness; Psychedelics; Mind and Body
- Effects of psilocybin mushrooms microdoses: Questionnaire

Project Structure

This project is based on Telegram, a cross-platform social media messenger that does not limit the size of data and allows you to exchange messages and media files of many formats. In August 2019, using Telegram, I circulated a public survey questionnaire and a collection of reports. Telegram has the ability to provide support for private channels and social theme chat rooms free of charge. Equipped with bots, the messenger performs third-party applications to serve users' needs. It is easy to control bots that run inside Telegram by sending commands and requests. I used Votebot and Pollbot to create questionnaires on four subjects: marijuana addiction, psilocybin mushrooms miscrodoses effects, *Amanita muscaria* miscrodoses effects, and sport fighters and *Amanita muscaria* microdosing. The applications inside Telegram allowed me to quickly, easily, and effortlessly collect public-opinion data. Telegram also connects people with similar interests and proximity. It allowed me to automatically process information and automate interaction among participants. Information processed by bots is presented as a percentage and is easy to read. These applications allow only one response from one profile, so the ability to manipulate the poll is minimal.

Four platforms for research on effects of microdosing AM were created: a channel with a questionnaire for polling, a feedback channel on the effects of AM microdosing, and two AM microdose chat-support rooms. Use reports of *Amanita muscaria* varied from 0.1 g to 50 g.

I created the questionnaire with 107 detailed questions based on my medical experience, professional knowledge of collecting data, physiology, etiology, nosology, pathogenesis, pathological physiology, pharmacology, and medical terminology. Some questions were repeated deliberately in different forms to identify inconsistencies. The questions were based on several hundred reviews I had received earlier on the effects of AM microdosing. Questions were added as the project unfolded and information arrived. If new, unexpected effects were identified (as in the case of psoriasis, nail fungus, hypertension, and asthma), a new question was added to the questionnaire. In this regard, the number of responses on different issues varied. In the process of researching, I discovered information about AM's impact on more than seventy nosological units, health conditions, and body and mind performance. Negative or inconclusive experiences were also reflected in the questionnaires, which were designed in a specific way in order to track all possible negative effects. Each negative experience microdosing AM was personally evaluated in chat rooms with microdosers' discussion and support. As a result of the general analysis of negative effects by chat participants, abuse, violation of AM dosing, and the acquisition of unidentified powder on the internet were revealed.

This study also used information from two public AM microdosing support group chat rooms—mine and my associate Thomas's. The number of participants in the two chat rooms was 6,200 on January 1, 2021. Thomas has been living in the forest for several years, practicing with *Amanita muscaria*. He has collected a huge amount of unique information on the effects of the fungus—effects on the hunting, identification, procurement, and manufacture of medical preparations based on fly agaric. Thomas's public articles with photographs of *Amanita* can be found (in Russian) on Telegram, where his channel is https://t.me/BCE_O_MYXOMOPE.

The number of subscribers following the development of the data on the questionnaire channel was 5,600 on January 1, 2021. The channel is active and information is updated in real time (in Russian) at https://t.me/bMasha_Amanita. The individual AM microdoser reports channel had 5,900 subscribers on January 1, 2021, and is available to the general public at https://t.me/bMasha_AmanitaM. More than two thousand reviews on effects of microdosing AM are collected on that channel. The feedback also includes information from the comments on my two YouTube channels, which had 7,200 subscribers on January 1, 2021.

In addition, at the request of a group of athletes, a channel was created for questions about the effects of dosing AM in wrestling. This information is presented in chapter 7 of this book. I also offered free consultations on AM microdose intake and the answers to questions in a private Telegram format and published in reviews. There were livestream discussions of *Amanita muscaria* microdosing on Telegram.

The electronic annual report was published in June 2020 in Russian. It included information about AM microdose individual calibration, Thomas's articles, recipes, poll data, and personal reports to that date. There were 15,000 downloads in four days and 45,000 in the first month. In September 2020 a printed AM microdosing report was published in Moscow per participants' requests, and two thousand copies of the book were sold in three months. I then received more information about new effects on various conditions and added them to the questionnaire. An expanded section on addictions was added to include designer drugs, amphetamines, cocaine, opiates, nicotine, and caffeine. The number of individual reports doubled after publication.

In the scientific world "fear" is usually called "skepticism."

JAMES FADIMAN,
THE PSYCHEDELIC EXPLORER'S GUIDE

PART TWO
Amanita muscaria
Microdose Effects
Summary Data

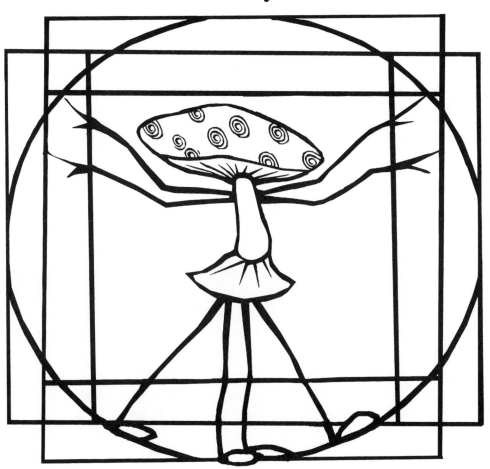

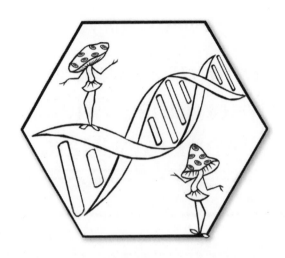

Introduction to Part Two

The following chapters present information received from project participants regarding the use and effects of *Amanita muscaria* microdoses. The data I show have many limitations that separate this book from scientific literature.

First, the data are based on varieties of individual experiences with *Amanita muscaria* collected in different geographic zones from all continents of our planet. The biogeochemical study of *Amanita muscaria* confirmed that elemental distribution in different geographic zones is variable and may change according to soil properties, climate, and time of harvesting. Also, the method of harvesting, preparation, and storing affects chemical specificity and may all contribute to the various types of elemental distribution. This study is not based on a double-blind, placebo-controlled clinical trial, a medical study involving human participants in which neither side knows who's getting what treatment and a placebo is given to a control group. This study was not based on the same active substance following statistical evaluation.

Second, the data were collected over a period of time, which would limit its quantitative analytic value because not all survey respondents replied to the same questions.

Third, the available quantitative data are mostly appropriate for reporting descriptive information such as the number and percent of survey respondents who experienced a variety of symptoms and how those symptoms are associated with AM microdose use. All these factors suggest that the results have limited potential for generalization.

Despite this, the data are highly consistent, and I believe these data are useful. They act as a record of how individuals might follow a course of AM microdose and provide a framework for what questions would be valuable for our further investigation. These analyses also capture the variety of applications people have found for microdosing with AM.

Throughout the remainder of the book, I will present descriptive statistics to aggregate AM microdosers experiences. It should be regarded as a qualitative examination of individuals' experiences with AM microdosing and as a preliminary survey and opinions of random *Amanita muscaria* microdosers.

Creativity is intelligence having fun.
ALBERT EINSTEIN

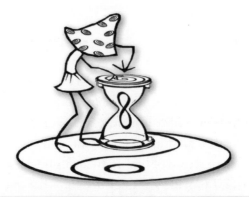

I designed a project questionnaire that contains 107 detailed questions with optional answers. The questionnaire covers over seventy health conditions, negative effects, various drug addictions, and sport fighters' performance outcomes.

Questions were added as the project unfolded and new information arrived. When new effects were identified, the list of questions was immediately updated for participant response. In this regard, the number of responses on different issues varies.

Participants' General Information

Of those who provided this information, most participants (91%) were 18–50 years old (1,501 of 1,642). No detailed breakdown by age was made as that was not important in this study. Most of the project participants (77%) were men (758 of 983), with females making up only 19% (182) (see fig. 1 and fig. 2).*

---

*The gender question was added once the study was underway.

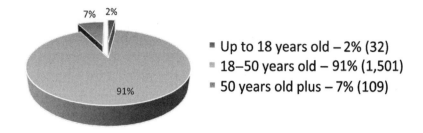

Fig. 1. Participants' ages (total 1,642)

- Up to 18 years old – 2% (32)
- 18–50 years old – 91% (1,501)
- 50 years old plus – 7% (109)

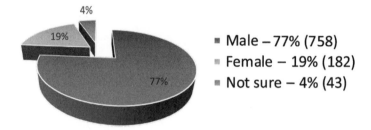

Fig. 2. Participants' genders (total 983)

- Male – 77% (758)
- Female – 19% (182)
- Not sure – 4% (43)

Psychedelic experiences prior to an AM microdose course are reflected in figure 3. About 53% (266 of 499) of the participants had prior psychedelic experiences, 40% (197) did not, and 7% (36) reported psychedelic experiences only with *Amanita muscaria*. Participants' geographic locations are presented in figure 4 (p. 30). Eastern Europe had 47% (881 of 1,872), the European Union had 10% (180), Asia had 20% (378), North America had 8% (152), South America had 2% (45), and 13% (236) responded as other.

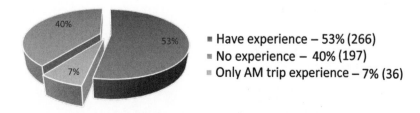

- Have experience – 53% (266)
- No experience – 40% (197)
- Only AM trip experience – 7% (36)

Fig. 3. Participants' psychedelic experiences (total 499)

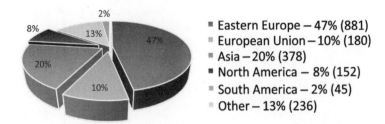

- Eastern Europe – 47% (881)
- European Union – 10% (180)
- Asia – 20% (378)
- North America – 8% (152)
- South America – 2% (45)
- Other – 13% (236)

Fig. 4. Participants' geographical location (total 1,872)

Sources and Species of
Amanita muscaria

Amanita muscaria mushrooms were collected and prepared personally by 46% (508 of 1,102) of users. Purchase of a reliable quality of *Amanita muscaria* was reported by 25% (275); 25% of participants (279) reported purchasing *Amanita muscaria* of unknown quality; and 4% (40) were unsure of the AM source (see fig. 5).

This project is based on the use of *Amanita muscaria,* which is familiar to us from the illustrations in children's fairy tales. Most participants (94%, 567 of 604) used the *Amanita muscaria* species for AM microdosing consumption. Both *Amanita muscaria* and *Amanita pantherina* species were used in microdosing in 5% (30) of participants. Only 1% (7) used *Amanita pantherina* (see fig. 6). *Amanita pantherina* requires its own investigation due to its stronger effect and different chemical compounds.

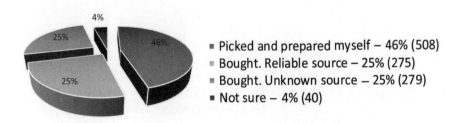

- Picked and prepared myself – 46% (508)
- Bought. Reliable source – 25% (275)
- Bought. Unknown source – 25% (279)
- Not sure – 4% (40)

Fig. 5. Sources of Amanita muscaria
(total 1,102)

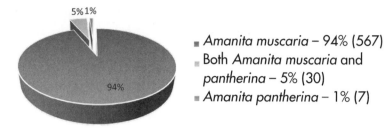

5% 1%

94%

■ *Amanita muscaria* – 94% (567)
▪ Both *Amanita muscaria* and *pantherina* – 5% (30)
■ *Amanita pantherina* – 1% (7)

Fig. 6. Amanita species used for AM microdosing (total 604)

Later in the project development, at the request of participants, two questions were added to compare the positive effects during AM microdose course with purchased *Amanita muscaria* and mushrooms that were collected personally (table 1). There were positive effects with purchased AM (86%, 178 of 208); there were positive effects with personally picked AM (90%, 166 of 185). There were no effects with purchased AM (11%, 23) and no effects with personally collected (8%, 15), respectively. There were negative effects for 3% (7) and 2% (4) with purchased and personally collected AM respectively.

TABLE 1. EFFECTS AND AM SOURCE

SOURCE	NEGATIVE EFFECTS	POSITIVE EFFECTS	NO RESULTS
AM Bought (208)	3% (7)	86% (178)	11% (23)
AM Picked Personally (185)	2% (4)	90% (166)	8% (15)

Preparation and Procurement Methods

AM preparation is still ardently discussed in the support chats. The question remains open since the essence of the controversy boils down to the decarboxylation of ibotenic acid to muscimol. The drying process increases decarboxylation, and the final dried form provides stronger psychoactive effects. There is an opinion among participants that procuring the fungus and storing it for two to three months in a cool, dark place without access to air (curing process) stimulates the decarboxylation of ibotenic acid to muscimol. A lower level of nausea was reported by some participants with use of cured mushrooms.

However, a study led by K. Tsunoda titled "Change in Ibotenic Acid and Muscimol Contents in *Amanita muscaria* during Drying, Storing or Cooking" shows a correlation between the concentration of ibotenic acid and muscimol depending on different procuring and storage methods.[1] This study also shows no change of concentration in ibotenic acid and muscimol during ninety days of storage. The comparative spectrographic method was used in this study.

The question remains open. There are positive medicinal effects of dried AM (fresh dried or cured). There are also positive medicinal effects of using *Amanita muscaria* alcohol tincture in which decarboxylation of ibotenic acid does not occur. There is an obvious difference in the individual effects of fresh-dried and cured AM used for microdosing according to the survey. The difference was also confirmed by reports of several families using the same AM prepared different ways for microdosing. The next step in our research is to measure the ratio of ibotenic acid and muscimol with liquid chromatography and mass spectrometer in the samples of *Amanita muscaria* prepared in different ways.

Amanita muscaria Microdose Forms

Figure 7 reflects the opinions of users as to the most popular forms of AM microdose reception—dried mushroom, powder, tea form, and alcohol tincture. The preferred form of AM microdose by 38% of participants was a powder (283 of 740); dried AM cap pieces was preferred by 36% (267). The tea form was less popular, favored by 22% (166), and the consumption of *Amanita muscaria* alcohol tincture was the least preferred at only 3% (24).

Figure 8 shows participants' choices of the *Amanita muscaria* procurement form—fresh dried AM was used by 66% of participants (465 of 704), cured AM by 25% (177), alcohol tincture by 6% (41), and raw by 3% (21).

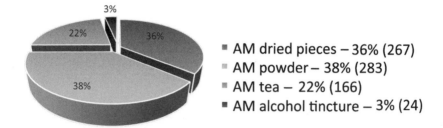

- AM dried pieces – 36% (267)
- AM powder – 38% (283)
- AM tea – 22% (166)
- AM alcohol tincture – 3% (24)

Fig. 7. Forms of AM microdose consumption (total 740)

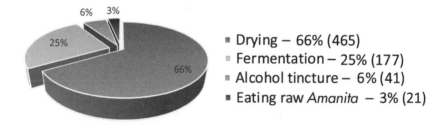

- Drying – 66% (465)
- Fermentation – 25% (177)
- Alcohol tincture – 6% (41)
- Eating raw *Amanita* – 3% (21)

Fig. 8. Methods of AM microdose preparation (total 704)

After publishing the report of AM microdose effects for the first year of our project in Russia in June 2020, there were more questions proposed by participants for public discussion. Two more questions were added to the questionnaire for further investigation. It was proposed to compare discomfort (light nausea) and positive effects of fresh dried and cured methods of *Amanita muscaria* preparation. The results are reflected in figures 9 and 10.

The majority (57%, 109 of 192) of AM microdosers did not have any discomfort with either preparation method of AM. Discomfort with fresh dried AM was reported by 34% (66) of participants. Discomfort with any form was reported by 4% (8), and cured AM by 5% (9) (see fig. 9, next page).

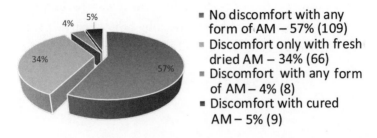

- No discomfort with any form of AM – 57% (109)
- Discomfort only with fresh dried AM – 34% (66)
- Discomfort with any form of AM – 4% (8)
- Discomfort with cured AM – 5% (9)

Fig. 9. Discomfort and AM curing methods
(total 192)

Figure 10 shows that positive effects were higher with fresh dried *Amanita muscaria* compared to cured mushrooms in 41% (83 of 202) and 26% (53) of participants respectively. Positive effects with both forms of *Amanita muscaria* preparation were confirmed by 33% (66) participants.

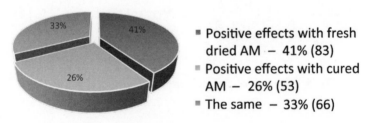

- Positive effects with fresh dried AM – 41% (83)
- Positive effects with cured AM – 26% (53)
- The same – 33% (66)

Fig. 10. Positive effects and AM curing methods
(total 202)

Overall Opinion on
Amanita muscaria Microdose Intake

Stability

The presence of various illnesses and their severity was not taken into account when assessing AM microdose intake. Surprisingly, a preliminary general evaluation of the results showed highly positive and stable effects. The overall rating of the AM microdose course was evaluated positively in 92% (938 of 1,018) of the cases (see fig. 11). A negative

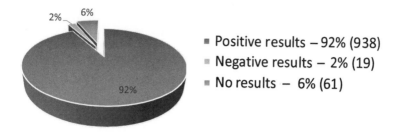

- Positive results – 92% (938)
- Negative results – 2% (19)
- No results – 6% (61)

Fig. 11. AM microdose overall opinion
(total 1,018)

outcome after the AM microdose course was expressed by 2% (19) of users. An outcome with no results was noted in 6% (61).

Dependency
Stable effects of AM microdosing were reported by 74% (163 of 219) of participants (see fig. 12). The effects lasting only during reception, with no dependency, was reported by 21% (46). We did not investigate the reason for the return to the previous state. It could be the presence and

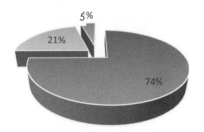

- Stable effects after course, planning to continue – 74% (163)
- Effects are stable only during the consumption – 21% (46)
- Dependency, unstable condition without AM microdosing – 5% (10)

Fig. 12. AM microdose stability, dependency (total 219)

severity of illness, the quality of the *Amanita muscaria,* the duration of the intake, or the AM microdosage. Dependency and an unstable condition without AM microdosing were reported by 5% (10) of the participants. Due to low indicators, an investigation of preexisting body and mind health in that group was not performed.

Withdrawal

Withdrawal symptoms after an AM microdose course were absent in 74% (214 of 291) of the participants (see fig. 13). According to reports, withdrawal was determined as unbalanced mood in 17% (51), insomnia in 6% (17), and other in 3% (9) of participants.

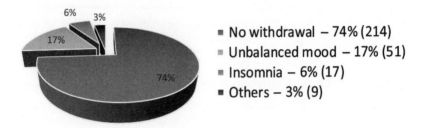

Fig. 13. Withdrawal after AM microdose course (total 291)

Through joint efforts in the discussion chats, it was determined that the cause of a withdrawal syndrome was usually abuse and violation of the optimal AM microdosage. Figure 14 shows the condition after the AM microdose course. About 75% (184 of 245) of participants described their condition after an AM microdose course as great. The condition returned to the previous in 22% (54), and 3% (7) of participants reported the condition was worse than before the *Amanita muscaria* microdose course.

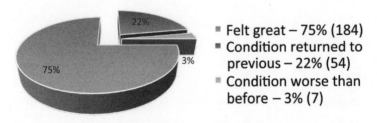

Fig. 14. Condition after AM microdose course (total 245)

Optimal *Amanita muscaria* Microdose Parameters

AM weight cannot be standardized. Each user will have his or her own individual response to the same weight of the same fungus. Individual sensitivity is the most important criterion, which has been proved by the thousands of reviews submitted.

Professor James Fadiman, who has been studying the effects of psilocybin mushrooms for a long time, proposed an effective method for individual calibration of the fungus in *The Psychedelic Explorer's Guide*.[2] I decided to use Professor Fadiman's method for calibration of individual microdose weight, and it worked perfectly for *Amanita muscaria*. The weight of AM cannot be determined per kilogram of the user's weight or fit into a common conditional unit that is right for everyone.

Subsequent findings are based on information from two chat support room discussions on this topic, personal contacts with participants, feedback, and responses on the proposed questionnaire.

The optimal individual AM microdose is the weight of the dried fungus chosen empirically. With a properly selected weight, there are no changes in perception, consciousness, or behavior. The occurrence of euphoria, hysterical laughter, uncontrolled behavior, hallucinations, fractals, dizziness, drowsiness, sudden weakness, apathy, and aggression are signs of an incorrectly selected dosage.

Weight

It varies according to the obtained data since the study is based on various *Amanita* sources with variations in chemical composition and quality, which depends on the territory of growth, the method of harvesting, drying and preparation conditions, storage duration, and individual sensitivity.

According to the data obtained, microdosing AM is most effective when taken in a dosage of 0.5–2 g of dried fungus. The optimal dosage of *Amanita muscaria* should not cause any changes in perception, lack of motivation, insomnia, emotional differences, aggression, irritability, depression, or low energy level. For more detailed information on taking *Amanita muscaria,* see part 4 of this book.

A personal approach is proposed in calibrating individual AM microdoses similar to Fadiman's method of calibrating psilocybin microdoses.[3] Each new *Amanita muscaria* batch is subject to new personal calibration. For example, thoroughly dried *Amanita muscaria* absorbs moisture directly from the air, loses crispiness, becomes elastic, and increases in weight. For instance, 0.5 g crispy dried *Amanita* left without vacuum packaging could almost double its weight, depending on the humidity of the air. As the experiments showed, the weight of *Amanita muscaria* powder, the equivalent of a heaping teaspoon, varies from 1 g to 3 g, depending on the dryness of the fungus.

During this project it was proposed to start with 0.5 g of dried *Amanita muscaria* in the morning thirty minutes before breakfast and, depending on the effect, move toward lowering or increasing the weight of the microdose for the next intake. The most popular dosage according to a poll was 1–2 g of dried *Amanita muscaria* (41%, 476 of 1,168), then up to 1 g in 31% (364), and finally 3 g or more in 17% (198) (see fig. 15).

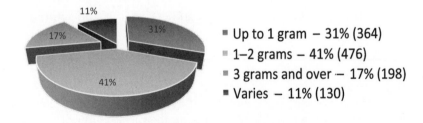

- Up to 1 gram – 31% (364)
- 1–2 grams – 41% (476)
- 3 grams and over – 17% (198)
- Varies – 11% (130)

Fig. 15. Optimal AM Microdose weight (total 1,168)

Intake Frequency

Once a day frequency of AM microdose was the most optimal and effective according to participants' feedback and responses to the poll

(45%, 512 of 1,150). The next most effective frequency was twice a day, in the morning and evening (35%, 403); followed by 1–3 times a week reported by 10% (121); and the least popular was taking *Amanita muscaria* doses irregularly (10%, 114) (see fig. 16).

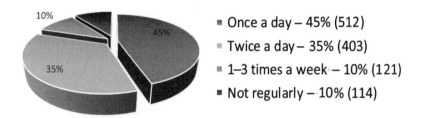

Fig. 16. AM Microdose intake frequency (total 1,150)

Intake Timing

An interesting observation was revealed in the process of collecting information. As it turned out, the reception time of the AM microdose gives a specific polar result. Therefore, choosing a time for use has different goals.

After taking an AM microdose in the morning, participants indicated a tide of energy and physical strength, a mood rise to a positive level, ease of communication, calmness, effectiveness during the day, cheerfulness, a feeling of well-being, and the disappearance of irritability and a mental chatterbox.

Taking an AM microdose at night resulted in quickly falling into a deep, even sleep with amazing, realistic, and fantastic dreams. The following morning, there was a state of vigor and the sensation of a well-rested body.

Figure 17 (next page) presents participants' reported AM microdose intake time—morning, evening, or both. The most popular time was in the morning, thirty minutes before eating (34%, 419 of 1,229). The next most popular time was in the evening, confirmed by 16% (190). Taking *Amanita muscaria* microdoses in both the morning and evening

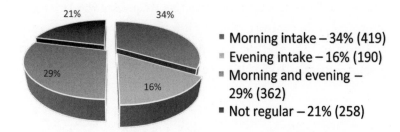

Morning intake – 34% (419)
Evening intake – 16% (190)
Morning and evening –
29% (362)
Not regular – 21% (258)

Fig. 17. AM microdose intake time
(total 1,229)

was favorable for 29% (362). More detailed information of morning and evening AM microdose intake is provided in chapter 4 and part 4 of this book.

Duration

The information from this study revealed the optimal duration of AM microdose reception was up to one month with a subsequent break of up to ten days. During the break, the host then has the ability to determine the effectiveness and stability of the effects. Further microdosing was chosen based on personal evaluation.

The optimal period was determined to be up to one month according to the questionnaire data (67%, 665 of 999), and then up to three months (11%, 114), and lastly up to six months (8%, 82). Microdosing

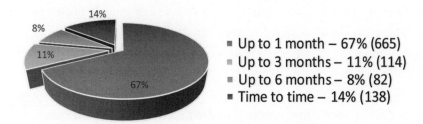

Up to 1 month – 67% (665)
Up to 3 months – 11% (114)
Up to 6 months – 8% (82)
Time to time – 14% (138)

Fig. 18. AM microdose optimal duration
(total 999)

from time to time was reported by 14% (138) (see fig. 18).

Most project participants pointed to the cumulative effects of AM microdosing and the continuation of the effects of microdosing AM after a week, two weeks, and even more.

The only way to make sense out of change is to plunge into it, move with it, and join the dance.

ALAN WATTS

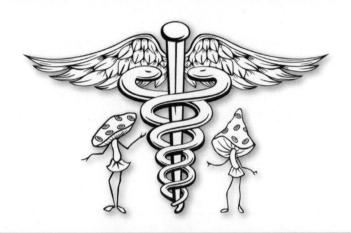

CHAPTER 4 *Amanita muscaria* Microdose Effects on Various Conditions

Among the topics addressed in the AM microdosing surveys was the effect of *Amanita muscaria* on a wide range of conditions. The results are impressive and are presented here in detail.

Allergy

Allergy is a chronic disease caused by an inadequate, undesirable, and unexpected reaction of the immune system to the effects of substances that usually do not lead to a disease and do not harm a person (things like food, medicines, plant pollen, insect venom, etc.). The causes and types of allergies were not considered in questionnaires but were addressed in general. There are more detailed data in the participant reviews in part 4 of this book.

Figure 19 presents *Amanita muscaria* microdoses' effects on allergy. There were 59% (61 of 104) positive results with allergy symptoms; 41% (43) indicated no results.

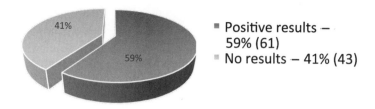

■ Positive results –
59% (61)
■ No results – 41% (43)

Fig. 19. Allergy and AM microdosing (total 104)

Appetite, Diet, and Digestion

A sufficient number of participants reported that *Amanita muscaria* microdose intake changed diet habits, food cravings, and appetite. That gave me a reason to further investigate those factors.

Appetite

The question of microdosing AM and its influence on appetite also was raised at the request of James Fadiman. He was surprised by the speed of the response of the project participants; over two weeks, there were more than three hundred responses to this question.

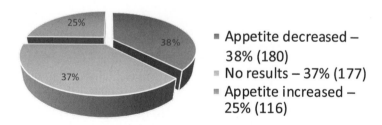

Fig. 20. Appetite and AM microdosing (total 473)

Figure 20 reflects an appetite decrease in 38% (180 of 473) of cases, no changes in 37% (177), and an appetite increase in 25% (116).

Diet Habits

Diet habit changes during an AM microdose course occurred mostly in meat and sugar consumption. Change to a vegetarian diet was reported by 12% (60 of 485) participants, less meat consumption by 31% (151), and no results by 57% (274) (see fig. 21). According to the posts in the chat support rooms, there was an observation that appetite and sugar consumption were increased in the first two weeks of AM microdose intake, followed by a decrease of both. Participants connected that effect to body cleansing from a variety of parasites. For instance, I have multiple reports about detecting worms in excrement during AM microdosing and alcohol tincture intake. Complete rejection of sweet products was reported by 10% (50 of 501) of participants, and decreased consumption of sugar products was noticed by 38% (190). No results were experienced by 52% (261) (see fig. 22).

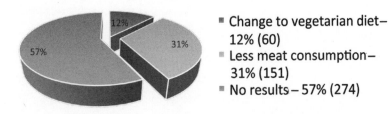

Fig. 21. Meat consumption and AM microdosing (total 485)

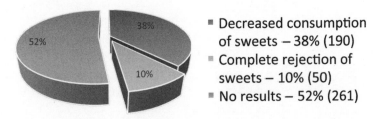

Fig. 22. Sugar consumption and AM microdosing (total 501)

Heartburn

The sensation of burning in the esophagus as a result of irritation of its mucosa is how heartburn manifests. Sometimes heartburn is a relatively harmless consequence of eating inappropriate food, but it could be a symptom of a condition that requires treatment. The medium of a healthy stomach is acidic due to the action of hydrochloric acid, the main component of gastric juice. In the esophagus, acidity is close to neutral. Normally, the reverse movement of food is hindered by the circular muscle, the sphincter. When it weakens for one reason or another, the acidic contents of the stomach escape into the esophagus. This process is called reflux. Stomach walls are lined on the inside with a protective mucus film. Thus, they are not susceptible to the aggressive action of acid. But there are no glands in the esophagus that produce protective mucus. Therefore, acidic gastric contents can corrode the lining of the organ, and a chemical burn of the esophagus can be observed. This is manifested by a sense of burning, sometimes pain, in the chest area.

In this study 53% (35 of 66) of participants noticed that AM microdosing eliminated heartburn (see fig. 23). Heartburn increased with AM microdosing for 15% (10), and there was no change in 32% (21).

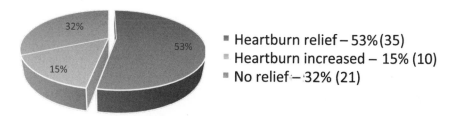

- Heartburn relief – 53% (35)
- Heartburn increased – 15% (10)
- No relief – 32% (21)

Fig. 23. Heartburn and AM microdosing (total 66)

Tongue Plaque

Since childhood we have all been familiar with a doctor's request to open the mouth and show the tongue. Doctors say that the tongue is an indicator of the whole body's health. Indeed, this seemingly simple examination speaks of many pathologies that require further diagnoses. The reasons for tongue plaque may be due to the following: oral diseases (candidiasis, stomatitis, glossitis), GI diseases (gastritis, colitis), infectious diseases, reduced immunity, organ pathology, drug intake, and smoking. The purification of the tongue from plaque was noted

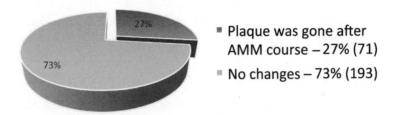

- Plaque was gone after AMM course – 27% (71)
- No changes – 73% (193)

Fig. 24. Tongue plaque and AM microdosing (total 264)

in 27% (71 of 264) of participants, and no changes were noted in 73% (193) (see fig. 24).

Stool Regulation

Constipation often occurs due to an unhealthy diet (inadequate intake of fiber) or an inactive lifestyle, and thus it can be easily corrected. AM microdose intake reduced constipation and made the stool more regular in 58% (111 of 192) of participants, and there were no changes in 42% (81) (see fig. 25).

There were four posts in the chat support rooms that AM microdosing stopped diarrhea from short-term to persistent cases that had no success with common medications. This information is reflected in part 4.

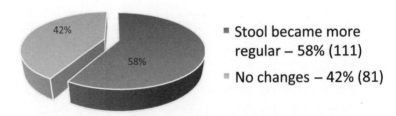

- Stool became more regular – 58% (111)
- No changes – 42% (81)

Fig. 25. Constipation and AM microdosing (total 192)

Asthenia, Depression

Asthenia is a nervous mental state manifested in increased fatigue and mood swings with the presence of capriciousness, tearfulness, discontent, loss of self-control, impatience, sleep disturbance, irritability, and increased excitability. The etymology of asthenia is mental and somatic diseases, infections, overstrain, and prolonged conflicts.

Depression is a mental health disorder. Depression has different types—mild, medium, and severe. Over a long time, depression can lead to psychosomatic disorders. Depression can be expressed in a variety of problems, from negative emotional states to mental health disorders. The cause of depression can be diseases such as thyroid dysfunction, hormonal changes, dementia, and ingesting drugs and narcotic substances, including alcohol. Depression can also be due to endogenous causes such as nutrition, lifestyle, or even prolonged lack of sunlight. The main symptoms of depression are fatigue, dissatisfaction, depressed mood, constant self-criticism, low self-esteem, sleep disorders, reduced concentration, thoughts of death and suicide, arousal, and retardation.

In this project the cause of asthenia or depression was not studied. However, a high improvement rate, regardless of the etiology, is reflected in figure 26, and a detailed description of the subject is discussed in part 4 of this book. Stable positive effects were reported by 79% (790 of 999) of the participants; temporary relief was seen in 8% (84); there were no results in 10% (100); and there were negative results in 3% (25).

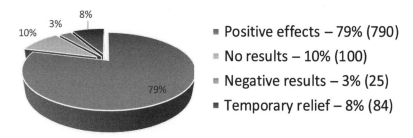

Fig. 26. Asthenia, depression, and AM microdosing (total 999)

Participants noted an increase in positive emotions and feelings, including the following:

- desire to live
- balance and harmony
- calm joy of being
- strengthening of the voice of the inner observer
- increase of the life tonus
- reduced criticism and envy
- reduced aggression to oneself, to the environment, and to people
- reassessment of priorities
- disappearance of fears
- study and rethinking of mental traumas
- normalization of criticism and control
- paradigm shift
- rethinking of worldview attitudes
- change in style of thinking
- exit of spiritual crisis
- increasing self-interest
- improved communication
- reduced sense of inflated ego and self-importance
- disappearance of sadness and guilt for any reason
- increased self-esteem and self-confidence
- good and respectful attitude toward oneself and one's own existence

Substitution of Antidepressants with AM Microdosing

After publishing the AM Microdosing Annual Review in Russia, I received new information related to the substitution of antidepressants with AM microdosing. Respondents described the method of switching from antidepressants (AD) to AM microdosing and the results obtained after the course. The data are presented in the following diagrams. Figure 27 shows that 60% (35 of 58) of participants quit AD cold turkey with positive results, 19% (11) quit AD gradually with positive results, 7% (4) quit AD cold turkey with negative results, and 14% (8) quit AD gradually with negative results.

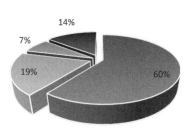

- Quit AD cold turkey, positive effects – 60% (35)
- Replaced AD gradually, positive effects – 19% (11)
- Quit AD cold turkey, negative effects – 7% (4)
- Replaced AD gradually, negative effects – 14% (8)

Fig. 27. Substitution of AD with AM microdosing (total 58)

Figure 28 reflects the positive results of substituting different AD brands with AM microdosing: Zoloft (sertraline) 35% (24 of 69) of participants; Prozac (fluoxetine) 14% (10); Cipralex and Lexapro (escitalopram) 12% (8); Paxil (paroxetine) 10% (7); others, including Wellbutrin (bupropion), 29% (20).

Figure 29 shows that 89% (42 of 47) of microdosers who substituted AD with AM microdosing had great results, and only 11% (5) had no results from the substitution and returned to AD.

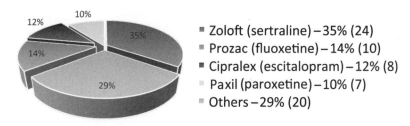

- Zoloft (sertraline) – 35% (24)
- Prozac (fluoxetine) – 14% (10)
- Cipralex (escitalopram) – 12% (8)
- Paxil (paroxetine) – 10% (7)
- Others – 29% (20)

Fig. 28. AD Brands Substituted with microdosing (total 69)

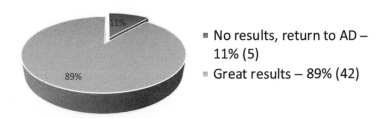

- No results, return to AD – 11% (5)
- Great results – 89% (42)

Fig. 29. AD Results of substituting AD for AM microdosing (total 47)

Asthma

Asthma. Allergic asthma is the most common type of asthma. Exposure to inhaled irritants, or triggers, can cause the walls of airways to become inflamed and the muscles around the airways to tighten up. That makes the airways narrower, leaving less room for air to flow.

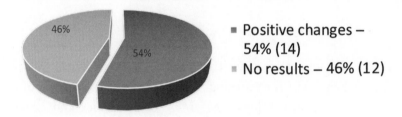

46%

54%

- Positive changes –
  54% (14)
- No results – 46% (12)

Fig. 30. Asthma and AM microdosing (total 26)

Figure 30 shows that positive changes to asthma symptoms during an AM microdose course were experienced by 54% (14 of 26) of participants; there were no results for 46% (12).

Autism

Autism is a developmental disorder, neurological in nature, that affects a person's thinking, perception, attention, education, behavior, social skills, interaction, and communication. The poll on autism was added in response to participants' requests later in the project's develop-

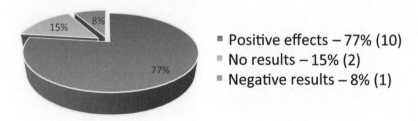

8%
15%
77%

- Positive effects – 77% (10)
- No results – 15% (2)
- Negative results – 8% (1)

Fig. 31. Autism and AM microdosing (total 13)

ment after publishing the AM Microdosing Annual Review in Russia. Information submitted is reflected in figure 31. Positive results were reported in 77% (10 of 13) of participants. There were no results in 15% (2) and negative results in 8% (1).

Cold

Cold is a viral infectious disease of the upper respiratory tract. Most common symptoms are nasal congestion, chills, watery eyes, headache, and throat irritation. AM microdosers reported that their cold was quickly resolved in 24–48 hours in 44% (81 of 186) of cases after taking *Amanita muscaria* microdoses. Symptoms were elevated in 34% (64), and there were no results in 20% (38) (see fig. 32).

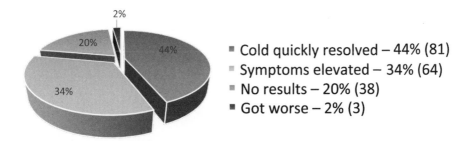

■ Cold quickly resolved – 44% (81)
■ Symptoms elevated – 34% (64)
■ No results – 20% (38)
■ Got worse – 2% (3)

*Fig. 32. Cold and AM microdosing
(total 186)*

Color Perception and Vision

The effects of microdosing AM on improving color perception and vision acuity were discovered by users and proposed for the poll. No change in vision or perception of the color scheme was observed by 63% (222 of 354) of participants (see fig. 33, next page). Improved color perception was seen by 18% (62), improved vision acuity by 5% (18), positive results of both were observed by 11% (41), with negative results in vision acuity by 3% (11).

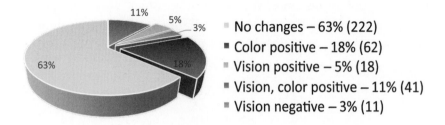

* No changes – 63% (222)
* Color positive – 18% (62)
* Vision positive – 5% (18)
* Vision, color positive – 11% (41)
* Vision negative – 3% (11)

*Fig. 33. Color perception, vision, and AM microdosing
(total 354)*

Conditions of the Skin

Eczema

Eczema is a chronic skin disease based on inflammation. Eczema symptoms are itching and redness of the skin with the formation of small vesicles filled with fluid. The vesicles resemble air bubbles that form during the boiling of water, which explains the name of the disease ("boil" from the Greek word *eczeo*).

The positive effects of AM microdosing on eczema symptoms were discovered by project participants, and a question was added to the poll per their requests after publishing the AM microdosing project's annual report in Russia. Positive effects of AM microdosing on eczema symptoms were noted by 51% (23 of 45) of participants. Positive effects with topical application of AM products were seen in 17% (8) of cases. There were positive effects with AM alcohol tincture taken orally in 16% (7) of cases and no results in 16% (7) (see fig. 34).

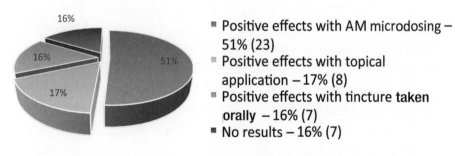

* Positive effects with AM microdosing – 51% (23)
* Positive effects with topical application – 17% (8)
* Positive effects with tincture taken orally – 16% (7)
* No results – 16% (7)

*Fig. 34. Eczema and AM microdosing
(total 45)*

Warts and Skin Pigmentation

I combined the effects of AM microdosing on clearing the skin of warts, growths, and pigment spots because this question was proposed by the participants almost at the end of the project and I did not want to inflate the already huge questionnaire on the effects of microdosing AM. However, in part 4 of this book, in individual reviews, there is a more detailed description of the effects and application methods. Figure 35 shows positive results with AM microdose consumption in 40% (52 of 128) of participants. Positive results with topical application of AM products were noted in 9% (11), and there were no changes in 51% (65).

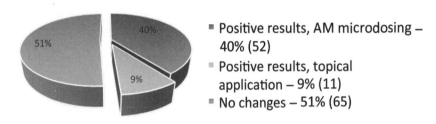

- Positive results, AM microdosing – 40% (52)
- Positive results, topical application – 9% (11)
- No changes – 51% (65)

Fig. 35. Warts, skin pigmentation, and AM microdosing (total 128)

Psoriasis

Psoriasis is a skin disorder that manifests itself in noninfectious inflammatory lesions of the skin cells. It is not contagious and cannot be passed from person to person. The etiology of psoriasis is not well understood. Autoimmune, genetic, stress, neurosis, reduced immunity, and psychosomatic causes of disease development are suggested. Psoriasis can be localized to any part of the body and is expressed in rashes, scales, and red patches accompanied by itching and pain. The positive effect of AM microdose intake was discovered by project participants, and on this basis, the question was put to further investigation. Two diagrams present the effects of an AM microdose course on psoriasis. Improvement in psoriasis with the use of AM microdose was detected by 65% (35 of 54) of questionnaire responders, no changes

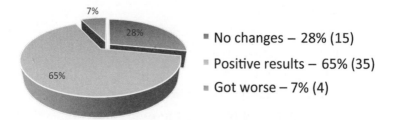

No changes – 28% (15)

Positive results – 65% (35)

Got worse – 7% (4)

Fig. 36. Psoriasis and AM microdosing (total 54)

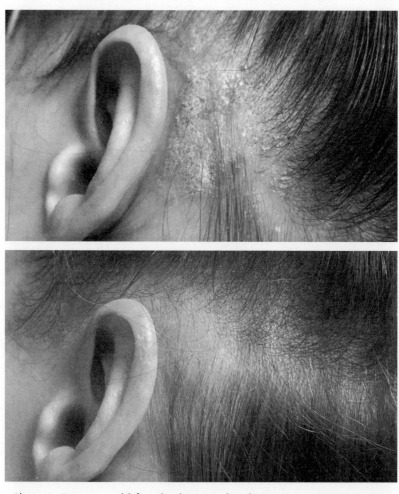

Photo 1. Forty-year-old female diagnosed with psoriasis seventeen years ago. Treatment with different prescription drugs was not successful. Morning intake of Amanita muscaria *microdose 0.35 g daily and local application* Amanita muscaria *lotion for forty days showed great results.*

occurred in 28% (15) of cases, and negative results were seen in 7% (4) (see fig. 36).

Figure 37 presents a direct comparison of positive effects with the various forms of *Amanita muscaria* that were used to treat psoriasis symptoms. Positive effects for an AM microdose course were observed in 64% (45 of 70) of cases; AM tincture consumption was seen in 19% (13); AM tincture topical application accounted for 6% (4); and AM ointment was used by 11% of participants (8). Details on the psoriasis treatment duration with *Amanita muscaria* products are presented in individual reviews and can be seen in the photos on page 54.

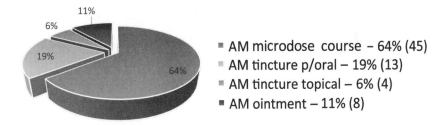

Fig. 37. Psoriasis and AM forms (total 70)

Onychomycosis (Nail Fungus)

Onychomycosis is a fungal infection of the nail. The symptoms include changes in the appearance of nails such as discoloration, thickening, and separation of the nail from the nail bed. Currently, there are about fifty species of fungi that can infect the nail plate. The spread of onychomycosis is highly dependent on climatic and social conditions, age, sex, profession, comorbidities such as diabetes, peripheral angiopathy, obesity, immunodeficiency conditions, endocrinopathy, oncology, diseases of the gastrointestinal tract, diseases of the nervous system, blood diseases, drug intake (cytostatic drugs, hormonal drugs, etc.), chemical factors, wearing cramped shoes made of synthetic materials, and other factors. The introduction of the fungus is usually preceded by nail injury, a violation of the body's natural resistance associated with immunodeficiencies, or dysfunction of life support systems leading to neurotrophic changes in the nail bed. Due to the presence of favorable conditions, the pathogenic fungus is introduced and begins to multiply, giving rise to the infectious process. Taking *Amanita muscaria* microdoses alone does not improve the disease without further eliminating the causes.

After a course of *Amanita muscaria* microdose, a complete cure was observed by 20% (49 of 245) of participants; an improvement in the nail plate condition was seen by 33% (81); and there were no results in 47% (115) of cases (see fig. 38). Further information on this topic is available in part 4 of this book.

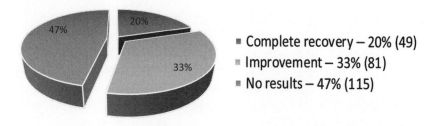

- Complete recovery – 20% (49)
- Improvement – 33% (81)
- No results – 47% (115)

Fig. 38. Onychomycosis and AM microdosing (total 245)

Burns

Burns treated with AM ointment showed great results. Photos of treating third-degree burns with mukhomor ointment are shown on page 57. The patient was treated in the hospital for a month using Levomekol without success. When amputation was suggested, the patient refused. My associate Thomas suggested a recipe for an ointment made with 200 g of bear fat and two heaping tablespoons of ground, dried *Amanita muscaria*. At night, a bandage with plenty of the ointment was applied. It was changed in the morning.

Usually, Thomas insists on preparing the ointment at least two weeks in advance, but there was no time to wait, and use of the ointment began immediately.

Figure 39 (p. 58) reflects the respondents' experiences treating burns with AM products. Great results were reported by 77% (17 of 22) of participants, and no results were noted by 23% (5).

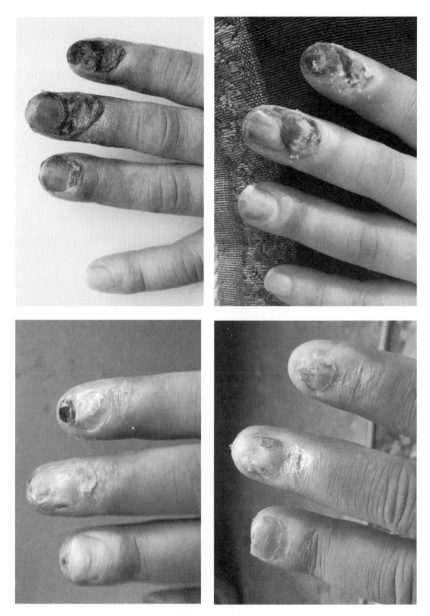

Photo 2. Left to right, top to bottom:
progression of burns treated
with AM ointment

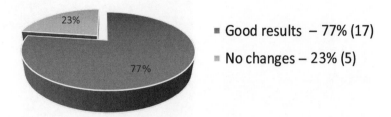

Fig. 39. Burns and AM microdosing (total 22)

Creativity

The influence of AM microdosing on creativity was also proposed by the project participants and added to the poll. A positive impact of AM microdosing on creativity was revealed in 63% (166 of 262) of participants, and no changes were seen in 37% (96) (see fig. 40).

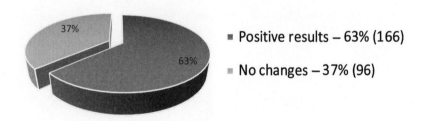

Fig. 40. Creativity and AM microdosing (total 262)

Epilepsy

Epilepsy is a brain disease characterized by attacks of repeated seizures in the form of motor, sensitive, or mental function disorders. In the period between attacks, the patient may feel normal and no different from other people. Questions on this condition were added recently, and we do not have a lot of data. However, the collection of information is ongoing, and we have more and more information. Positive results were noted by 77% (17 of 22) of participants; no changes were seen in 14% (3) of cases; and negative results occurred in 9% (2) (see fig. 41).

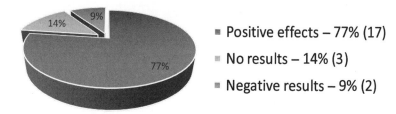

- Positive effects – 77% (17)
- No results – 14% (3)
- Negative results – 9% (2)

Fig. 41. Epilepsy and AM microdosing (total 22)

Gingivitis

Gingivitis is an inflammatory gum disease. The causes of gingivitis are multiple, including insufficient oral hygiene, smoking, avitaminosis, systemic diseases, and exposure to some drugs and heavy metals. Symptoms of gingivitis are inflammatory process in the gum area, bleeding, redness, and changing contours such as receding gums. Taking an AM microdose alone cannot improve the disease unless there is some elimination of the causes. This question was added at the suggestion of the participants. The results are shown in figure 42. Improvement with AM microdosing was observed by 37% (17 of 46) of participants; no changes were seen by 46% (21); and there was an improvement with the topical application of AM alcohol tincture in 17% (8) of cases.

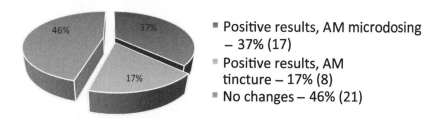

- Positive results, AM microdosing – 37% (17)
- Positive results, AM tincture – 17% (8)
- No changes – 46% (21)

Fig. 42. Gingivitis and AM microdosing (total 46)

Goiter

A goiter is a persistent tumorlike enlargement of the thyroid gland, visible to the eye and accompanied in some cases by a disorder of its function and disorders of the general state of the body. A goiter commonly develops as a result of iodine deficiency or inflammation of the thyroid gland. External manifestations include swelling on the front surface of the neck.

I added a poll on goiter after witnessing the great effects of AM microdosing. I was testing my English skills while writing this book alongside my sixty-two-year-old female friend who had been diagnosed with goiter and had visible symptoms. After reading a couple hundred letters from the study's participants, she asked me to give her some *Amanita muscaria* to try to improve her mood and appetite, as well as help with nicotine addiction and a sleep disorder. In three weeks we discovered changes in the size of the goiter and photographed her neck. I am proud to present the photos below.

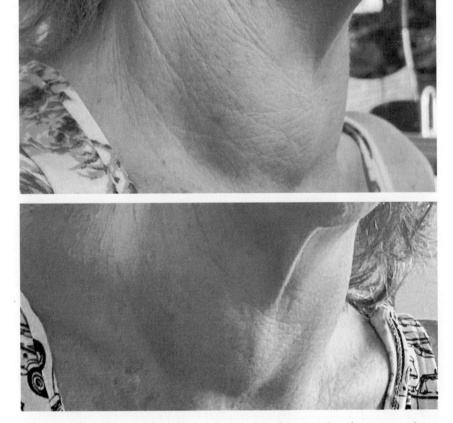

Photo 3. Top: the condition of the goiter after three weeks of AM microdose intake; Bottom: the result after three months of AM microdose consumption.

Figure 43 reflects the information I received from the program participants relative to the effect of AM microdose on goiters. There were positive effects for 88% (15 of 17) of participants and no changes for 12% (2).

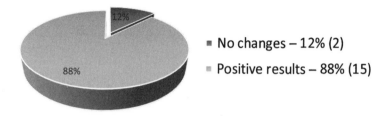

> ■ No changes – 12% (2)
> ■ Positive results – 88% (15)

Fig. 43. Goiter and AM microdosing
(total 17)

Hormonal Imbalance

Hormone imbalance in the female body most often leads to a number of gynecological diseases and pathological conditions. In addition, with hormone failure, emotional and physical well-being changes. If a woman has hormonal disorders, it can be evidenced by the presence of disorders of the menstrual cycle. The causes and types of previously diagnosed hormonal dysfunction were not considered in the questionnaires. The questions were general, although more detailed data can be found in participant reviews in part 4 of this book. Figure 44 reflects that no changes were noted by 49% (26 of 53) of participants. There were positive effects for 47% (25) and negative effects for 4% (2).

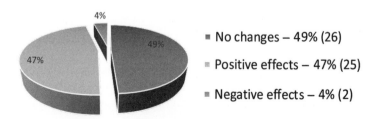

> ■ No changes – 49% (26)
> ■ Positive effects – 47% (25)
> ■ Negative effects – 4% (2)

Fig. 44. Hormonal dysfunction and AM microdosing
(total 53)

Libido

Libido is a person's general sexual drive or desire for sexual activity. Figure 45 and figure 46 show the effects of AM microdosing on libido. Libido improvement was reported in 43% (165 of 384) of men and 48% (48 of 100) of women. Libido was unchanged in 52% (198) of men and 41% (41) of women. Negative effects were seen in 5% (21) of men and 11% (11) of women.

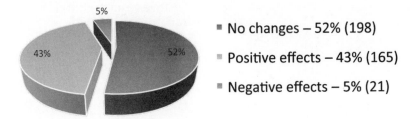

- No changes – 52% (198)
- Positive effects – 43% (165)
- Negative effects – 5% (21)

Fig. 45. Male libido and AM microdosing (total 384)

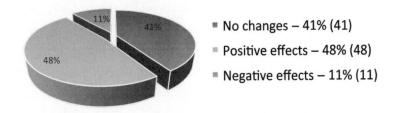

- No changes – 41% (41)
- Positive effects – 48% (48)
- Negative effects – 11% (11)

Fig. 46. Female libido and AM microdosing (total 100)

Hypertension

Hypertension is a condition where the force of blood pressure on blood vessels exceeds the norm. Hypertension is persistently elevated blood pressure. Blood pressure that is higher than 140/90 is considered hypertension. The reasons for the development of hypertension include smoking, alcohol use, heredity, sedentary lifestyle, overeating, excess weight, osteochondrosis, atherosclerosis, age-related hormonal changes, systematic stress, overstress, overload, negative emotions, and diabetes. This study did not take into account the etiology and degree of hypertension.

Figure 47 reflects the effect of microdosing AM on hypertension. Improvement was observed by 73% (46 of 63) of participants; no changes were reported by 19% (12); and there were negative results for 8% (5).

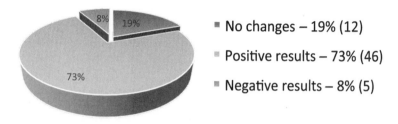

No changes – 19% (12)

Positive results – 73% (46)

Negative results – 8% (5)

Fig. 47. Hypertension and AM microdosing (total 63)

Mood Enhancer, Energizer

Project participants indicated that an AM microdose is a great mood stabilizer, especially if it is taken in the morning (see fig. 48, next page), according to 88% (868 of 981) of respondents. Sleepiness was observed in 12% (113) of users. Participants describe the morning intake effects as follows:

- balance
- bliss
- body tone
- boost of cheerfulness
- burst of energy
- calmness
- creativity
- deeper appreciation of nature, world, self, and life
- desire to act
- disappearance of irritability and mental chatterbox
- disappearance of past and future worries
- ease of communication

- effectiveness of the day
- endurance
- enhanced self-awareness
- feeling of well-being
- firmness of intent
- great mood uplift
- greater emotional connection and empathy
- happiness
- improved focus and concentration
- increased physical strength
- mental clarity, optimism, stamina, and motivation increased
- peacefulness
- purity of thoughts
- reduced anxiety
- virility
- vitality

Participants noted that morning intake sometimes caused sleepiness, which was gone after switching to the evening intake for a week and switching back to the morning intake after that.

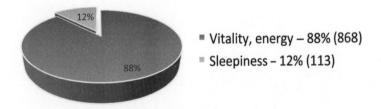

■ Vitality, energy – 88% (868)
▪ Sleepiness – 12% (113)

Fig. 48. AM microdosing as mood enhancer (total 981)

Pain Relief

This section presents the analgesic property of *Amanita muscaria* used in different forms, including dried fungus, lotion, and alcohol tincture. The subjects of research were joint pain, pain in the musculoskeletal system, menstrual pain, migraine pain, and neuropathic pain.

I fully confirm the analgesic long-term effects of *Amanita muscaria* tincture from my own experience. I have tested all possible alternative and conventional medicinal forms to treat my back pain, and none of them gave me effective, long-term pain relief. I have been using *Amanita* tincture for about five years, reducing the amount every year. The effect is prolonged and persistent, although *Amanita muscaria* does not treat the primary condition itself and the cause of the pain (age-related disorder of the spinal musculoskeletal system). The recipe for alcohol tincture can be found in chapter 9 of this book.

Arthritis, Rheumatoid Arthritis, and Muskuloskeletal Pain

Program participants confirmed the analgesic properties of *Amanita muscaria* in the form of microdoses, tincture, and lotions as well. Figure 49 presents the results of AM microdosing to alleviate arthritis pain. Positive effects were observed by 70% (333 of 477) of participants. No results were seen in 30% (144).

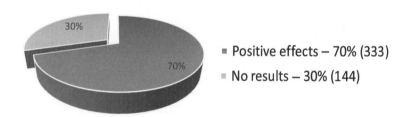

Fig. 49. Arthritis and AM microdosing
(total 477)

Participants proposed separating rheumatoid arthritis after publishing the annual AM microdosing report in Russia, and these results are presented in figure 50 (next page). Pain relief after using AM microdose and tincture was observed by 39% (9 of 23) of participants; pain relief with tincture only was seen by 22% (5); relief was noted with AM microdose only use in 30% (7) of cases; and no results were observed in 9% (2).

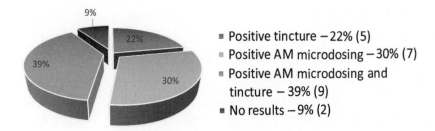

* Positive tincture – 22% (5)
* Positive AM microdosing – 30% (7)
* Positive AM microdosing and tincture – 39% (9)
* No results – 9% (2)

Fig. 50. Rheumatoid arthritis and AM microdosing
(total 23)

Figure 51 reflects the effectiveness of *Amanita muscaria* alcohol tincture when used for pain relief on arthritis and musculoskeletal pain. Positive effects were observed by 81% (93 of 115) of participants, and no results were seen by 19% (22).

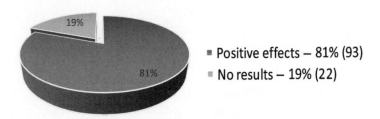

* Positive effects – 81% (93)
* No results – 19% (22)

Fig. 51. Pain Relief and AM tincture
(total 115)

Menstrual Pain

As outlined in table 2, positive results of pain relief during a menstrual period were registered by 52% (39 of 75) of participants; no changes were noticed in 36% (27); and negative effects were perceived by 12% (9).

Migraine

Migraine pain relief was reported in 65% (72 of 110) of the reports; no results were observed in 35% (38).

Neuropathic Pain

Pain relief with chronic neuropathic pain was noticed by 86% (55 of 64) of participants, and no results were seen in 14% (9).

TABLE 2. PAIN RELIEF

CONDITION/ EFFECTS	POSITIVE EFFECTS	NO RESULTS	NEGATIVE EFFECTS
Menstrual Cramps (75)	52% (39)	36% (27)	12% (9)
Migraine (110)	65% (72)	35% (38)	
Neuropathic Pain (64)	86% (55)	14% (9)	

Perspiration

Some participants in the project noticed a change in sweating during the use of AM microdose. The changes consisted of the amount of sweating and a change in smell. The question was proposed for an additional survey.

The results are shown in figure 52. No perspiration changes were registered in 67% (248 of 369) of participants. An increase in perspiration was reported by 16% (60) of participants and a decrease in

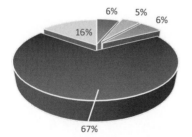

6%   5%   6%

- Perspiration decrease – 6% (22)
- Perspiration and smell increase – 5% (17)
- Perspiration decrease and smell increase – 6% (22)
- No changes – 67% (248)
- Perspiration increase – 16% (60)

Fig. 52. Perspiration and AM microdosing (total 369)

perspiration was noted in 6% (22). Perspiration and smell increased for 5% (17) of participants, while perspiration decreased with an increase in smell for 6% (22) of participants.

Prostatitis

Prostatitis is an inflammation of the prostate gland that manifests itself in an acute or chronic form. The causes of prostatitis may be bacterial infection, congestive phenomena of the pelvic organs, hypodynamic lifestyle, and so on. Symptoms include difficulty urinating, groin pain, pain in the pelvic area, genital pain, sometimes flulike symptoms, and others.

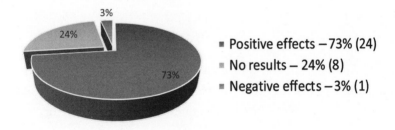

- Positive effects – 73% (24)
- No results – 24% (8)
- Negative effects – 3% (1)

Fig. 53. Prostatitis and AM microdosing
(total 33)

The effect of AM microdosing on prostatitis is reflected in figure 53. Improvement was noticed by 73% (24 of 33) of participants, no results were noted in 24% (8), and negative results were observed in 3% (1).

Sleeping Aid

Sleep is extremely important for human health. During sleep, the human body regains its strength. On average, a person needs from 6–10 hours of sleep. People spend a third of their lives in a dream, which is completely justified. A person will not survive for more than two hundred hours without sleep. They become lethargic, their emotions disappear, their reactions decrease, and immunity decreases.

The causes of insomnia are numerous. They include conditions such as Parkinsonism, hyperthyroidism, depressive disorders, neurosis, pain, mental disorders, endocrine system pathologies, apnea, increased emotional experiences, side effects of drugs, bad habits (alcohol, tobacco, drugs, overeating before bed), neurology, external irritants, night work, and changing time zones, as well as individual characteristics such as age, temperament, current state of health, and lifestyle.

Insomnia manifests itself in trouble falling asleep, restless sleep with frequent awakenings after which it is difficult or impossible to sleep, daytime apathy, and fatigue. During the day, signs of insomnia appear in the form of irritability, lethargy, reduced level of attention, distractions, and mood swings. All that leads to human social dysfunction since insomnia symptoms cause a decline in motivation for anything. People suffering from insomnia feel constant drowsiness during the day. Often, they have headaches and problems with their gastrointestinal tract.

Many participants taking an AM microdose at night reported that it enabled them to quickly fall into a deep sleep with amazing, realistic, and fantastic dreams. In the morning, they woke with a feeling of vigor and the sensation of a well-rested body. Figure 54 shows successful use of an AM microdose as a sleep aid in 73% (719) of the 980 participants with no dependency. The effects were long-lasting after the course ended. There were no changes in 17% (168), and insomnia was observed by 10% (93) of participants.

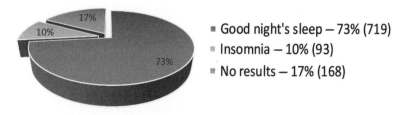

Fig. 54. AM microdose as sleep aid
(total 980)

Stroke and Cardiac Arrest Recovery

The effects of AM microdosing on stroke and cardiac arrest recovery require a closer, more detailed consideration of the effects and severity of the condition. In the framework of the project as a preliminary study, the results are enough to warrant such further investigation, especially given the small amount of information received.

There were 35% (6) positive results among the seventeen participants during stroke recovery and 66% (12) positive results from eighteen participants in using AM microdosing during cardiac arrest recovery. There were no changes in 53% (9) of participants for stroke recovery and 17% (3) for cardiac arrest recovery. Negative effects were observed by 12% (2) and 17% (3) of participants, respectively (see fig. 55 and fig. 56).

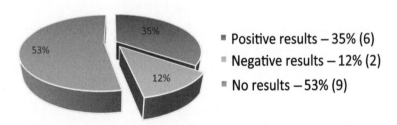

Fig. 55. Stroke recovery and AM microdosing (total 17)

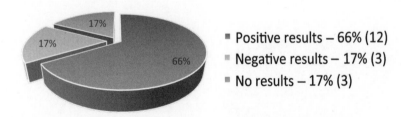

Fig. 56. Cardiac arrest recovery and AM microdosing (total 18)

Swelling of the Lower Extremities

Swelling of the lower extremities is expressed by the accumulation of fluid in the tissues as a result of damage to the lymph nodes or blood circulation. Symptoms are expressed in swelling of the legs, vascular asterisks, fatigue in the legs, cramps, and so on. The reasons vary, including hypodynamic, or immobile lifestyle; excessive salt consumption; smoking; force loads; uncomfortable shoes; trauma; bruises; pregnancy; cardiovascular, kidney, adrenal conditions; and so on. In this regard, it is necessary to determine the cause of the swelling and make a lifestyle correction before taking an AM microdose. Figure 57 shows the effects of AM microdosing on swelling of the lower extremities. There was an overall positive effect from both delivery forms, AM microdose and AM alcohol tincture, for 83% (39 of 47) of participants. There were no results for 17% (8).

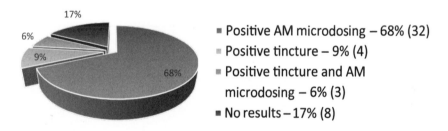

- Positive AM microdosing – 68% (32)
- Positive tincture – 9% (4)
- Positive tincture and AM microdosing – 6% (3)
- No results – 17% (8)

Fig. 57. Swelling of lower extremities and AM microdosing (total 47)

Data Summary Effects of *Amanita muscaria* Microdosing

The following table (in alphabetical order) reflects the data summary effects of AM microdosing on nosological units that were researched in this study. I added more polls to the questionnaire per participants' requests in October 2020. The questions for discussion cover the effects of AM microdosing on nosological units, including Alzheimer's disease, chronic cystitis, coronavirus, *Helicobacter pylori,* HIV, Hunter syndrome, multiple sclerosis, and Parkinson's disease. The results are reflected at the end of table 3. There is more information in the reports about quick relief from tick and mosquito bites and poison oak symptom relief.

TABLE 3. DATA SUMMARY EFFECTS OF AM MICRODOSING

CONDITION	POSITIVE EFFECTS	NO RESULTS	NEGATIVE EFFECTS
Allergy (104)	59% (61)	41% (43)	
Antidepressants Subst. (47)	89% (42)	11% (5)	
Appetite (473)	25% (116) increased	37% (177)	37% (180) decreased
Arthritis (477)	70% (333)	30% (144)	31% (151) decreased
Asthenia, Depression (999)	87% (874)	10% (100)	3% (25)
Asthma (26)	54% (14)	46% (12)	
Autism (13)	77% (10)	15% (2)	8% (1)
Burns (22)	77% (17)	22% (5)	3% (25)
Cardiac Arrest Recovery (18)	66% (12)	17% (3)	17% (3)
Cold (186)	78% (145)	20% (38)	8% (1)
Constipation (192)	58% (111)	42% (81)	
Creativity (262)	63% (166)	37% (96)	
Eczema (45)	84% (38)	16% (7)	
Epilepsy (22)	77% (17)	14% (3)	9% (2)
Gingivitis (46)	54% (25)	46% (21)	
Goiter (17)	88% (15)	12% (2)	7% (4)
Heartburn (66)	53% (35) relief	32% (21)	15% (10) increased

CONDITION	POSITIVE EFFECTS	NO RESULTS	NEGATIVE EFFECTS
Hormonal Dysfunction (53)	47% (25)	49% (26)	4% (2)
Hypertension (63)	73% (46)	19% (12)	8% (5)
Libido, Men (384)	43% (165)	52% (198)	5% (21)
Libido, Women (100)	48% (48)	41% (41)	11% (11)
Meat Consumption (485)	Change to vegetarian 12% (60)	57% (274)	31% (151) decreased
Menstrual Cramps (75)	52% (39)	36% (27)	12% (9)
Migraine (110)	65% (72)	35% (38)	8% (5)
Mood Enhancer (981)	88% (868)	12% (113)	
Nail Fungus (245)	53% (130)	47% (115)	
Neuropathic Pain (64)	86% (55)	14% (9)	
Prostatitis (33)	73% (24)	24% (8)	3% (1)
Psoriasis (54)	65% (35)	28% (15)	7% (4)
Rheumatoid Arthritis (23)	91% (21)	9% (2)	
Sleeping Aid (980)	73% (719)	17% (168)	10% (93)
Stroke Recovery (17)	35% (6)	53% (9)	12% (2)
Sugar Consumption (501)	48% (240) decreased	52% (261)	12% (2)
Swelling (47)	83% (39)	17% (8)	17% (3)
Tongue Plaque (264)	27% (71)	73% (193)	
Warts, Skin Tags (128)	49% (63)	51% (65)	

TABLE 3. DATA SUMMARY EFFECTS OF
AM MICRODOSING (not discussed in this book)

CONDITION	POSITIVE EFFECTS	NO RESULTS	NEGATIVE EFFECTS
Alzheimer's Disease (11)	73% (8)	18% (2)	9% (1)
Chronic Cystitis (25)	48% (12) stable remission	52% (13)	
COVID (48)	44% (21)	52% (25)	4% (2)
Helicobacter pylori (18)	56% (10) stable remission	33% (6)	11% (2)
HIV (18)	61% (11)	22% (4)	17% (3)
Hunter Syndrome (7)	43% (3)	57% (4)	17% (3)
Multiple Sclerosis (21)	52% (11)	38% (8)	10% (2)
Parkinson's Disease (9)	45% (4)	33% (3)	22% (2)
Postchemotherapy (12)	58% (7)	34% (4)	8% (1)
Chronic Cystitis (25)	48% (12) stable remission	52% (13)	

Nothing will come of nothing.

WILLIAM SHAKESPEARE,
KING LEAR, ACT 1, SCENE 1

Comparison of
Microdosing Effects of *Amanita muscaria*
and Psilocybin Mushrooms

I want to briefly address the differences and similarities of the micro-dosing effects of two mushrooms: *Amanita muscaria* mushroom and psilocybin mushroom. I collected my own data on psilocybin mush-room microdosing using the Telegram media platform with the help of built-in polling bot programs.

According to my survey, AM microdoses have a wide range of effects on an extensive variety of pathologies of different etiologies, or causations, including hormonal, endocrine, immunological, bacterial, and viral infections. The use of psilocybin mushrooms does not cover somatic diseases. That information is correlated with other research, and psilocybin mushroom microdosing is not effective in combating diseases or physiological symptoms such as pain.[1]

According to my research, psilocybin mushroom microdosing is not showing sleep aid quality, and it is not showing results in the treatment of skin pathologies such as psoriasis, eczema, warts, or skin pigmentation.

There was no analgesic property of psilocybin mushrooms when compared to *Amanita muscaria* that was used in various forms such as dried fungus, lotion, and alcohol tincture. The treatment subjects were joint pain, pain in the musculoskeletal system, rheumatoid arthritis, menstrual pain, and migraine.

The majority of my respondents microdosed with psilocybin mush-rooms primarily to enhance performance such as increasing energy, creativity, study, motivation, and concentration, and alleviating psycho-logical symptoms such as asthenia and depression. Most reports revealed a general increase in reported psychological functioning—well-being, mystical experiences, personality and mood traits, as well as a reduc-tion in negative emotions, dysfunctional attitudes, neuroticism, anxiety, aggression, frustration, relationship problems, fear of communication, and panic attacks. These effects are very similar to *Amanita muscaria* microdosing as presented in chapter 4.

There are some similarities between AM microdosing and psilocybin mushroom microdosing. Psilocybin microdoses are proving effective at treating addiction to alcohol, nicotine, and amphetamines. Addiction to drugs (alcohol, narcotics, prescription drugs, and nicotine) was recurrently said to be effectively treated by a microdosing practice.[2] Researchers from Johns Hopkins found that 80% of smokers who took psilocybin as part of cognitive behavioral therapy were able to quit tobacco completely.[3]

Psilocybin microdoses have also been found to have comparable or better results in treating cluster headaches than most conventional medications. Many people have experienced extended periods of remission after treating their headaches with psychedelic substances.[4] The intense desperation described by sufferers of treatment-resistant cluster headaches and how microdosing cured or lessened the frequency of pain episodes were other noteworthy testimonies of experienced health benefits.[5]

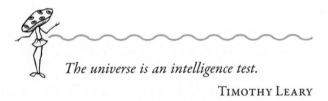

The universe is an intelligence test.

TIMOTHY LEARY

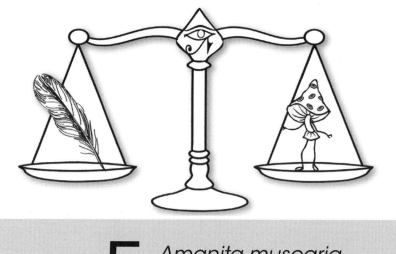

5 *Amanita muscaria* Microdose Negative Effects

Contraindications

Contraindications for taking AM microdoses according to my data are:

1. Mental illness (bipolar disorder, schizophrenia, and so on). I received quite negative feedback from those taking AM microdoses with this pathology.
2. Pregnant mothers and those who are nursing newborns.
3. Presence of urolithiasis (kidney stones). As it turned out, AM microdoses activate the removal of stones from the bladder and kidneys. (This information was confirmed in the 2021–2022 period and is not reflected in the reports or negative effects chapter.)

Overall Negative Symptoms of *Amanita muscaria* Microdose Intake

This project is a preliminary study without extensive physical examination data for the presence and severity of pathology or preexisting conditions. However, as shown in figure 58, rejection of AM microdosing due to negative effects occurred in only 7% (36 of 552) of cases, and 93% (516) of AM microdosers successfully finished the course and were planning to repeat it in the future.

Figure 59 reflects the diversity of these possible AM microdosing negative effects: 7% (46 of 679) experienced discomfort in the kidney area; 3% (22) had pancreas discomfort; 3% (21) had liver discomfort; 10% (69) experienced headaches; and 5% (34) had other negative effects. However, these numbers do not indicate the incidence of pathology in this group.

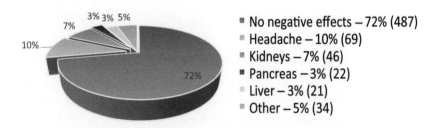

■ Continue AM microdosing, plan to repeat it – 93% (516)
■ Quit AM microdosing because of negative symptoms – 7% (36)

Fig. 58. Overall opinion on AM microdose course (total 552)

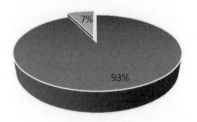

■ No negative effects – 72% (487)
■ Headache – 10% (69)
■ Kidneys – 7% (46)
■ Pancreas – 3% (22)
■ Liver – 3% (21)
■ Other – 5% (34)

Fig. 59. Negative symptoms and AM microdosing (total 679)

For instance, 10% (42 of 419) of participants reported pain in the kidney area, while 90% (377) had no pain; 6% (22 of 399) reported diagnosed renal pathology, 16% (64) were not sure if they had renal pathology, and no renal pathology was reported by 78% (313) (see fig. 60 and fig. 61).

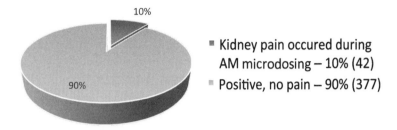

Fig. 60. Kidney pain and AM microdosing (total 419)

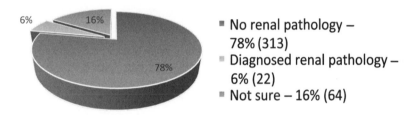

Fig. 61. Presence of renal pathology (total 399)

Individual reports in part 4 of this book indicate that most negative symptoms were light and went away shortly after the course continued.

When the AM microdosing annual report was published in Russia, I received participants' requests to add five more questions for polling. These conditions were acne, diarrhea, exacerbation of chronic diseases, body temperature, and urine color during an *Amanita muscaria* microdose course. The following numbers were collected in a couple of months and show the high activity of the participants in this project.

There was no acne observed during an AM microdose course in 92% (234 of 253) of cases. Acne appeared at the beginning of the course and disappeared quickly for 6% (14), and 2% (5) of users quit AM microdosing because of acne (see fig. 62, next page).

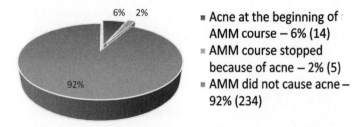

- Acne at the beginning of
  AMM course – 6% (14)
- AMM course stopped
  because of acne – 2% (5)
- AMM did not cause acne –
  92% (234)

Fig. 62. Acne and AM microdosing (total 253)

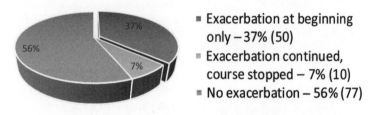

- Exacerbation at beginning
  only – 37% (50)
- Exacerbation continued,
  course stopped – 7% (10)
- No exacerbation – 56% (77)

Fig. 63. Exacerbation of chronic diseases (total 137)

There was no exacerbation experienced during an AM microdose course in 56% (77 of 137) of questionnaire responders with chronic diseases. There was short-term exacerbation at the beginning of an AM microdose course, and it was gone shortly in 37% (50) of participants. The AM microdose course was stopped because of exacerbation of chronic diseases by 7% (10) of participants (see fig. 63).

Body Temperature, Urine Color

Two more questions—body temperature and urine color during an AM microdose course—were included in the poll at participants' requests. The results are reflected in figures 64 and 65. Body temperature during the AM microdose course was normal in 94% (258 of 277) of the cases. No changes in urine color during the AM microdose course were reported in 95% (298 of 315).

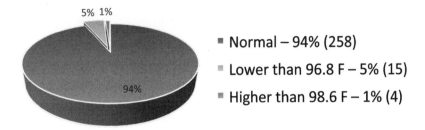

5% 1%

94%

- Normal – 94% (258)
- Lower than 96.8 F – 5% (15)
- Higher than 98.6 F – 1% (4)

Fig. 64. Body temperature during AM microdosing
(total 277)

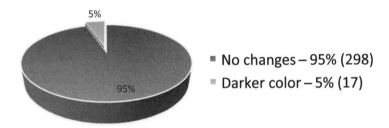

5%

95%

- No changes – 95% (298)
- Darker color – 5% (17)

Fig. 65. Urine color during AM microdosing
(total 315)

Diarrhea

Figure 66 reflects that 75% (202 of 270) of participants did not have diarrhea during AM microdose intake. In 21% (57) of cases diarrhea occurred only at the beginning of the AM microdose course and quickly disappeared; and the AM microdose course was terminated because of diarrhea in 4% (11) of the cases.

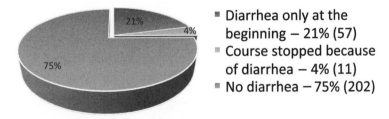

21%
4%
75%

- Diarrhea only at the beginning – 21% (57)
- Course stopped because of diarrhea – 4% (11)
- No diarrhea – 75% (202)

Fig. 66. Diarrhea during AM microdosing (total 270)

Digestive System, Nausea

The following pie charts illustrate the effect of AM microdosing on the gastrointestinal tract, including nausea and other uncomfortable conditions. More information is available in part 4 of this book.

There was no discomfort observed in 63% (443 of 702) of participants while microdosing AM. Nausea was observed in 22% (153); burping, rumbling, and gas were seen in 14% (99); and abdominal cramps occurred in 1% (7) of participants (see fig. 67).

The questionnaire revealed that nausea correlated with the way the AM microdose was consumed. In 67% (265 of 394) of cases, nausea was not observed with any form of AM microdose reception. The presence of nausea when taking dry AM was 18% (72); nausea when taking AM in the form of tea was seen in 11% (43); and nausea when taking AM was observed by 4% (14) of participants (see fig. 68).

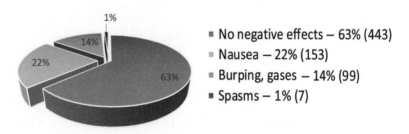

- No negative effects – 63% (443)
- Nausea – 22% (153)
- Burping, gases – 14% (99)
- Spasms – 1% (7)

Fig. 67. Digestive system and AM microdosing (total 702)

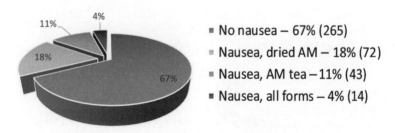

- No nausea – 67% (265)
- Nausea, dried AM – 18% (72)
- Nausea, AM tea – 11% (43)
- Nausea, all forms – 4% (14)

*Fig. 68. Nausea and AM microdose form
(total 394)*

The correlation of the presence of nausea with the method of harvesting the fungus is reflected in figure 69. Nausea with an unknown method of preparation (purchased AM) was noted in 49% (76 of 156) of cases. Nausea with cured AM was 13% (20), and for fresh dried AM, it was 38% (60).

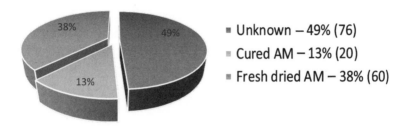

- Unknown – 49% (76)
- Cured AM – 13% (20)
- Fresh dried AM – 38% (60)

Fig. 69. Nausea and AM microdose preparation (total 156)

There is a clear correlation to the presence of nausea when the AM microdose weight is increased, as shown in figure 70. At up to 1 g, nausea was observed in only 12% (24 of 202) of participants; with 1–2 g, nausea was reported in 16% (32); and for 3 g and above, nausea was observed in 72% (146).

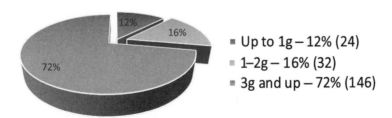

- Up to 1g – 12% (24)
- 1–2g – 16% (32)
- 3g and up – 72% (146)

*Fig. 70. Nausea and AM weight
(total 202)*

Nausea also was not a permanent effect of taking 1 g of AM or less. Sometimes nausea was observed at the beginning of the course but ceased to be an issue later on; this was the case with 16% (78 of 493) of respondents (see fig. 71). Other times, nausea disappeared after a decrease in dosage or by changing the intake form, as was seen in 5% (24) of cases, and there was no nausea with 1 g of AM in 79% (391) of participants.

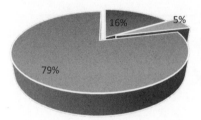

- Nausea only at the beginning of the course – 16% (78)
- Nausea was gone with change of AM form – 5% (24)
- No nausea with 1g – 79% (391)

Fig. 71. Nausea with 1g AM microdose
(total 493)

Heartburn

Figure 72 shows that AM microdosing caused heartburn in 15% (11 of 75) of reports; 49% (37) of participants noticed relief of existing heartburn; and 36% (27) reported no relief of existing heartburn.

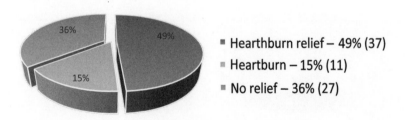

- Hearthburn relief – 49% (37)
- Heartburn – 15% (11)
- No relief – 36% (27)

Fig. 72. Heartburn and AM microdising
(total 75)

Salivation

Salivation is a reflex release of saliva by the salivary glands located in the oral cavity when stimuli affect the nerve endings of the oral cavity. Increased salivation was observed during the AM microdose course, and it was proposed for questioning. The result is shown in figure 73. As you can see, normal salivation was observed in 78% (356 of 458) of reports, and increased salivation was seen in 22% (102).

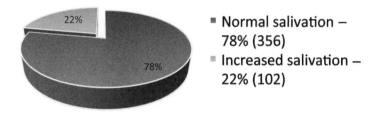

Fig. 73. Salivation and AM microdosing (total 458)

Correlation of AM Weight with Intoxication and Consciousness Changes

In the questionnaire I stated that AM poisoning is called severe intoxication, accompanied by spasmodic abdominal pain, vomiting, frequent liquid stool, drop in blood pressure, comatose state, confusion, and salivation. Particular attention was given to poll responders whose symptoms developed on a dosage of less than 3 g (see fig. 74). Four users

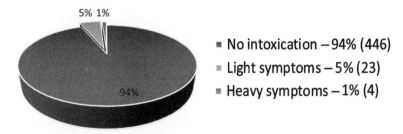

Fig. 74. Intoxication and AM microdosing (total 473)

reported poisoning and the need to consult a doctor. My calls to these participants to discuss the situation privately were unsuccessful. But 94% (446 of 473) of participants reported no intoxication signs with up to 3 g of AM microdose intake.

Correlation of AM Dosage with Change in Perception

This part reflects information on the correlation between the AM dosage and the appearance of changes in perception. Symptoms of change in perception and consciousness are visions of fractals and color patterns; loss of control over physiological functions of the body; auditory, tactile, and visual hallucinations; change in the perception of time; change in the sequence of real events; the transition of perception from visual-sensual to verbal images; changes in existing values; change of concentration and attention; depersonalization and derealization; speech disorders and difficulty verbalizing; lack of critical thinking; and more. These were observed mainly after receiving more than 3 g, according to the participants' reports. A change in perception when taking an AM microdosage of up to 1 g was observed in 6% (13 of 228) of cases; at dosage of 1–2 g, a change was seen in 7% (15); at 3–5 g, change was seen in 22% (50); and at 5–10 g, change was seen in 65% (150) (see fig. 75).

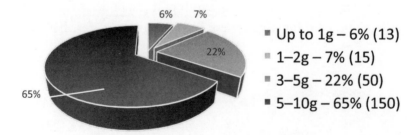

6%   7%

22%

65%

- Up to 1g – 6% (13)
- 1–2g – 7% (15)
- 3–5g – 22% (50)
- 5–10g – 65% (150)

Fig. 75. Perception change and AM weights
(total 228)

The correlation between the increase of trip effects with an increase in the weight of the consumed AM is reflected in figure 76. The increase in trip effects when taking more than 10 g was 61% (123 of 200) of participants, compared to 20% (39) at 5–9 g, and 19% (38) at AM microdose up to 5 g.

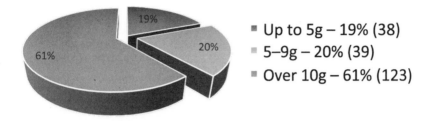

- Up to 5g – 19% (38)
- 5–9g – 20% (39)
- Over 10g – 61% (123)

Fig. 76. Trip effects and AM microdosing
(total 200)

Data on Consumption of AM Stems

The use of twice-boiled and then fried AM stems for food has repeatedly been addressed in support chats since the experiments were ambiguous. My personal experience with eating twice-boiled AM by the recipe given me by participants was unsuccessful, although I finally figured out a good way to take away all the unnecessary substances and prepare a tasty, mouth-watering dish with AM stems. I present that recipe in chapter 9 of this book.

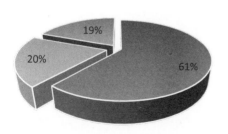

- Normal reaction, no changes – 61% (70)
- Obvious changes in perception – 20% (23)
- Slight changes in perception – 19% (22)

Fig. 77. Consumption of AM stems (total 115)

At the request of the participants, the question of stem consumption was included in the questionnaire. The results are reflected in figure 77 (previous page). Trip changes in consciousness when eating the cooked AM stems were noted in 39% (45 of 115) of AM stem eaters, and no reaction was seen in 61% (70).

No army can withstand the strength of an idea whose time has come.

VICTOR HUGO, *LES MISÉRABLES*

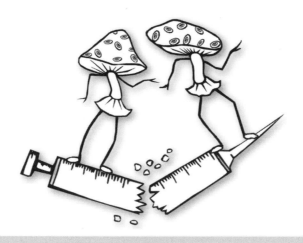

6 Amanita muscaria Microdose Effects on Various Addictions

Alcohol, Caffeine, Marijuana, Nicotine

Alcohol is a toxic psychoactive substance, a depressant that inhibits a human's central nervous system.[1] It is a legal drug with a high probability of the user developing an addiction. Ethyl alcohol is also used as a fuel, a solvent, and a disinfectant. Since I grew up in a country where this so-called rocket fuel was absorbed in immeasurable quantities by the entire population with no exclusions, I've seen the obvious influence of alcohol on the human body. My medical practice also proved that.

Ethanol is a hemolytic poison.[2] Alcohol has a toxic effect on metabolism and human organs such as the brain, gastrointestinal organs, the cardiovascular system, and the genitourinary system. There is practically no organ that does not suffer from the toxic effects of ethanol. According to observations from 1990 to 2001, more than half of Russian males ages 15–54 died from causes directly related to alcohol abuse.[3] Ethyl alcohol consumption holds the leading place among household poisoning in the absolute number of deaths.[4] The International Agency for the Study of Cancer classifies ethanol in alcoholic beverages as a proven carcinogen that can cause cancer in humans.

There is a statistically significant reduction in the risk of impaired brain cognitive function associated with moderate alcohol consumption compared to total alcohol abstinence in various countries.[5] Parental alcoholism significantly affects the development of the mental sphere of preborn children and is one of the reasons for the formation of undifferentiated forms of mental retardation.[6] Adult children of alcoholics are a fairly vast, highly autoaggressive layer of society. These people are the most susceptible in terms of frequency of development of various kinds of addictions, as well as attempted suicide.[7]

Figure 78 reflects the effects of AM microdosing on alcohol consumption. According to the responses, it was noted that AM microdosing decreased alcohol consumption in 50% (192 of 385) of participants, and 35% (136) of participants stopped drinking alcohol. No results were observed in 15% (57). There is more detailed information about the severity of alcohol dependence, the effects obtained, and the duration of the AM microdose course in part 4 of this book, which is devoted to individual reviews of project participants.

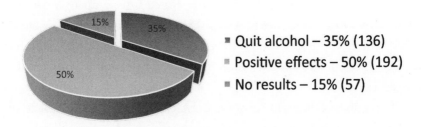

- Quit alcohol – 35% (136)
- Positive effects – 50% (192)
- No results – 15% (57)

Fig. 78. Alcohol addiction and AM microdosing
(total 385)

Figure 79 shows respondents indicated a prolonged and stable result of the anti-alcohol effect of AM microdosing with 89% (184 of 207)

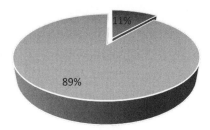

■ Return to previous level of alcohol consumption after AMM course – 11% (23)

■ Stable effect – 89% (184)

Fig. 79. Stability of AM microdose on alcohol consumption (total 207)

of participants. A return to the previous level of alcohol demand was observed only in 11% (23).

Table 4 shows the total positive effects of AM microdosing on the use of caffeine for 40% (83 of 210) of participants and no results in 58% (122). Total positive effects on the use of marijuana were 57% (96 of 169) of users, and there were no results for 40% (67). Total positive results on the use of nicotine were 49% (96 of 196) of contributors, and there were no results for 45% (89).

TABLE 4. ADDICTIONS AND AM MICRODOSING

SUBSTANCE	QUIT	POSITIVE RESULTS	NO RESULTS	NEGATIVE RESULTS
Caffeine (210)	14% (29)	26% (54)	58% (122)	2% (5)
Marijuana (169)	13% (22)	44% (74)	40% (67)	3% (6)
Nicotine (196)	18% (36)	31% (60)	45% (89)	6% (11)

Amphetamines, Cocaine, Designer Drugs, Salts, Mixes, Spice, Opioids, Heroin, Methadone, Oxycodone, Fentanyl, Opium

Substance abuse can cause organ damage, hormone imbalances, gastrointestinal diseases, fertility issues, and other illnesses. Many of these medical problems come with long-lasting consequences. The discovery of the positive effects of *Amanita muscaria* microdoses on various drug addictions during project development was a really good surprise. *Amanita muscaria* microdoses also challenge unhealthy thoughts and behaviors associated with drug abuse according to collected data.

Table 5 shows the positive effects of AM microdosing on the use of amphetamines for 78% (61 of 78) of participants; the use of cocaine for 74% (28 of 38); the use of synthetic drugs such as designer drugs, salts, mixes, and spices for 88% (65 of 74); and the use of opioids, heroin, methadone, oxycodone, fentanyl, and opium for 68% (23 of 34). The effects of AM microdosing on other addictions (e-cigarettes, computer games, etc.) can be found in part 4 of this book.

TABLE 5. DRUG ADDICTIONS AND AM MICRODOSING

SUBSTANCE	POSITIVE RESULTS	NO RESULTS	NEGATIVE RESULTS
Amphetamines (78)	78% (61)	14% (11)	8% (6)
Cocaine (38)	74% (28)	26% (10)	
Designer Drugs, Salts, Mixes, Spices (74)	88% (65)	12% (9)	
Opioids, Heroin, Methadone, Oxycodone, Fentanyl, Opium (34)	68% (23)	17% (6)	15% (5)

Only the madman is absolutely sure.

ROBERT ANTON WILSON

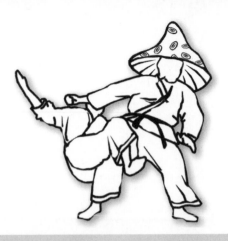

CHAPTER **7** *Amanita muscaria*
Microdose and Sport
Fighters' Performance

Sport performance is a multiple combination of different factors that include biomechanical, neuromuscular, mental, psychological, and other aspects. The discovery of positive effects of *Amanita muscaria* microdosing on sport performance was made by project participants. They noticed improvement in the ability of the body to respond to external stimuli in sports, elevated mental control, focus, self-motivation, confidence, discipline, and advanced relationship between the nervous and musculoskeletal systems.

Amanita muscaria microdosing improved mental toughness and helped athletes to overcome the anxieties around performance, physical pain, fear of an injury, or even embarrassment and humiliation related to not performing well enough. These factors significantly helped athletes reach the heights of their full potential.

A group of sport fighters approached me during the *Amanita muscaria* microdosing research and proposed collecting information about the impact of AM microdosing on wrestling. A new questionnaire addressing eight new elements was designed.

The questions proposed for research were coordination, endurance of the fighter, fighting intelligence (reading the opponent, preparing for the attack, misleading the enemy about their actions), general effects on the central nervous system (CNS) during sports, integrated impact (combat mindset and using proven fighting techniques and strategies), neuromuscular function (major adaptive system that facilitates and controls movement and stability), reaction rate, and sense of distance.

The data is reflected in table 6. The number of participants was small, but nevertheless, the data gives us a general idea of how the AM microdose course affects sport fighter performance. Improvement was indicated for all proposed indicators provided by a group of athletes who voluntarily tested the following AM microdosing effects as they trained.

TABLE 6. SPORT FIGHTER PERFORMANCE AND AM MICRODOSING

SPORT FIGHTER PERFORMANCE	POSITIVE EFFECT	NO RESULT	NEGATIVE EFFECT
Coordination (51)	72% (37)	22% (11)	6% (3)
Endurance (153)	85% (131)	12% (18)	3% (4)
Fighting Intelligence (51)	76% (39)	20% (10)	4% (2)
General Effects on CNS during Sports (90)	81% (73)	7% (6)	12% (11)
Integrated Impact (78)	86% (67)	10% (8)	4% (3)
Neuromuscular Function (73)	69% (50)	30% (22)	1% (1)
Reaction Rate (52)	60% (31)	38% (20)	2% (1)
Sense of Distance (45)	56% (25)	40% (18)	4% (2)

It is the time you have wasted for your rose that makes your rose so important.

Antoine de Saint-Exupéry,
The Little Prince

PART THREE

Amanita muscaria
Preparation

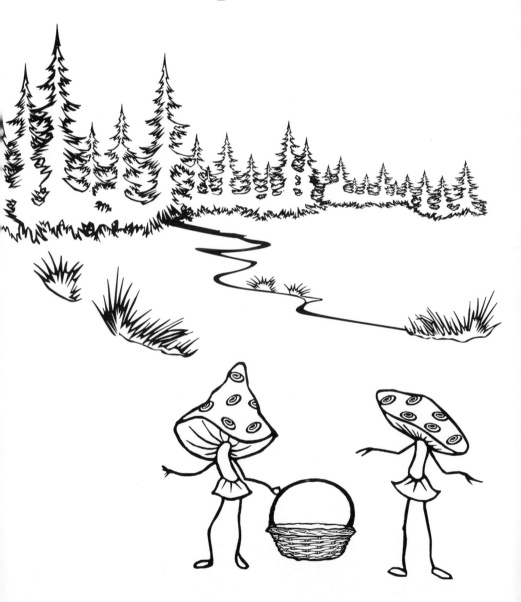

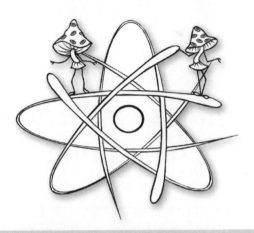

CHAPTER 8 Hunting, Preparing, and Storing *Amanita muscaria*

A journey of a thousand leagues begins beneath one's feet.

LAO TZU

Hunting *Amanita muscaria*

Hunting season for *Amanita muscaria* starts at the moment ordinary mushrooms appear. In Northern California the season starts in late October and ends in February. *Amanita muscaria* grows mainly under birch and pine trees, sometimes under alder, willow, aspen, and oak. For growth and development, *Amanita muscaria* needs a symbiotic mycorrhizal relationship with its host trees. Mushrooms are highly dependent on rain and soil moisture preceding fruiting.

When *Amanita muscaria* emerges, it is covered with white dots. As the fungus expands, the dots distribute, and the red cap shows through. The white gills are not attached to the stalk. The stalk is white to off-white with a bulbous base. The spore print is white. The color of the mushroom cap depends on the composition of the soil, the climate, and where it grows. On dry sunny spots among pines,

Amanita muscaria has a yellow or orange tint. In the lowlands with high humidity, the caps are cherry red. Strong, dense mushrooms are best suited for drying. You should not collect old or damaged mushrooms that have been eaten by worms or animals. The main concentration of active substances is in the cap or, more precisely, in the skin of the cap and in the yellow-white layer under it. For AM microdosing we collect *Amanita muscaria* caps only.

Drying and Preserving *Amanita muscaria*

There are certain rules for drying and preserving an *Amanita muscaria* crop. The mushrooms should be processed as soon as possible, especially if they are collected in damp places or during rainy weather, which may result in losing part of the crop while processing the fungus. The caps should not be washed before drying because the fungus' chemical compounds are water-soluble. However, any sand, dirt, or foliage should be removed with a damp cloth or napkin. It is much more difficult to clean the mushrooms once they have been dried, and sometimes it is simply not possible.

Amanita muscaria caps should be cut like pizza into several pieces with a plastic knife. It is more likely that the mushrooms will not deteriorate with that process. Anything metal such as knives, lids, or cans should not be used in processing or storing AM products.

Amanita muscaria can be dried in several ways. The most common method is in a dehydrator. The optimal temperature for drying is between 45°C and 55°C (109°F and 131°F). Below 45°C the mushroom can deteriorate before it dries, especially if it was collected after a rainfall and filled up with excessive moisture. Even if worms were not detected prior to harvest, there is still a possibility that worms will eat the fungus if the drying is done at a low temperature.

Another common method of drying mukhomor is to string them with a thread, not touching each other, and hang them in the kitchen above a source of heat. The worst drying method is in the oven because the temperature is too high, the caps will burn or bake, and they will lose their juice and become useless. My associate, Thomas, who collects large quantities of *Amanita muscaria,* has found that the most effective drying method is an infrared dryer that he built with infrared professional film used in housing construction to warm floors.

The mushroom caps should be dried until they are crisp. When mushrooms are dried correctly, they will sound much like the cracking of a potato chip when pressed. I use a two-stage drying process. After drying the AM caps until they are crisp, I put the caps together in a large glass jar and let it sit overnight. In the morning the caps are no longer crunchy and dry on the outside since moisture from inside the caps rehydrates the outer portions. I then dry the caps again in the dehydrator.

With proper drying the weight ratio of the dried to raw fungus is 1:10. The mushrooms are then stored in airtight containers. Mushrooms should avoid moisture, light, oxygen, and high temperatures. I keep mushroom pieces in the refrigerator in small glass jars with a tight lid for only up to six months.

According to collected data, the mushrooms can be used right away after drying. I use AM right after the drying process. Thomas, however, has a slightly different process. He likes to cure *Amanita muscaria.* After drying the mushrooms, he places them in a dark, cool place without oxygen for further fermentation. He uses ziplock bags, removes the air, and keeps them in a cool, dark place at a temperature of about 10°C (50°F) for two to three months. In Thomas's experience the mushrooms retain their properties for a year.

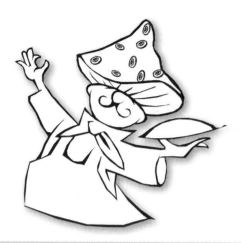

CHAPTER 9 *Amanita muscaria* Recipes

Be kind to people whether they deserve your kindness or not.

James Fadiman, *Essential Sufism*

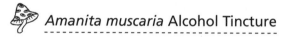

Amanita muscaria Alcohol Tincture

<u>Uses:</u> *Amanita muscaria* tincture can be used both externally and internally.

In external application the tincture is used to relieve pain in the musculoskeletal system by rubbing or as a compress. External application is effective for relief of arthritis; arthrosis; osteochondrosis; radiculitis; inflammation of the sciatic nerve; pain and inflammation in muscles, ligaments, and joints; bruises; sprains; inflammatory processes; redness; and itching (mosquito and tick bites, poison oak irritation).

For internal application the tincture is administered in drops according to a certain protocol. For each disease the regimen is different. We did not study the effects of AM tincture via oral intake, and it is not considered microdosing. Chemically, AM tincture is closer to raw mushroom and causes a lot of negative effects according to my observations.

Ingredients:

2 pounds *Amanita muscaria* caps

250 ml 160 proof food-grade ethanol (or vodka)

Tips: There are quite a few recipes for *Amanita muscaria* tincture. It can be made with vodka or a high-percentage food-grade ethanol. It can be made from fresh, dried fungus or from juice squeezed from fresh caps. I experimented with the methods and found that the most effective tincture was made from fresh AM caps and 75–95% food-grade ethanol. The highest quality alcohol should be used for AM tincture since the quality of the tincture is directly related to the quality of the alcohol. Vodka can also be used, but there is a possibility that green mold may appear in the tincture, even if it is refrigerated, because the final alcohol concentration is reduced by 50% or more by the end of the process. The concentration of the final product depends on the amount of *Amanita muscaria* and how wet the mushrooms are.

The color of the tincture depends on the original color of the mushrooms. From the classic red caps, the tincture is scarlet. If the mukhomor is a lighter shade—yellow, peach, orange—then the tincture is light. Accordingly, if we gather dark caps, then the tincture will be ruby dark. The color of the tincture can also change—become lighter or darker—during storage and often precipitates. According to Thomas's observations, those changes do not affect the healing properties of the tincture.

Directions: I make AM tincture as soon as possible after a harvest. I thoroughly clean a glass jar and place the *Amanita muscaria* mashed caps in it. I then pour ethanol into the jar enough to cover the mushrooms by about one inch. I cover the jar with a plastic lid. The jar must be stored in a dark place at 4°C (40°F) for 40–45 days. The jar can be wrapped with foil and stored in the refrigerator for 40 days, but since I currently live on a farm on a small, unpopulated island, I prefer the old-fashioned method of burying the jar in the ground three feet deep. Thomas uses his own well instead of the refrigerator to store the jar. There is a constant temperature and complete darkness in a well, which makes it a perfect place to store the tincture. After the 40–45 days, I strain the contents of the jar, pouring the liquid into convenient containers, and throw the rest away.

Storage: In my experience AM alcohol tincture can be effective up to four years. I keep the tincture in the refrigerator in a glass jar with a plastic lid.

Alternate Method: An alcohol-free method can be used as well. The glass jar is filled densely with crushed, fresh *Amanita muscaria* caps, covered tightly with a plastic lid, and stored in a cold, dark place for 40–45 days and then mixed with ethanol 50-50. This method is not very useful because AM juice can be infected by mold.

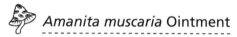 *Amanita muscaria* Ointment

Uses: Relief from arthritis; arthrosis; osteochondrosis; radiculitis; inflammation of the sciatic nerve; pain and inflammation in muscles, ligaments, and joints; bruises; sprains; treatment of skin diseases of various etiologies, namely dermatitis and neurodermitis; fungal diseases; inflammatory processes; redness; itching; and damage to the skin such as cuts, burns, and abrasions.

Ingredients:
cold-pressed coconut oil or petroleum jelly (e.g., Vaseline)
ground, dried *Amanita muscaria* caps

Directions: Thomas's recipe calls for mixing the AM cap powder 50-50 with the fat (either coconut oil or petroleum jelly). Keep it at least two weeks in the refrigerator before using—the longer the better, but a couple of weeks is the minimum. Add the ointment to a warm bath, mixing it well.

Storage: Store it in the refrigerator. Do not strain the solid particles from the ointment.

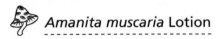 *Amanita muscaria* Lotion

Uses: I experimented with AM lotion for a few years and came up with this recipe to remove age spots.

Ingredients:
dried *Amanita muscaria* powder
AM tincture
homemade marijuana coconut butter (recipes available online)
black walnut tincture

Directions: Mix two parts dried AM cap powder with two parts marijuana butter, 50-50 by volume, in a glass jar. Add one part black walnut tincture and one part AM tincture. Store it 2–3 weeks in the refrigerator, and then it is ready to use. For difficult age spots, apply the lotion topically for 2–3 days, covering the skin with soft plastic and an adhesive bandage. Do not reuse the same bandange.

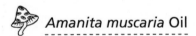 *Amanita muscaria* Oil

Uses: Thomas uses this oil to treat skin abrasions, cuts, rashes, inflammation, and burns. It can also be used for softening, restoring, and improving the structure of the skin. It smooths wrinkles, improves complexion, nourishes, and moisturizes.

Ingredients:
Amanita muscaria cap powder
sea buckthorn oil or any good-quality cold-pressed oil such as
coconut, jojoba, or grapeseed oil

Directions: Mix the dried *Amanita muscaria* powder and the chosen oil 50-50 by volume, and infuse it for about a month. Then strain the oil to separate it from the coarse particles.

Storage: *Amanita muscaria* oil should be stored in the refrigerator. It will stay good forever until it is used up.

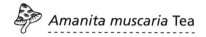 *Amanita muscaria* Tea

Ingredients:
One gram *Amanita muscaria* coarse powder
One cup of warm water

Directions: To make *Amanita muscaria* tea, the mushroom should be dried and broken into small pieces or ground. One gram *Amanita* coarse powder and one cup of warm water should steep for 20–30 minutes and then be strained. The mushroom bits should be discarded. The recommended water temperature is 45°C–55°C (113°F–131°F).

Storage: *Amanita muscaria* tea can be stored for a day in a thermos without losing its power.

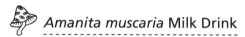 *Amanita muscaria* Milk Drink

Uses: The *Amanita muscaria* milk drink—called Soma in Russian-speaking territories—is used to reach an alternate state of mind. Users drink it slowly, one or two sips at a time, which allows them to monitor their condition and avoid any complications or overdoses.

Ingredients:
Amanita muscaria powder
milk
honey
water

Directions: Boil 0.5 liter (17 ounces) of water, then allow it to cool off a little. Add 2 tablespoons honey, stirring until it dissolves. Add 3 heaping tablespoons dried, ground mukhomor. Stir until the fungus powder becomes wet and puffed up. Add 0.5 liter (17 ounces) of milk; heat and stir until it bubbles. Turn the stove off, cool the mixture, and then strain it through gauze. Consume only the liquid and discard the rest. It is a powerful drink and must be used with caution by taking only 1 to 2 moderate sips then waiting one hour to adjust the amount and find the desirable effect.

🍄 *Amanita muscaria* Extract

The therapeutic properties of the mukhomor extract were discovered by one of our project participants. By chance, he extracted 20 g of dried Amanita muscaria *as an experiment. The effects of the extract were positive, both for external use and microdosing.*

Ingredients:
A Soxhlet extractor was used
High-proof alcohol was used as a solvent
The size of your extractor will determine the amount of solid and solvent needed

Extraction could also be achieved using a water solution. The participant who described this noted, "This extraction process has a number of advantages." He instructed, "There is no need to follow the AM drying protocol. The extract does not need to be infused and fermented as a tincture, and it is ready for use immediately after production."

🍄 Cooking *Amanita muscaria*

Uses: There are no health benefits from eating *Amanita muscaria,* because all the chemicals are water soluble and they will be washed out. What remains is just like any other edible mushroom.

Tips: The common way to prepare AM stems as regular food is to boild them twice for 15 minutes and then fry, mash, or cook into a soup or sauce. My personal experience with this method was not successful, and it did not work well for many others according to the poll. Over 50% of people experienced light psychedelic effects or tremor. But I figured out a very safe method for turning *Amanita muscaria* stems into delicious dishes.

Directions: By experimenting I found that soaking small pieces of AM stems for forty-eight hours in lightly salted water, changing the water 2–3 times, takes away all water-soluble AM substances, and the stems become just regular mushroom bodies ready to be used in any way possible—fried, soup, pâté, and so on. AM stems have a very strong structure, and after forty-eight hours of soaking, they keep their firm texture. A lot of my friends and family members ate AM stems prepared this way for years with no side effects or complaints.

Other Application Methods

Smoking, Inhaling, and Applying *Amanita muscaria*

A few dozen participants (including myself) reported smoking *Amanita muscaria*. The red cuticle of the AM cap was peeled off, dried, and then smoked. I tried this method using the water bong out of curiosity. The first couple hits gave me a very light sedative effect. With further use a loss of concentration and a sleepy state were observed. I am not sure how safe smoking *Amanita muscaria* is for the lungs.

I also have a report from enthusiasts who powdered dry *Amanita muscaria* to the size of 5 microns with professional equipment. Two female workers were distributing AM powder into gelatin capsules without safety masks and apparently inhaled invisible AM dust. In three hours one of the women had strong effects similar to alcohol consumption (the champagne effect). She was chatty, laughing, and dancing, and then she was sent home. The effect lasted six hours. The second woman had a strong energetic effect that lasted thirty-six hours in a no-sleep state with no tiredness or exhaustion.

The 5-micron AM powder mixed with lotion and applied on the skin of two men caused heavy psychedelic effects with signs of disorientation and the inability to walk and speak clearly.

The following *Amanita muscaria* uses were not proposed or planned in the *Amanita muscaria* microdose project frame. However, I received a couple dozen reports from volunteers, and I would like to present a short abstract of that to demonstrate the dedication and enthusiasm of the participants.

Amanita muscaria Enema

Several brave volunteers wrote me reports about using AM-infused water for an enema. The solution was prepared by the same recipe as

AM tea. Surprisingly, the effects were the same as using an AM micro-dose orally. Results included energy, motivation, productivity during the day, a great mood in the mornings, a good night's sleep, and a rested body after an evening intake.

Amanita muscaria Urine

I'd like to share a report I received about AM urine from one participant. "Masha, I tested my urine after mukhomor consumption as it was described in some books. Tell everyone that this is nonsense. I personally tried it. I immediately realized after one gulp that mukhomor pushes out all the poisons and all the slags from the system, including viruses and microbes. My urine tasted and smelled like acetone, chlorine, and sewage. I took just a couple of sips for analysis and could not keep it down. I threw it up. Never be sure until you try it yourself. Debunk the myths!"

PART FOUR

Collection of
Participant Reports

Life is really simple, but we insist on making it complicated.
CONFUCIUS

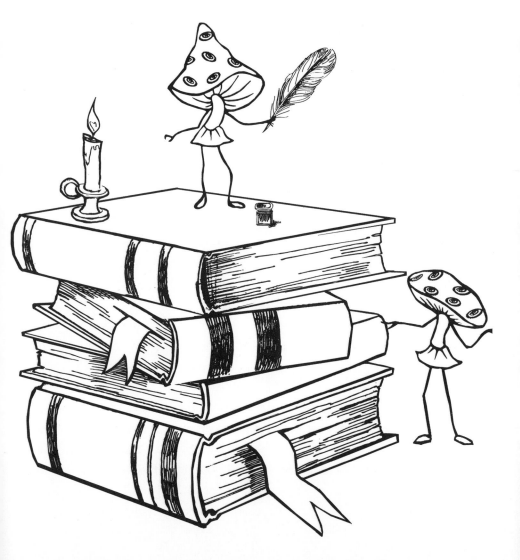

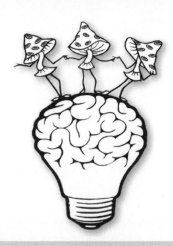

CHAPTER **10** *Amanita muscaria* Microdosers' Individual Reports

They always say time changes things, but you actually have to change them yourself.
ANDY WARHOL, *THE PHILOSOPHY OF ANDY WARHOL*

Over the years of my broadcast, I have collected more than three thousand reports on *Amanita muscaria* use, from doses of 0.5–50 g in various forms and for different purposes. The good news is that no one died, no one suffered organ damage or any type of physical harm, and no one ended up in a psychiatric ward from that "poisonous" *Amanita muscaria* mushroom. I have talked personally with many users and have had a few public interviews on the topic on my channel.

In this chapter I present participants' personal letters and reports on *Amanita muscaria* effects that were compiled over a period of two years. Personal letters are more than a list of effects received from the reception of AM microdosing. Since an AM microdose is not a pharmacological pill with a certain amount of chemicals and is not calculated per kilogram of the weight of the user, the potency of *Amanita muscaria*

varies depending on the place of growth, the season of collection, preparation, and storage. The selection of individual dosage is very important,
and the submitted personal reports show a range of effects depending
on the above data.

The participants specifically described,

how they prepared and stored AM,
how much they took,
how long they took it,
what problems they met with bigger doses,
which form of reception suited them better (dry AM or in the form
   of tea),
how time of intake (morning, evening, or both) worked for them
   individually, and
what kind of preparation worked better for them.

All participants were divided into three groups depending on effects
of storage time of a mushroom. The first group took the dried-up AM
immediately after drying. Taking an AM microdose immediately after
drying caused the following effects in this group: unpleasant metal taste
in the mouth, slight nausea and discomfort in the stomach, mild tremor
of the body muscles. The second group took mushrooms immediately
after drying and also after fermentation without variation in effects.
They did not find a difference in action. The third group took only
fermented AM (2–3 months of storage in the dark place without air
access). Reception of the fermented AM caused drowsiness and apathy. This shows how the same doses work on different people, and how
people react to different methods of storage and preparation. It shows
how important it is to find the individual dose. This provides even
more important information than just saying, "Oh, I took *Amanita* and
it improved my sleep."

I could dissect, systematize, and present the reports in condensed
form, but I have not done so because I want you to get the full picture of the effects of AM microdosing by reading the participants' own

reports. Each story presents unique facts, individual history, a variety of preconditions, and specific reasons for microdosing AM. I gave people freedom to express and write about the experience of microdosing AM as they felt it, and so I did not want to take away from the quality of their reports by dissecting them or attempting to organize them thematically. However, I have bolded the key words pertaining to specific positive effects in each report not to overstate the positive but to aid your reading experience and analysis. Specific conditions are also bolded. Many reports also comment on finding the individual dose and many share side effects discovered while on that journey. The index at the back of this book should be used as a resource to help you sort through the reports of interest to you.

While some participants shared reports about *Amanita pantherina,* only reports about *Amanita muscaria* are shared in this chapter.

Reading these informative stories and reports will provide you with firsthand, real-life information. These reports are not just dry statistical data with diagrams and tables. They come from real people with real-time individual histories of AM microdosing, and their reports are the most valuable part of the book. By sharing them I hope you'll see that *Amanita* does not serve only one purpose but instead improves several aspects of life and may balance the bodily systems as well as the mind in one use.

This information came from four sources and was posted on my Telegram channel, *"Amanita muscaria* Microdoses Reports." This channel, which is available to the public, currently has more than six thousand subscribers. The original Telegram channel reports are labeled with day, time, and source, which makes them easy to verify. Source labeling starts from Report No. 169, October 24, 2019, when I began to receive indignant comments suggesting that I wrote the reports.

The reports were translated from Russian as closely as possible to the original users' words. Punctuation was edited for greater clarity, and any words inserted for clarity have been placed in square brackets to signal their addition. Reports were either posted anonymously or names were removed in compiling this book. The reports originate from the following sources:

1. Personal letters from people who do not use social media public messengers.
2. Comments from two YouTube channels with more than seventy thousand subscribers.
3. Support group *Amanita muscaria* Microdosing Live Telegram Messenger Chat, managed by my associate, Thomas, with over three thousand subscribers. The information is available to the public.
4. My own Psychedelic Plants Live Chat on the Telegram Messenger platform, with over 3,400 subscribers. The information is available to the public.

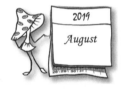

Report No. 1: Two people reported the following after two months of *Amanita muscaria* microdosing.

Condition before AM microdosing: apathy, asociality, aggression, prolonged depressive state, lack of aspirations, discomfort, lack of comfortable state in general, lack of all that is connected to **positive feeling of self, life, and society**.

Condition after AM microdosing: The result was mega positive. Both came to life, lit up like new. The **quality of life** had changed completely. After 3–5 months, the results diminished slightly, but not to the previous condition.

Additional information: I treated a **flu** successfully with AM microdosing, although not immediate. The temperature dropped after the AM microdose. I had long-term problems with **menstrual irregularities** after taking contraceptives for one year. After AM microdosing everything is fine now.

Report No. 2: I am a long-distance driver. My morning before AM microdosing looked like this: I woke up "dead," irritated and sluggish with ache in my bones. I began taking 0.33 g AM microdose before bed. Now I **wake up healthy and refreshed**. My **vision** and **reaction** are incredible. I feel like I am god of the roads!

Report No. 3: I had huge problems with **depression**. My search for a cure led me to the mukhomor (*Amanita muscaria*). After completing the AM microdose course, it was as if I had found myself again. I found who I once was. Unfortunately, the season is over, and here I am waiting for next year's harvest.

Report No. 4: Super effective six months of *Amanita muscaria* microdosing. My **alcohol** consumption is gone down to zero. I quit **smoking** cigarettes. My brain switched "on," and that internal egocentric dude is dead. I hope this knowledge becomes available to the world. Peace and kindness.

Report No. 5: Three weeks of *Amanita muscaria* microdoses. I have a lot of positive results similar to what I read in AM microdosing live chats.

Report No. 6: Hello. I picked *Amanita muscaria* mushroom and prepared it myself. I use from half a mushroom cap up to two of them (5–8 cm diameter). I had a pinched (bruised) nerve on my spine. It was painful for a week. After intake of half a mushroom cap, the **pain** passed without any echoes!

My friend had a bad ankle sprain. He took the whole cap of *Amanita* the first day and half a cap for the next three days. Additionally, he used alcohol tincture topically on his ankle the first day. Result—this treatment brought everything to normal in three days! *Amanita* also is a great tonic, ideal for long driving trips.

Report No. 7: I am taking an AM microdose twice a day—morning and night—one mid-size *Amanita muscaria* cap, dried like chips consistency. I chew it and drink water after that. This intake works for me. I wake up early in the morning around 6:30–7:00 a.m. [and feel] very **vigorous**. Physically, emotionally, and literally shit began to move. **Anger released**, feels like flipping a wasp nest. All this is realized and observed. It passes naturally, delivering some discomfort, and I wish it worked faster.

Report No. 8: My microdose of *Amanita muscaria* is up to 1 g every day in the form of dried powder. I am comfortable to drive with this dosage; it works great during my job duties as well.

Report No. 9: If I use about 1 g of dry *Amanita muscaria*, I am **cheerful**. The main thing to me is the oddly wonderful effect: I clearly distinguish the difference between "me" and "the useless chatterbox" of my **internal dialogue**. It's a very cool feeling. I am like **an observer** of my thoughts and reactions. I am the sky, and my thoughts and feelings are the clouds! This is the most important thing to me. There are more facets of change in me. I smile at strangers, **spontaneously [take] brave actions, [express] coolness on the opinion of others**. I completely disregard that pal inside me who whispered in my ear that I am unworthy or must justify my misconduct. Now my driving is bold, fast, confident, and nice with other drivers. **Sex**, it feels like I grew by 19 cm! Increased operability. Now I **sleep** for five hours, falling asleep instantly. **Dreams** are fire! I began to tell the truth, and I like it! I desire to live.

Report No. 10: I've microdosed about three weeks, 1 g in the morning. Man, I **smoked** a pack a day for twenty years, now I do not wish to smoke! Every weekend I got wasted [**alcohol**]! Not anymore now. I could not dream of anything like this, using any legitimate or natural substance without a side effect!

Report No. 11: Everything is super! I began to take AM because of health problems. I've used AM microdosing straight for six months already. I just chew dry pieces like chips before bed every night. In half an hour, the yawning begins. I go to bed immediately, and the **sleep** is very strong. I can ask Spirit Amanita to realize my dream, then I clearly feel that I am inside a lucid **dream**. It looks like I watch myself as an **observer**. I can ask in my dream to show my problems, and I can get a direction for its resolution.

A lot of miracles happened to me during AM microdose intake. **Intuition** unfolds more and more; I have gifts of **foresight**. It helps with **creativity**. It gives me a lot of ideas that I definitely could not have thought of in my "normal" state. General **irritation** was drastically decreased. My **energy level increased**, my time "stretched," and I **get more done** through the day. I feel **more holistic, more joyful, and happy**. My position as an observer in my life events is stronger than ever. The nonstandard solutions come more often. AM microdosing is very helpful in my activities. I am a psychologist, and AM microdosing improved my **communication skills**. I have a better understanding of people's problems and **empathy**. I observe constant **synchronicity of events**, clues, and signs of the universe. My life is saturated with events and impressions.

Report No. 12: Results of AM microdosing. As funny as it sounds, I just stopped buying **alcohol**. There were alcohol problems, too! I haven't had a drink in three months. Amen. The further away, the easier. Confidence and determination not to drink grows every day. I think in three months I will stop thinking about it at all.

Report No. 13: I microdose mukhomor every day. I take an AM microdose in the morning, from half an hour to two hours before meals, depending on whether I work or not. I've been a negative person all my life, and now I am a "yes" man. I feel **clear, vigorous with an absence of depression**. With mukhomor I became **more cheerful**. Before I experienced an apathy and constant lazy couch potato state for hours. Now it is gone. My habit of **alcohol** consumption is gone as well for two months for now. I have had alcohol problems all my life, and AM microdosing removed the residual pull of the poison (alcohol), to the point that I can have alcohol at my nose and I am totally not attracted to it. Yesterday I went shopping and noticed that everything around me was interesting, **colors were brighter, familiar landscapes looked more interesting**, as if I was there for the first time. I have the feeling that I am a third-party **observer** who emphasizes the unusual nature of the ordinary. I noticed that my movements while walking became **strong and assured**, as in a well-working mechanism, and before, I was stumbling a lot. Sometimes I think, "How do I look from the outside?" And suddenly I am becoming clumsy but then I understand that all is normal and let it go.

Before, I was possessed by an unattractive habit of lost awareness of clarity! By the way, yesterday it was very slippery on the streets, and it did not affect my walking speed and I was just fine, feeling connected to the icy ground with invisible roots, like *Amanita* is saying to me, "Brother, you have completely lost your connection to nature without me, and I will bring you back."

Report No. 14: I have taken mukhomor for four weeks. Everything is cool. When I miss a day or two, I have an internal reminder—take it. Everything became **more interesting** with *Amanita* microdoses. I have problems with my business now but understand—everything is possible, and with the mukhomor there is **energy** to solve the problems. **Thoughts are clear**. I am not fixating on the problems. I feel great **positive pressure** boiling inside me. Microdosing of *Amanita muscaria* is a very positive thing.

Report No. 15: I am taking a half teaspoon AM powder before bed. I **sleep** very well, wake up with light euphoria, **rested**, and get up from the bed really easily. Before, it was difficult to wake up. My day is charged with energy, a flurry of **energy**. Bad thoughts have left me alone. I lost my habit of negative thinking. I am **calm**, and nothing annoys me. Even my two children could not break my **peaceful mood**. Now I can sit down quietly and talk to them and discuss the situation. So far, everything is fine. I started a diary for monitoring the health benefits of *Amanita muscaria.*

Report No. 16: I have a great help with **depression** in my microdosing experience. I was taking antidepressants, but it could not control my behavior, and soon depression came back and I was getting in my nervous state. While I microdosed for five days, I could see the results immediately. I've become **calmer** about certain things that I used to be acutely responsive to. I continue intake of microdoses, and I absolutely love it!

Report No. 17: Microdosing effects: I have **better communicability**. In the morning, I get up **rested** and in a nice calm condition. My **appetite** is unusually good.

Report No. 18: My microdosing experience: I take 1 g or 1.5 g every morning before food. In the beginning of my microdosing sessions, I took a dose before bed. My **dreams** were amazing. But I like morning intake more than night. One day after AM microdosing, I slept all day. After that I felt **cheerful, energetic** all day long, and I have had these effects for three weeks. I observed the **changes in my diet** as well—more fruits and vegetables. I do not crave meat during these last three weeks. My dreams became bright and colorful, and I travel through other worlds. My dreams before AM microdosing intake were flat, boring. I have had a great experience with *Amanita.*

Report No. 19: Yes, I can confirm from my experience that mukhomor has a very fruitful influence on **food behavior**. My food has changed, too. I did not give up meat completely, but I began to eat it much less. I more turned to cereals and vegetables. I can't eat store food full of chemicals at all. And yes, it happened very naturally and painlessly for the psyche, of course. There are also bursts of shit-mood, but they became **much easier to cope** with!

Report No. 20: I want to share a personal story of recovery, thanks to the mukhomor. There was extremely **unhealthy skin** of my face and head, strong exfoliation, red spots, sometimes itching. For several years no ointments, no pills, no shampoos, no infusions, nothing helped. Probably a fungus that was spreading harder and harder. When mukhomor knocked on my door, I decided to use it for treatment—stirred with butter and made a paste and applied for two hours. Twice was enough for me to get rid of 90% of such a terrible problem, which I had almost accepted as impossible to treat.

Report No. 21: *Amanita* microdose is an incredible surprise for me. I suffered for many years with **cystitis** and problems with the urinary system. All traditional treatment was not effective, so I had settled to live with it all my life. I got a cold and drank AM tea for three days, twice a day by 5 g. Astonishingly, a week later I realized that my **urinary problems** were simply gone. Mukhomor is a miracle.

Report No. 22: Mukhomor microdosing: I had brain trauma with 70% hematoma of the brain, epilepsy. I take 2–3 g in the morning before meals. Four weeks of reception. A **state of vigor** comes over me. I have unlimited faith in myself and my capabilities, **scars are healing**, having bright wonderful **dreams**. No **alcohol** urge while taking the fungus. So far, everything going well.

Report No. 23: It's been four weeks since I started microdosing with mukhomor. There was about 40 g of this wonderful substance for three and a half weeks. Before, I was in prolonged **depression**, sluggishness, apathy. I had interest in nothing. The first two weeks of intake, I experienced heightened emotions, a tide of strength and **energy**, bright dreams, mood swings from happiness to depression. Periods of vacillation when I could not remember the state of almighty and feeling that everything will turn out, I can do anything, materialization of desires. Now my state is stabilized—**dreams**, **energy**, **power**, **positive mood**—all this outweighs negative emotions. It became **easier** to experience external troubles and difficulties, easier to treat things, [and easier to] **change priorities** in pleasure.

Report No. 24: I have taken *Amanita* microdoses with my husband for a week. We take 0.5 in the morning. About 8–8:30 a.m. My husband goes to work, and I'm getting knocked out, like a night **sleep**. In my dream, the mukhomor **pulls out all my fears**. **I see things from a different angle** that are poisoning my life. When we microdose for the night, I fall asleep quickly, but dreams are the same in different interpretations. I want to note that I have been in a very stressful situation for the past year.
  1. The **mood improved**.
  2. I like **beer**, but now I look at the bottle, and I don't get involved.
  3. Husband was diagnosed with **psoriasis**. There was inflammation; now the crusts have fallen off.
  Maybe it's a coincidence, maybe not. Regardless, I like the results. We had no psychedelic experience prior to microdosing. Thank you for you. I will continue to write you.

Report No. 25: My AM microdosing report: I take twice a day, in the morning and in the evening at 1.5 g. My spouse too. We collected AM ourselves this season. You know, I am very surprised, our **youth came back** to us! Although we have been together for a long time with grandchildren. We are **laughing** a lot; we became more **friendly** to each other. Before AM microdosing, we were irritated and disgusted with each other, we couldn't stop being crazy for no reason, mainly about the future. **Alcohol** intake goes down—although we have taken only three weeks of AM microdosing—the beer is not winning over us anymore! Our brains have been cleaned up. It's not an inexplicable thrill but a **quiet pleasure** in life. I'll keep you informed. Continue AM microdosing!

Report No. 26: I want to share the joy. All my life I was plagued by **psoriasis**, and after a month of AM microdosing, I saw the light in the window! I take for the night less than 2 g or so. I **sleep** like a stone; I haven't slept like that in a long time. I've been tormented with negative thoughts. No side effects. Thanks to you, dear.

Report No. 27: Masha, I collected and dried *Amanita muscaria* mushrooms myself. I persuaded my grandma to take AM microdoses. She's seventy-eight, in bad condition, [and] barely walking. I gave her 1.5 g in the morning, 2 g for the night. My grandmother **came to life**, **laughs**, she began to go out in the garden. She sits on the bench and **smiles**. She is not so tormented with **pain** anymore because of **arthritis**. Yesterday she even cooked a meal for us! I will add more in a month.

Report No. 28: I continue my reports. I picked and prepared AM myself this time. The AM I used before was probably old, [but] I am not sure because I bought it online. The first two weeks were stormy with nausea, and then once and again, just like you say, the worms are dead inside my guts. I feel super **energy** blasting out of me. I want to **love** everyone. I developed a nonchalant **attitude**. It was difficult to persuade my husband to take an AM microdose because he suspected that I wanted to poison him. But when he tried and after a week, **sex** is awake. Yahoo! Now he asks me for *Amanita muscaria* microdose every morning! Big gratitude to you with all my heart for everything that you have done for us "energy sponges."

Report No. 29: Masha, you are our savior. We have an **autistic child**, eight years old. Doctors fed us with tons of pills, and at our own risk this year we collected and dried *Amanita muscaria* and tried AM microdosing.

Immediately from the first week we saw improvement. Our son became **calmer**; attacks are coming less and less; he **sleeps** well. There seems to be **increased communication** between us. I give him a little bit, started from 0.5 g twice a day—in the morning and evening before bed. We are microdosing almost a month. I take an AM microdose myself too. I see how my nervous condition has **calmed**. Before that, the psycho attack could start from nothing to disaster. Now, I believe that it is not a placebo. The child does not know. My gratitude to you is huge, and I will keep you posted.

Report No. 30: Masha, I have been microdosing AM for six months, and since we talked, I have a lot of changes. Finally got rid of **depression**. I have not taken pills since the beginning of AM microdosing. I increased the dose to 2 g per night. Dreams feel like I am in a movie with **passionate feelings and emotions**. I realized that **joy** is in life itself. I got a job. Everything is getting better in my family as well. My mother is asking for *Amanita muscaria* microdoses too. I am getting more AM soon. Last week I brought more from the woods. It hurts a lot to think about our conventional medicine: it harasses and treats us as slaves. The doctors kept me with pills as a suicidal zombie for many years, and I'm ashamed of those thoughts now. I pray for you, and I wish all the happiness.

Report No. 31: I like to take AM microdoses in the morning, or maybe the mukhomor likes it. I experience a tide of **energy** and **positive mood**. I find it very **easy to communicate** with people. During the process of taking *Amanita muscaria,* I gave up **eating meat** for six months. It happened naturally with no struggle. I feel a lot of **energy** and a permanent state of **pleasure** from life. And my **dreams**, a lot of people have talked about unusual dreams during AM microdosing. I confirm, they are incredibly real.

Report No. 32: Microdosing of mukhomor gives me so much **energy**. It helps me in my life chores and choices. **Love** for life itself appeared suddenly. I appreciate what I have and I stopped craving for more.

Report No. 33: Yes, the **quality of life** with the mukhomor has increased big time, and I experienced the **thrill**. Euphoria state.

Report No. 34: My wife's **vision** improved when microdosing, sharpness increased, and **color perception** improved. When the microdosing stopped, everything returned to its previous state, nearsighted (-4). I have great vision. While taking a mukhomor I register that sometimes there are more highlights, and sensitivity to the sunlight increased very much. Sometimes, I cannot go outside without sunglasses.

Report No. 35: My father is a communist to his core. His head lives inside a TV, but I broke it. The second month he is on AM microdoses he became more **kind**. **Vodka** is not the attraction for him. He **smokes** less and less. He stopped being rude to my mom and all of us in the family too. There has appeared some clearance in our dialogue and **communication**. All my family, including my spouse, are taking AM microdoses. Individual doses up to 3 g. Gee! It's some kind of magic! The whole village is watching us. At first they laughed like horses. Now I see villagers here and there picking *Amanita* in the forest. Divine comedy! I see how **life force** comes back to me. Joints became drier, no puffiness, **pain** goes away. My daily **mood** reminds me of a constant birthday when I was a child. Thank you. If you need anything, please write to me.

Report No. 36: I am reading the reports on your channel. And I feel my **energy** is bursting from inside my body. I'm at work now. Usually, I always feel sleepy at work. I am on [a] microdose now, and all I want is to run and jump!

Report No. 37: Hello. I am taking AM microdoses for four months. I keep a calendar and write down reports. There's a lot to tell. Here is my outcome of AM microdosing. There was a feeling and understanding that something was wrong with me. Now I **think differently**, I talk to people more often, and they strangely became attracted to me. When I did not get enough sleep and felt **lack of energy**, I took about 3 g of *Amanita*, and everything was great for six hours or so. My **dreams** were always very colorful with a presence effect, and with AM microdosing it became brighter with some hidden meaning. Under an AM microdose, ideas for business came easily, my **creativity and imagination** in drawing improved. Also used AM microdosing before work. But the dose was greatly overestimated, and I could not work well. I got lazy to do regular work, but it was positive with desire to create, write, enjoy rather than routine work like building a house. I noticed that people and children treat you differently, smiling as if they see something special in me. **Communication** with children is cheerful, they understand me easier, and I kind of fall to their level and understand their desire and behavior. I gave an AM microdose to my sister. I wanted to pull her out of negativity. But she is closed and unavailable. I tried big doses of AM, about 10 g. I use it with honey 1:1 to reduce strong disgust and vomiting; this is not a pleasant bonus. As soon as the trip started, I got into a loop. I felt like Jesus and tried walking on water. I experienced and understood how this world got created. The orgasm of explosion—Big Bang. I felt that I am a part of god, the whole world, all people are god, all in one. It was beautiful. I asked myself the question of how to live with that, and in response, there followed emotions, feelings, and thrill of realization. High on life! Enjoy every event. But sober, I forbid myself all of that! Then the catch, entering the dream I saw the future, but half I do not remember, only what came true at once, namely. When I got in the loop and everything was repeated again and again, I laughed and laid down on the floor, and I was waiting until it passed. I woke up understanding with laughter that if I said it to all the people—what I understood now—I would be taken to the nut house. I smiled wildly from this assumption. There were not many visuals, or I don't remember.

Report No. 38: My purpose of AM microdose intake: to get rid of the illusions with which I packed my head because of the endless thirst for information. That got me to this condition, with no strength and no desire to do anything. I refused to move on. I gave up on my development. I experienced **depression** and an apathy to everything.

Actions: I decided to take AM alcohol extract for a month, increasing daily from one drop up to fifteen, then go back one drop less each day.

Results: Now I am always in the **good balance** and **great emotional state**. My **mood** is not jumpy like before. It's difficult to get into an emotional hole. I am motivated to study. **Dreams** became less emotional. The **delusions** on which I based my future plans for life are gone. For a while, I felt internal void, and I had to work with it. I asked myself a lot of questions and sought answers that helped me not to collapse into depression. I realized what I want, not what someone wished for me. I lit up with my intentions. It gave me **strength**. I see now my past life as someone else's experience. At the same time, it is sad and joyful, but more **joyful**. It's like the **new world opened** up in front of my eyes. I begin to understand what is really valuable and how to spend my time and energy without unnecessary waste. Can I say I've gotten better and **happier**? Definitely YES!

Report No. 39: My review: I microdosed almost eight months. The changes are as follows: very strong, great night **sleep**. I hear nothing, although I used to wake up from any little sound. I easily fall asleep, easily wake up, there is no desire to stay in bed in the morning anymore. I literally jump out of bed. I got a strong wave of **energy**. **PMS** has completely passed. My **immune system** is stronger. I do not catch colds anymore like before. My **mood** changed; I became calmer. I **stopped controlling** my loved ones. I am more **engaged** in myself. I am more **peaceful**. My joints have ceased to hurt completely. The herniation of my spine sometimes worries, but rarely and only after hard physical work. I seldom get annoyed and **do not worry** anymore; there is a youth in my soul. **No pain**. I do not want to write about mystical experiences, [but] there were so many! I had a break after eight months, and now I started microdosing again. It's all super. Operability at high altitude. Now I only have **creative modes**. It is very difficult to piss me off now. You really have to try hard. Also, I noticed that I have **less floaters** in my eyes.

Report No. 40: Hi! I have had some **allergic reaction**—itchy, watery eyes. The pills just took the symptoms away for a couple days, that's all. And then I decided to try microdoses AM. My intake was one full teaspoon powdered AM mixed with a half teaspoon of honey for nineteen days, every morning. *Effects:* **psychological state** was good, noticed better **ability to concentrate**, and **elevation of general mood** all day. Physical sensations and digestion are normal. No bad side effects. And just today I discovered that my **allergy is gone**! This is the most interesting effect of microdoses of AM to me.

Report No. 41: I thank you, Baba Masha! And in response to your work, I want to share with the whole universe my recipe for happiness. After I drink a smoothie with mukhomor, I am ready to turn the mountains over. I am jumping and running, I have a sea of **strength** and **energy**. I fly over the earth. Seriously, I fly! Recipe: I soak flax cannabis and oats seeds overnight. In the morning, rinse with water a couple of times, put in a blender, add honey, cocoa, and you can add dried fruits. I sometimes add raisins or dates for sweetness. Add some water. You can also add a banana, favorite nuts. Be creative. And now add mukhomor. The amount is individual (I use 2–3 teaspoons). Whip it in the blender, add more water, if needed. Before I came up with this recipe, I took three months of mukhomor microdosing, and I didn't like the effect. I took it in the morning with salt. I was sweating like an elephant; I could not feel my fingers; I felt sick. My mom said I was out somewhere else flying. Everything changed when I started cooking this drink of happiness. I began to feel a lot **more confident** in myself. Little things **did not irritate** me. I began to talk to people normally, not screaming crazy. I started to exercise: stretching, swimming, biking, running. Sometimes I am afraid of so much **power and energy**.

Report No. 42: BM, I finally decided to share my experience with you. It's just tearing me apart—how come people do not know about AM microdosing? I took 2 g dried powder of AM every morning for thirty-five days, in the morning. I didn't write you before just to be sure it is not just my imagination. I started to get confirmations from others that I am **lit up and smiley**, standing straight with great posture. **Communication** became **easy and free**. I surprised myself. I got back to long-abandoned dreams and desires. I began to truly fulfill what I sought and always wanted. Burst of **energy**. Time stretched. People asking me if I won a lottery! Exactly—I did win the lottery—it is *Amanita!* Since childhood I didn't feel that way. Life hit me hard and put my face to the ground. Now I realized that life is a great **pleasure**. My life is not luxurious, but I have everything I need. My beloved is with me. I realized now that I have to live to make them happy, without criticism, fights, and proving myself to them. These are great insights! I am taking a break from AM microdosing. The **new condition is stable**. I will start AM microdosing with a new harvest. Thanks to you, and I bow.

Report No. 43: Mukhomor microdoses give me great night **sleep**. I am over sixty and use alcohol tincture as topical application on the surface of my skin in generous quantities. This way I have very energetic mornings and a lot of **energy** during the day.

Report No. 44: Masha, after three months of AM microdoses, joint **pain** is gone, my sense of smell is sharper. I quit **sweets** and **alcohol**: thank you, dear, for your presence.

Report No. 45: I have right eye vision -2.5, left eye -1.5. I prefer to not wear glasses. After AM microdose intake, my **vision** improved, more **contrast**, and I can see now very clearly even the smallest details. Before *Amanita muscaria* microdoses I could see only by squinting my eyes. This really shocks me!

Report No. 46: Me, my mom, and a friend took an AM microdose at the same time. We picked *Amanita muscaria* in the forest, then prepared and dried it at the lowest temperature in the oven. *Effects:* **Excellent and stress-resistant mood**; increased **activity**; etc., as many write here in reviews. But all three began slight discomfort at the kidney's projection after about a week of consumption. We stopped.

Discomfort was gone in two days. I read that the transition of ibotenic acid to muscimol takes place in about 2–3 months. We will do that and try again.

Report No. 47: Since it's only a week of AM microdosing, it's too early to say anything. The main thing is that there are no problems. The first days I felt sleepiness, as well as my friends, who also took an AM microdose at very first days of intake. That comes after 6–8 hours. But these six hours were great, **energy** is markedly increased after.

Report No. 48: Week of AM microdosing. The *Amanita muscaria* caps are dried and not fermented. Intake before bed. First four days at 0.5 g. Fifth, sixth at 1 g and seventh day at 2 g. *Effects:* I fell **asleep** much more easily. My morning condition: body was **relaxed** but the mind was awake and **cheerful**; 2 g intake kept me awake. In the morning felt as a hangover. The mood is neutral/good. I noticed that I caught flashes of anger at the growing peak of emotions and during this, thought in my head, "what a stupid reaction." Feeling barely visible dissociation in the early days. It's like I'm an outside **observer** inside my body. After switching to 1g of dry *Amanita muscaria*, this effect stopped. Less "noise inside my head," it is **easier to focus**. There is no desire to think about past or future. Taking a break. I will continue soon.

Report No. 49: Baba Masha, after course of AM microdose I feel just fine, and the shit comes out from the mind visibly. After only a few AM microdoses I quit **alcohol** and desire of **marijuana** intake decreased greatly. *Amanita muscaria* mushroom is a great thing.

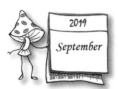

Report No. 50: I started microdosing in the morning from small doses and slowly reached 2 g of dry mushroom mukhomor. I have a week of microdoses. Flight is normal. **Clarity** and **concentration** of the mind. No intoxication. Driving sometimes all day even better. No sluggishness. **Focus** and **attention** improved. All day **good activity**, less tired. Sports are high, too. By the way, I don't go very much on the night because I don't fall asleep very quickly, the brain is active all night, **sleep** is intermittent and superficial, and all night there are breaks of incomprehensible dreams, as in comatose. Heart rate and pressure are normal. Pulse is 60–70 beats. The intestines' reaction is also in complete order. It turned out that AM is also tasty. In short, no side effects.

Report No. 51: I've had **sleep disorders** for years. I started AM microdosing instead of the drugs prescribed by doctors that made me vomit. I microdosed about eight months. Now I fall asleep immediately. Also, I've been on a **methadone** program for almost ten years. Mukhomor helped to lower the methadone dosage by three times. I consider that a very big plus. I take AM one teaspoon powder in the morning and one teaspoon at lunch.

Report No. 52: Only three days of *Amanita muscaria* microdoses. And I noticed improvements—feeling of **well-being, elevated mood**. My **daily performance has improved**. I started remembering a lot of **pleasant** things from childhood.

Report No. 53: The effect of night intake of AM microdose—the same as your statistics; but morning intake does not give me energy but **relaxation and feeling of happiness**. Also, it is hard for me to drive.

Report No. 54: Thank you for publishing *Amanita muscaria* microdoses data. After AM microdosing I completely refuse **alcohol**. It also improved my **sleep**. My **cannabis** addiction is gone.

Report No. 55: Day four of AM microdosing. I feel **vigorous**! Thank you! My ego specifically **calmed** down. I am eating more **vegetables and fruits** than before. **Portions of food** have become much smaller! It's cool. My **thoughts** became **organized**. The only downside was the unpleasant smell of my sweat.

Report No. 56: I am a forty-eight-year-old male. I've had **alcohol** addiction for twenty-eight years. Today is exactly a year since I completely gave up alcohol. I take an AM microdose regularly six months at a time. Then the body tells me to stop. My **weight dropped** from 102 to 84 kg [225 to 185 pounds]. I am a height of 186 cm [6 feet, 1 inch]. My beer stomach is gone. The carbuncle on my back, also known as a boil, a **painful infection** that I have had all my life, **is gone**.

Report No. 57: I completed two courses of AM microdose. It **cleaned my consciousness** and **removed the negative flow of my thoughts**.

Report No. 58: In the last five years I have plunged into the deepest **depression. I saw great improvement** just in two days of AM microdosing—one small dry AM cap. I want to continue and prolong that state of lack of emotional tension. I suffered with **PTSD** for years, and it is gone. **Resentment, anger**, the **EGO trips** are dissolving.

Report No. 59: After one course of *Amanita muscaria* microdoses I have lost **sluggishness**. I have **better performance** and **less anxiety**!

Report No. 60: Very good news! Short report on my AM microdosing. In January I had a **stroke**. I am thirty-three years old. I quickly got back to the normal rhythm of life after AM mushrooms. I recovered **speech**, **sleep**, head **stopped hurting**, etc. Maybe a coincidence?

Report No. 61: Tried AM microdoses for about a week, about 3 g in the morning, but better for the night. I discovered a very interesting effect! The **length of intercourse** has increased a lot, and it is definitely from this mushroom! I also do not believe everything that is written and said. So, I tried myself and felt only positive results. Now I cannot understand why people are convinced that *Amanita muscaria* is poison.

Report No. 62: The **pain** in my ligaments of the elbows was gone in two weeks of AM microdosing. Before that, no ointment, no anti-inflammatory injections helped. And my **sexual intercourse** increased.

Report No. 63: Microdosing AM a second month. *Effects*: excellent **sleep** aid. I recommend a mushroom to everyone who is tormented by **insomnia**. I consume up to 2 g during the day.

Report No. 64: Six months of AM microdosing. Clear improvements: Given up **alcohol** by 100%. Rejection of artificial **sugar**. I began to eat **less meat**. **Cheer, energy, positive attitude**. Dropped 15 kg [33 pounds] in six months (from 97 to 82) [from 213 to 180 pounds]. I recommend it very much to all my friends. Of course, it is not a panacea for everything. However, there is no medicine that can give you similar effects. The pharma business is nervously smoking on the side. Especially, I am impressed by how AM microdosing **activates the brain**. No comparison to any Nootropic Products. Why are they hiding it from us? Although the answer is clear and the question is rhetorical. . . . AM microdosing helped me to quit **smoking** and quit **alcohol**. It is a fact. I read the report here that AM microdosing **improves intercourse**. We also notice that—me and my wife.

Report No. 65: I've been eating dry mukhomor for almost a week in the morning and in the evening. From the first day, the effects appeared. **Feeling good**. Although I've never had anything to do with depression. Lazy only, and that got lessened. On day two to three I got constipated, hard stool, so I wrote right away here in this chat, and I was told that I was probably eating bad food. Well, I agree. I **changed my diet** by adding more fruits and veggies, everything got to normal. My condition is good.

Report No. 66: My usual condition is **hysterical workaholic**. After course of AM microdosing I am **calm** and **adequate**; of course, hysteria happens once in a while but not combustible. I **feel rested** and in **full of strength** in my nervous system.

Report No. 67: After AM microdosing I got a **great hard-on** every morning.

Report No. 68: Last year started eating mukhomors with my husband. We tried different doses. From mid-January until the end of March, I took 1 g per day and per night. The effects are as follows:

1. The **chatterbox** in my head has gone. No unnecessary thoughts, no **pain** about past or fear of the future.
2. My **sleep** improved. I sleep less but get up rested. I have had memorable and interesting dreams.
3. **Energy** rise, a lot of strength and desire to do something.
4. I stopped **excessive eating** while I had problems. I **lost weight** because I eat less. I gave up a lot of junk food.
5. My joints do not respond with **pain** to weather changes anymore. And I've suffered from it since I was a kid.
6. The **PMS** left. Menses are painless.
7. My **intuition** has risen.
8. I noticed that I do not remember some short-term and past events. At first, I thought it might be bad. But then I realized that it wasn't memory that deteriorated, but my **attention** began to work selectively. I stopped noticing and **focusing** on a lot of unnecessary things.
9. My **depression** and **apathy are gone**. I have **dealt with stress** situations much **easier**. I quickly recover from physical and mental overload as well.

Some results rolled back after the break. On August 24, I began taking microdoses of AM, 1 g per night. In a week my lumbar **pain** was gone; before, I couldn't sleep at night because of that pain. I will write you again after months of AM microdosing.

Report No. 69: I am sharing my experience of AM microdosing. First, I took AM microdose as tea. I felt nausea regardless of the dose. Switched to ground powdered dry AM intake. I also eat dry pieces. I felt less nausea, and if so, I ate ascorbic acid or a pinch of salt. It became more tolerable. Now I mix the powder with some sour juice. No nausea at all.

Report No. 70: Everything is wonderful, thank you. Two-week marathon with a cup of brew of AM microdose. Two weeks of great **sleep**, absolutely **calm** and **peaceful, cheerful, sociable**. In short—it's great.

Report No. 71: If I take an AM microdose every day, I don't see pronounced effects. With a break of a day or two, the effects are bright, more pronounced and expressed. At first, I brew 2 g of AM dried caps with boiling water in thermos. I add salt and black pepper. After a week I increase the dose from 2 g per day to 5 g per day.

Report No. 72: I take *Amanita muscaria* in dried powder, a tablespoon (4 g) every day for a week, and everything is super. Sometimes I feel dizzy, especially if I get up sharply, similar to dizziness that I have with a fasting diet. For the rest, a **state of fire in my veins**. My kidneys and liver are great. No side effects.

Report No. 73: I am taking an AM microdose 2–4 g a day since August (two months). I am forty-six years old. I used air-dried *Amanita* caps.

Results: I **achieve more** during the day. I have **less heartaches**. Everything seems good when I wake up, **negative thoughts** are gone. Sometimes if I do not take an AM microdose or take less, I feel like there is a small depressive pit, and it goes away after I take the right dose for me. I have **more understanding, crystal-clear thinking, less pain**. At the beginning of microdosing I felt a constant sense of some fairy-tale miracle or magic going around. AM microdosing gives me more **confidence in sex**. It's brighter and sweeter, **deeper feelings**, different state of consciousness, and a lot of changes that I cannot describe.

Because of AM mushrooms, I began to fulfill my life-long outstanding plans, ideas, and desires that I postponed for years. It makes my **life a better quality**; it is **easier to think**. I decided to microdose for a month and if everything will be good, for another month or a year.

Report No. 74: Thirteen days of microdosing. Weight by eye. Mostly one or two middle-size caps in the evening, sometimes in the morning. I **feel less tired** after work. Strange and sweet feelings. **Sharper attention and focus. Sharper eyesight**. My workouts are very **energetic. Communication** is more pleasant and more free than usual; nobody notices anything, but

I feel "good." I don't drink **alcohol** all this time. No desire but disgust with alcohol. I drink water or juice instead. **Brain activity** remains at a high level. The body is in **harmony**, nothing hurts or worries. **No anxiety or fear**, all as it should be. Head and **thoughts are clear**, nothing unnecessary. I **achieve more** and get **satisfaction** from work.

Report No. 75: Good day to everyone. I eat a tablespoon (5 g). I certainly felt good and high . . . but it was necessary to constantly control my speech and behavior in order not to cause suspicion.

Report No. 76: Twelve days I brew AM tea with 3–5 g in the morning and evening the same. During the day the efficiency and **ease of communication** is enhanced. Euphoria. **Sleep** is changing. By 10 p.m. I fall asleep. I sleep well. Quit **alcohol**. Less ego problems. One day I took a bigger dose. I did not like it. Not for me. Small doses rules.

Report No. 77: I noticed such a feature: If I eat an AM microdose and stay at home, then I see no effects. But when I go to work, walk outside, or am busy doing something, I see that I'm not lazy. I **feel well**, there is no such feeling as **frustration**, **neurotic state**, pressure, and desire to get rid of the subject I am working on. It feels sort of like a robot in a good way. A depressed man is so reluctant to do anything. I think that AM is good in business.

Report No. 78: Greetings! I read AM microdosing reports and observe that some people lost their **sleep**. The reason is the dosage. It is 100% confirmed with my own experience, repeatedly (three times). Night intake works well with dose of dry powder at the tip of a knife or the tip of a teaspoon. Like a pinch of salt. This dose knocks me out. My sleep is good, and in the morning, I wake up and feel the body is warm and soft. This is an unrealistically beautiful feeling!

Report No. 79: AM microdosing seven days. First, it was 2 g dry, now 1 g on empty stomach. Preparation: boiling water, add lemon juice, screening out mushroom body. **Easiness and purity of consciousness, positive state.** At the end of the week, I felt discomfort in pancreas and liver. I have chronic pancreatitis. I had to stop *Amanita muscaria* microdoses intake.

Report No. 80: Consumed five days of AM microdoses right after drying: 1 g. I had only 5 g of *Amanita*. Positive effects—less craving for **cigarettes**. Increased **working capacity**, **desire** to do something, desire to finish what I have started. **Less craving for food, normalized nutrition**. It was also quite easy to get up in the morning. After the termination all the positive effects went down. I began to eat like crazy again, I got wild desire to smoke, lack of desire to do something (in principle almost as before AM microdosing). Overall experience is **happy**. I am going to the forest to pick up more *Amanita*. Thank you for opening up the world of microdosing for me.

Report No. 81: Good time. My experience of two weeks AM microdosing: I consumed 2 g in the morning on empty stomach. My **psycho-emotional state** and **brain activity increased** twice in the positive direction. My character has changed—I have become a **calm** person. I am not steamed by small troubles or stupid people, although before it was very annoying. The **mood** is positive all the time, but it is not euphoric. It's just **fun**, and I treat everything with **humor**. The **mind is clear**, there are no garbage thoughts, and logic works in the right direction. I do a lot of intellectual activities, I am **not tired** by the evening, and I am ready to continue. Before AM microdosing I was baked by the evening and completely burned out. I experimented with different dosages. The dose from 2 to 6 g have **reverse effects**: entanglement of thoughts. Dose more than 6 g: the nausea appears, vomit calls, and discomfort in the stomach. These negative effects are gone in hour, and there is a state of mild intoxication and sleepiness, with good mood and euphoria added. It resembles the action of indica marijuana. I feel fresh in the morning without any side effects. The physiological level with AM microdosing: the body is filled with **energy** for the whole day, great **appetite**. Joint **pain** stopped; before AM microdosing I could not even lift a kettle without tormented paint in my elbow joints. I got **alcohol** disgust. I plan AM microdosing for couple more weeks, then I will take a break for a month. I want to check how long the positive effects stay without AM microdosing. Do I recommend it or not? I think it is a personal matter for everyone, and I believe that it is necessary to come to it on their own choice. There is no altered consciousness with small doses of AM! No side effects or poisoning! Would I go for *Amanita* trip—NO! It is wrong mushroom for a trip, and for that there is psilocybin mushrooms.

Report No. 82: By thirty years old I am almost a cripple with a bunch of diagnoses. Due to the static nature of the activity, I have an unhealthy back and **pain**. I overused various **alcohol** and **tobacco** poisons, as well as junk food. The second day AM microdosing by rubbing ointment (mukhomor) into trigger points, 1 g in the morning and 1 g in the evening, I had the most **lively**, **productive**, and **energetic** moments in ten years. Now I feel almost

healthy. There is some pain here and there, but nothing in comparison with how it was! AM microdosing helped me to get rid of **pain** from an old fracture. I also used AM tincture. Very **invigorating** and gives unrealistic **sex** drive.

Report No. 83: I am forty years old. One week of AM microdsing. Motivation for AM microdosing: improve my life, I mainly needed a cure for laziness, apathy, and help with alcohol consumption. Intake of dry quarter of a cap, twice a day. I had some **skin rash**; it went away in three days. In the beginning of the course, condition was unclear, confused consciousness, foggy thoughts. But I was able to drive, and reactions are **sharp** and less irritation by stupid drivers. In general, I felt much **calmer** and **uninvolved**. Later, everything got to normal and better—I was able to do much more than I planned, my speed and **motivation raised**. **Libido** is up! No more joint **pain** (five years of suffering), some **skin warts** disappeared. I cured two friends from **synthetic drug dependency** with *Amanita muscaria* microdoses. Microdoses are an amazing thing!

Report No. 84: Three days of AM microdosing: 1 g in the morning, and 0.5 g in the evening (thirty minutes prior to bedtime). What instantly became noticeable is an effect on morning awakenings: very **cheerful**, **healthy**, **and light mood**, **easy** to get up. A day-to-day transformation, in one word "**tonus**." **Less tired**, no sluggishness, there is **unity of body and mind**, here and now sensation. About night dose: if I take more, I have problems falling **asleep**. I am grateful for information on *Amanita muscaria* microdoses. Thanks to you, my **life became more pleasant**.

Report No. 85: Before AM microdosing: I had sluggish condition, no motivation, ate a lot of junk food, no interest in anything, apathy. After: better **choice of food** and less quantity. **Positive thinking**, discovered interesting activities, and I became **more social**.

Report No. 86: One month of AM microdosing—I got rid of my **depression**!

Report No. 87: Good afternoon! I live in St. Petersburg; I am a forty-three-year-old woman. After watching your videos, I tried AM microdoses. I collected it myself. For two weeks I consumed dry pieces of mukhomor (about 1/8 hat, 10 cm), on empty stomach. My observations: The action lasts a little less than a day, the peak comes in 4–6 hours. **Great feelings** are revealed. The Ego ceases to dominate, perception more through the heart.

First week I was up and down—strong sexuality turned to aggression. Later, aggression changed to quiet glide in the waves of feelings. **Love, kindness, mercy** is revealed. There was physical **energy**, body got flexible. I ate less, I became **slender** and **younger**! I feel love for my body. Several times more **powerful awareness** has occurred. Living has become **more interesting**. There was hope that I could cope with years of **depression** and longing. And my daughter and husband want to help. They are taking an AM microdose as well. Everyone is **happy**, we share our impressions with each other. Thank you for valuable information!

Report No. 88: Four days of AM microdosing: 1 g in tea form with lemon juice in the morning; 0.2–0.5 g at night. I fall asleep immediately. It gives me **great night sleep**, nice wake-up morning **mood**, philosophical **thoughts, healthy ignorance** to dark events.

Report No. 89: One week of AM microdosing: 1 g, dry flakes in the morning. **Harmony** and **happiness** simply went up. It is wildly pleasant for me to watch everything around. I **smile** and **sing**. Even now while I write, I have goose bumps. My **internal dialogue** prompts to me: "People need your help. Help them." I feel I have to be **kinder** and more useful to people around me. I never noticed before.

Report No. 90: I want to report a new effect of AM microdosing. I ate occasionally AM dry caps before bed and regularly use AM juice on problem areas—**joints and [areas that experience] muscle spasms**. Here's a new effect from the mukhomors. To my astonishment I recently found out that **prostatitis** was gone. I was diagnosed with it six years ago and no prescribed pill gave me any improvement. Simple observation of strong urine outcome, compared to few drops with pain before, pardon me.

Report No. 91: I want to report my own use of microdosing AM tincture. I discovered the effect of using tincture at the same time with oral administration of dry mukhomor microdoses. I used to rub AM tincture on my back **pain** areas. Later I used it on the acupuncture points on the face: between the eyebrows, at the base of the nose, in the pit under the lower lip, on the cheekbones. Also in the area of the thyroid. I got the same effects as of a dose of eaten dry mukhomors. The effect comes almost instantly. I feel the **invigorating effect** and the **antidepressant effect** lasting all day. After rubbing your neck and massaging acupuncture dots, you feel the **tide of vigor, calm, joy, and thrill** of just **being here and now**. In this state I am

resistant to stress. I talk **calmly** and **succinctly**. **Attention is increased** while driving.

Report No. 92: I tried AM microdosing, and it's not some nonsense! I suffer from **depression**, and my search for cure led me to the mukhomor. After taking an AM microdose course I got back to my senses, I found myself. I got **great relief**. I plan to continue with the new AM season.

Report No. 93: I am a twenty-eight-year-old man. Four months of AM microdosing 3 g per day, dry flakes. Up to 5 g on a weekend for fun. **Alcohol** intake surprisingly went down. **Marijuana** got down to once a week, not every day like before. Completely cured **stomatitis**. Before, it was a constant battle with new gum ulcers. The **mood** is always **good, vigorous and cheerful** all day, good **appetite**. **Libido** stabilized; **porn addiction** gone and actual sex more often. **Powerful awareness** has occurred. **Living has become more interesting**. I experimented with different doses. No more than 3 g at a time. Bigger amount makes me lazy, kind of drunk, and I do not want to do my household chores.

Report No. 94: I got rid of **heartburn** after a month of AM microdose intake.

Report No. 95: Age forty-three, weight 92 kg [203 pounds], height 186 cm [6 feet, 1 inch]. AM mushrooms were consumed in dry form, caps, brewed in water about 80°C [176°F] (in thermos), brew time—forty minutes. Dosage—one dried cap. Time of use—before bed. Duration of use—two weeks. Effects of AM microdosing met my objectives. Great night **sleep** and strong memorable dreams. During the day **great vigor, clearer consciousness, and easier concentration**.

Report No. 96: Eating raw mukhomors. Dosage: half a medium mushroom with a stem. The leg is delicious, has a nutty taste, the cap is just a mushroom taste. Before bedtime—good sleep, strong energy in the morning. High degree of cheer even with short 3–4 hours sleep. There is an impact on speech and logical centers. **Easy to communicate**, with **humor**, looking at things from a **different perspective**. If the dose is raised to one whole mushroom, mild intestinal cleansing—one-time diarrhea. My conclusion—the mushroom is instrumental; it can be set to specific tasks when taking. There is a **psychological adjustment** under the influence of an AM. Strictly positive assessment of the intake. The experiments with *Amanita muscaria* will continue.

Report No. 97: Fourteen days of AM microdosing. Intake in a form of tea with AM powder, lemon juice, and honey. Before, during six months endogenous **depression**, during six months with **suicidal thoughts** and total **apathy**, antidepressants did not help. Starting with day one, the **mood** got to normal for the first time in six months. I even managed to play volleyball—loved this since I was a child, but forgot how pleasant it could be. The next two weeks I got back my **appetite**, got to work without forcing myself, mood is normal, **pleasure from life**, so cozy. And most important **changes in my brain**: it seems that all the questions simply disappeared. I got all the answers I need. It was really cool, like a super brain turned on. Life decisions became **easier** to make. The **food habits** changed, stopped eating **sweets**. Now I have awareness of negative effects of flour products. *Amanita muscaria* microdoses help very much.

Report No. 98: Three months of AM microdosing, one-half teaspoon dry powder. Shoulder joint **pain** went away. I was tormented with it for six months. AM microdosing turned me away from **sweets** and **alcohol**. AM tincture has great effects as well; it instantly relieves any **pain**. Super mushrooms, I love them, the mukhomor works in a very positive way! Nausea with 3 g; no negative effects with 1–2 g.

Report No. 99: Hey, Baba Masha. I'm **allergic** to cats. I took an AM microdose for two weeks, I came home, there's a cat, allergy doesn't show up in any way. I took cat in my hands and nothing at all. Very surprised. Thank you for your useful information.

Report No. 100: Baba Masha, hello! Eight days of *Amanita muscaria* microdoses. I noticed that I **argue less** with people, with some I do not argue at all. **Sleep** well; dreams have become more realistic; sometimes I wake up in the morning and do not immediately understand whether it was a dream or real!

Report No. 101: AM microdosing for ten months. Dose from 0.25–0.7 g, 1–2 times a day. Before, I have had spring **allergy** attacks every year from May to July. I took allergy pills on constant basis. Not anymore after *Amanita muscaria* microdoses. I also used rappe tobacco mix as well. This combination took away my allergy.

Report No. 102: My experience of AM microdosing for a month. First three days, I took one tablespoon (appr. 5.5 g) in the morning and before bed:

sweating and feeling burning sensation of palms and feet, confusion of consciousness, joints chills, loss of sleep. It was accompanied by a sense of isolation from what was happening and a tangible immersion in itself during the day. NO pain was observed anywhere, nor were symptoms of liver damage, biliary system, intestinal disorders by clinic tests—blood test, general urine test, liver panel—all normal. After the first three days I took a break. By the end of day five, the condition had fully normalized. From day six I continued on half a teaspoon in the morning and overnight. A sense of **energy** rose, starting two hours after reception until the end of the day. Thought process is **harmonious**, quiet **determination**, **libido** not raised but normal, freely controllable. Present **pleasant detachment** from primary emotional assessment. I decide how to feel, not settle on reflex. The mukhomor ended—the course ended. I don't feel a big slide back because I remembered to analyze during the course why I don't feel like this without a mukhomor. I began to think the same as under *Amanita muscaria* microdoses: **calmly**, suspended, without doubt. I express my wishes calmly—it makes no sense to prove anything. I let myself be myself. Former **depression** at the same level, but I don't see it as a problem.

Report No. 103: Hi! Three days microdose with my wife: 1–2 g in the morning and 1–1.5 g in the evening for me. My wife's dose was 1 g. From observations of both: **less fatigue**, absolutely sober with **pure consciousness**, bright-colored **dreams, desire** to read and work, good **mood**, internal **calm**. Regarding the gastrointestinal system—no disorders at all.

Report No. 104: Hi. Thank you. I started AM microdosing after reading your information. I take 1 g a day in the morning. There is no intoxication nor euphoria, but a state of **calm, irritability has gone, a lot of energy**. It took away **alcohol and nicotine** cravings totally. I went to the store yesterday. I thought I'd buy chips and a coke. Before I got to the counter, I realized I didn't want them at all. I ended up buying pomegranate and juice. The meat dumplings I used to buy periodically are disgusting. Couldn't finish eating it and threw it out. I continue the experiment.

Report No. 105: Hello, Baba Masha. First of all, thank you for your educational spiritual activities and light in your voice! I've microdosed AM since September. It was interesting to compare by analogy with still fresh memories of psilocybin microdose for three months. First time, I ate a small piece of AM fresh in the forest. The effect **seems like revitalizing children's percep-**

tion of the world, like some fairy tale. It was an amazing palette of bright and magical sunset. Later on, my AM microdose is a teaspoon before bed. In twenty minutes there is a **pleasant sleepiness**, and I fall asleep with a smile. **Dreams** in the first few days of microdosing acquire specific motifs, bright, a little surreal. The experiment continues. I will regulate the dosage, and I will observe what will happen next.

Report No. 106: I'm forty-nine. After watching your videos, I started taking 2 g of mukhomor mushroom at night for fifteen days because of **back pain**. The first thing that I noticed: the **awakening**, the eyes opened, and the **brain is working clear**. After day three I found that my long-time sore on the ankle is healed. There are no negative feelings. Funny, but I noticed a change in my face, as if the wrinkles were gone. I have much **better skin condition**. This was confirmed by people around me. I feel **calmer** and more **balanced**. I stopped using **cannabis**, which I regularly used since 1991.

Report No. 107: Hi, I want to share with you my experience of taking mukhomor microdoses. I've been taking AM microdoses about three weeks. I started with very small dosages of 0.2 g and slowly increased to 1 g a day. After about 0.7 g, began to feel the effect. There was a huge **energy**. At the same time there was no rollback, no down time in comparison to other stimulants. In general, there is the effect of **transforming consciousness** to a level where you can control your **emotions**. It seems that you feel everything around, and there are no boundaries of power and thought.

Report No. 108: Hi, Baba Masha. Here is my AM microdosing experience with my wife for two weeks. We take an AM microdose in the morning and evening around 1.5–2 g. In the morning we get a lift of energy; sometimes there is also a failure, in a sluggish state, for an hour or two. Then lift again to the end of the day. We tried another dose of about 1.5 g at lunch. Did not work well. Switched to morning and evening. The other day, the wife got a **cold** and increased the dose to 5 g in the morning and 5 g in the evening. At the end of the second day of illness, the wife's condition improved significantly. In summary: **well-being**, **energy rise**. Food preferences have not changed much (I am a vegetarian for five years), but we have **less sugar urges**.

Report No. 109: Hi. I just read new reviews here on AM microdosing. I see that some people eat a tablespoon AM from the first days and are complaining of negative effects. I think it's because of excessive dose. I started with 0.2 g and reached 0.5 g. It is so **good and joyful, and my soul laughs**.

I do not remember the last time I felt that in general. I stopped **smoking** cigarettes a couple days ago as well.

Report No. 110: I take *Amanita muscaria* microdoses for a second month, in the form of tea with lemon in the morning before breakfast. The **positive changes** are felt after the second reception.

Report No. 111: I am thirty-five years old, married, with two kids. I am taking an AM microdose in 1 g dose (tea form with lemon juice) in the morning, sometimes at night. The positive effects: **bright dreams** and **restful sleep**, a more **balanced emotional state**, **increased performance and focus** on tasks, **raised mood** and **motivation**. I stopped because of increased sensitivity of my liver.

Report No. 112: I take *Amanita muscaria* mushroom by one dry cap, 3–4 cm in diameter, in the morning and evening. Positive effects—**calmness**, **balance**. It was hard to wake up in the morning sometimes. In general, after each intake I have an **ease**, **energy**, and increase in **libido**.

Report No. 113: My AM microdose is 0.5 g for four weeks. I have strong **sleep**; the **mood is cheerful** in the morning. I'm getting **calmer**. There is an **energy**, a **desire** to do something useful. I was diagnosed with kidney stones. To my amusement *Amanita muscaria* mushroom is crushing it. The sand is coming out. I had to drink diuretic. Generally, the **experience is positive**.

Report No. 114: AM microdosing for a month 1–1.5 teaspoons in a form of tea (thirty minute wait). There are obvious changes. I became more **reasonable**. On the one hand I became **calmer**, [but also became] more intolerant of negative people. **Sleep** has improved, dreams are very bright. Most of the time, the forest dreams.

Report No. 115: I took an AM microdose 1–2 teaspoons a day for a month. In the morning or evening, before the meal or after the meal, no difference was noticed. On the day of the intake there was a sense of **increased awareness and energy**. I forgot what laziness is. I do so much in a day that I wouldn't have done in a week, great help at my job. At the end of the month I noticed that my life-long **allergy** to animals is gone. Now I can easily play with dogs or cats and symptoms do not appear at all. Before, I couldn't be in a house where there are animals for even ten minutes.

Report No. 116: Three weeks of AM microdosing, half a teaspoon in powder form. Positive changes: **depression, disturbing thoughts disappeared** during the intake, **clarity in thoughts** appeared, decisions were made more **easily**, good **mood**. **Self-uncertainty has disappeared**. It became easier to get up in the morning. There was a wish to smoke less. **Cigarette smoke** became unpleasant.

Report No. 117: Two months of microdosing. No side effects were observed after fermentation and storage in vacuum. Preparation: dry in a dehydrator about 60°C [140°F]. Consumed differently, dry powder, tea with lemon, steamed with herbs and just boiling water. According to my feelings the best is dry, grated, and drinking warm water with a teaspoon of honey, 2–3 g, every other day. **Vigorous, fresh, clarity of thought, healthy sleep, lost a lot of weight.**

Report No. 118: Hi everyone! One week of AM microdosing, 1–2 g before bed. I have all similar effects that I read above. In addition to that, my **tongue has completely cleared** from white to pink. I'm shocked. Instant **sleep aid**, somewhere in 30–40 minutes after intake, and bright, interesting dreams, plus **good mood** in the morning. I am **motivated** to do a lot of things that I neglected before: clean up in the house with **pleasure**, walking, listening to music, working in the garden, drawing. I have **better communication** with colleagues and relatives. I do everything with pleasure, and at the same time I have no fatigue as before, and I'm in a good mood.

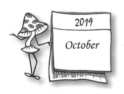

Report No. 119: AM microdosing during two weeks, 1 g per day. My **sense of smell increased**. I became **balanced and calm**. It became easier to hold **consciousness in the moment** (here and now). Less thinking about the past. I am not glued to the phone constantly as before; it was taking all my attention. There is some sense of **greater awareness**. Complete impartiality, not indifference to what's going on. It's when you just watch what's happening, without superimposing some of your accumulated beliefs on it. **Empathy** for people has increased. There comes an **understanding** that everyone has their own way, and that there is no right or wrong in peoples' actions. I started to **appreciate more** what I have. It was easier to understand my desired wishes and their reasons.

Report No. 120: Hi, Baba Masha. Great thanks to you for all the information you provided. Before microdosing: **depression, laziness, and constant eating.**

I started from 0.5 g and gradually increased to 1, 2, and 3 g. I report that 3 g is too much, I was unable to work, I **laughed** a lot and became too **relaxed**. My effective dose is 1–1.5 g. Preparation: I brew like tea with a spoon of lemon juice, wait 15–30 minutes. *Effects:* The laziness was gone. I became more **effective** and more **active** at my work, more **cheerful**. My inner voice is louder; it says that it is not necessary to eat too much junk food. I excluded **sugar and sweets**.

Report No. 121: I am thirty-five years old, male. One month of AM microdoses. I took it 1–2 times a day, morning and evening at 1 g. From the first days I noticed that I became **calm and balanced**. I stopped paying attention to external stimuli. At the same time I sort of didn't become a vegetable, but I just set priorities of important and secondary things. The **mood** is raised. Same about my **food addictions**. I eat much less **meat** and **sweets**. It used to be a tradition in the evening with my wife to drink tea with sweets— chocolate, cookies, or candies. There is no routine and monotony, every day some **fresh feelings**. I set **new priorities**. I became more **socially active** and took a **better grip** on my business. I am going to continue *Amanita muscaria* microdoses intake.

Report No. 122: Good evening, Baba Masha. My feedback on AM microdoses. The reason for intake: For ten years I have experienced problems with life activity. Three years ago I was diagnosed with **manic-depressive psychosis** and **insomnia**. My energy vacillated from strong, dropped down to painful high bursts. For a week I took 1–2 g, brewed as tea in boiling water. Hard to believe, but **normal sleep** is back, falling asleep at night is fast, waking up in the morning is easy. Dreams are very bright, as in childhood. Stopped **craving fat food**. **Meat** has a nasty taste. Craving for **alcohol** is gone. **Destructive thoughts went away**; I focus on the important things in my life. Tomorrow I will buy more mushrooms, and I will continue therapy. Surprised by the lies we live in, as a child we were taught to destroy mukhomors, and now we are ashamed of it.

Report No. 123: I am forty-three years old. My weight 90 kg [198 pounds]. Three weeks on *Amanita muscaria* microdoses. I have a break every weekend. My dose is 1–1.5 g once a day, in the evening. I brew a tea in a thermos with lemon for twenty minutes. There are no side effects. I tried to increase the dose; it did not feel right. The dose amount somehow became immediately clear.

Changes:
1. The inflammation of a sciatic nerve—the **pain** is gone.
2. **Tranquility**. I began to react **more calmly** to situations. In summer I wanted to break up with my wife, but we came to **peace** and some **understanding**.
3. **Alcohol**. I clearly see that alcohol makes me stupid, even the wine that I used to take a little bit of after work. I have no desire to drink it. I noticed it was an old habit or a social gesture—which is bullshit in itself. I am free from alcohol.
4. **Feelings**. I began to feel happiness in the moment! It is so healthy! At the same time it is a spontaneous state, a feeling of gratitude and harmony with others.
5. **Internal dialogue**. First, I began to notice it clearly. Second, there are significant declines of negative internal dialogue. It is very pleasant and peaceful.
6. **Dependence**. With my weekend breaks I notice an absence of dependency to *Amanita muscaria*.
7. **Activity**. I mentioned above the lack of energy. Now my "to do" list clears up quickly. I do as I planned, and I do not get tired.

Report No. 124: Month of *Amanita muscaria* microdoses. My opinion about the dose: 3–5 g is too much. I started with 0.5 then began to raise to 3.5 g, noted negative side effects with bigger doses. I have scattering, reduced emotional background, suppressed state of mind. I reduced the dose of AM microdose to 1.5 g and my **mood** became significantly better. *Amanita* microdoses made me quit **alcohol**! I confirm that AM is great medicine for alcohol addiction, but no one knows about that!

Report No. 125: I've been an **alcohol** lover for over ten years, suffering but drinking excessively. I have taken AM microdoses since August this year. There was both vomiting and aggression, but only in the first month of reception. Second month of practicing AM microdosing, I quit drinking. Alcohol is no longer for me. I don't need to relieve the tension anymore because my **tension is gone**. After a month and a half of AM microdosing, I **lost 10 kilos [22 pounds] of fat** from my body. Thank you, Baba Masha, that you brought this information in masses.

Report No. 126: I take mukhomor twice a day, one teaspoon. **Alcohol** is not desirable to me anymore, though before I was a steady drinker. Now it just turned off!!! A lot of **strength**, **energy**, even cleaning the house is pleasure! **Sleep** has improved, and dreams are very realistic and very colorful. I plan to take AM microdoses for three months, then pause for a month.

Report No. 127: My mukhomor microdose is about 1 g in the evening. First week, I took it in the morning, but it made me feel sleepy during the day, and I switched to evening intake. However, I tried morning intake after ten days of microdosing. Now it **feels great**, and I am **energized and in good mood**. Total course was thirty-five days. I am planning to collect mushrooms myself next season.

Report No. 128: Hi! I started mukhomor microdosing, and the **quality of my life** has improved considerably, and that's all thanks to your channel! Many thanks! For the last couple of days, two level teaspoons with a glass of water. Before I was taking 1.5 spoons. Now I don't know how I lived without AM microdosing; everything described by people is pure truth, it's like magic.

Report No. 129: My experience is with the mukhomor stems. My husband got into these mushrooms. We are vegans. I was not going to microdose or trip at all. I'm an ardent opponent of any drugs, psilocybin, or anything. It just my opinion; other adults can do what they desire. If my husband is interested in the fungus, I will support him because it is an interesting subject. Yesterday we went to the forest and collected about 150 pieces of *Amanita muscaria*. The caps were dried, and the stems were washed, cleaned, cut, and thrown into boiling water twice, then fried with onion, pepper, tomatoes, and lemon juice. I ate about ten stems, maybe less. An hour later I got a headache. I was reading these reports, and letters were jumping. I felt sleepy, we went to bed. I woke up and realized something was wrong with me. I had a dream, but it was not a dream. It's all hard to describe. Clusters of realities. Muscular twitching. I panicked, cried, and told my husband to call an ambulance. But the mushroom suddenly sheltered me with calm, and these clusters were removed. I calmed down quickly, realized that everything was fine. That I did not get poisoned and to carry this condition was a burden to me, and I asked the mushroom for sleep. Woke up with less sound ringing in the head, I calmed down, and I was able to more calmly "speak to the fungus."

Report No. 130: I boiled AM stems two times, then fried. I ate half a plate, and it smashed me seriously hard. My hands and legs were twitching on their own right after I ate some. My arm muscle tone went limp. Eating cooked AM stems is not funny at all. I tried three times. It was not the same effect as eating a dried AM microdose. It's the same harsh as eating raw AM mushrooms! AM microdoses are a bomb!

Report No. 131: Thank you for your work. I did not use any drugs, but the mukhomors found me. A couple of days I brewed a tea using one AM cap; the next couple weeks I used dried AM microdose. I used tea for the night. I am trying to find my daytime dose. **Alcohol** became bad news! I have **increased working capacity**, and I **sleep** well. I **crack jokes** all the time now.

Report No. 132: Hello, Baba Masha, thank you for your enlightenment! After two times microdosing AM, dry and tea forms, my body refused to eat **meat**. I love bacon, but yesterday I could not eat or smell it.

Report No. 133: Hi, Baba Masha. I am vegan, I do not smoke, no alcohol. We collected AM, with my husband, in early October. We dried AM in a dryer at 60°C [140°F] and started the course immediately after drying. We take the same amount. It is the fourth day now. I take one coffee spoon of mukhomor powder in the morning and the same amount at night. I brew it and drink the tea with lemon juice after thirty minutes. I feel lightness in my head in the hour after the reception, then it passes, at the same time my **condition is cheerful**. AM microdosing **lowered my appetite**. My **mood improved** and became **magnificent**: I started **singing** at home. I became more restrained with others, I do not ask—I do not answer, I **do not get involved** in any small empty discussions. I became **more affectionate** with my husband and son. **Sleep** is strong, I fall asleep quickly. I wake up easy, **rested**, though I can lie down late.

Another point: One day a **pimple** popped on my face. I mixed a pinch of mukhomor powder in the palm with a drop of apricot oil and put this on my face for the night. In a morning it was gone. I am very happy about this effect!

Yesterday my husband ate three AM fried stems; he said it was very tasty, no hallucinatory effects received. The initial result of AM microdosing is inspiring. At the end of the course, I will write about new results. I hope you are not tired of a lot of letters. Thank you, Baba Masha, you are my inspiration! Thank you for your contribution and education, for your positivity! Kiss, peace, and love!

Report No. 134: About us: we're a couple, thirty-nine and thirty-eight years old. We microdosed with AM caps for a month at 1 g, brewed at 7 a.m. and consumed in an hour. Our observations: AM mushroom creates a **working mood. Removes the wrong irritability.** Does not let go into resentment. We both became **more kind.** Now we treat other people with **great understanding,** and people do not piss us off. We ordered 200 more g. Waiting for the shipment.

Report No. 135: Hello. I am over sixty years old. After reading about AM, I picked some last summer in the forest. I ate one stem raw. The effect impressed me. I was working in my garden nonstop until it got too dark. I did not feel the slightest fatigue but just a **beautiful mood.** I made a tincture and took it by drops, increasing every day. With 7–8 drops I felt incredible **calm, healthy coolness and complete harmony** with the surrounding world. A state of **delight, balance, and happiness.**

I experimented with my **dog,** too. She had a huge breast **tumor** the size of a ball. I refused to put her to sleep. The poor dog almost didn't get up anymore, only to eat and go to the bathroom. I decided to give her the tincture. Started with ten drops. A couple of days later, dog got up, started walking, wagging her tail, behaving like a normal, healthy, young dog; she welcomed me near the gate, barked at passers-by, etc. The tumor didn't go away and it certainly created discomfort because of its severity. Anyway, she didn't die until earlier this summer. Only for the last three days the dog could no longer get up, eat, drink. Six months, I've been watching an absolutely cheerful, healthy, happy animal.

In brief: AM microdosing is not a placebo anymore; it's animal experiments, and I tried AM microdosing on my friends as well. The effect is always the same—**wings behind your back, peace, happiness.** Thanks to you. By the way, I cooked *Amanita muscaria* stems; it is not just food, that is a misconception. It gives a soft trip.

Report No. 136: Hello, Baba Masha! I am going to talk about the positive action of AM microdosing on my **teeth condition.** I have a bad situation with my teeth and cannot afford to do major work. I had constant swollen gums, inflammation in root canals. I was taking two teaspoons of AM powder per half glass of water before bed. I drastically **decreased inflammation and pain** in my mouth.

Report No. 137: Hi, Baba Masha! I am very glad that there is such an amazing person who has dispelled all my fears and helped me with a lot of conflicting information on psychedelics. Thanks to you! I want to tell you about the mukhomor microdoses. I ate a dry AM microdose, two weeks, 2 g in the morning, sometimes at night.

Effects: **Reduction of appetite**, for me it is a huge help, I could not stop eating. **Skin rash** on my back disappeared. My **menstrual cycle** passed without usual **pain**. Before I had to take 5–10 pills to take away the **cramps**. Coincidence? I don't think so. I became super **calm**. I do not have those moments when I shake and go out of my senses. I **laugh** more and have **fun**. I have **motivation and desire** to do something instead of living inside my phone. No side effects. I am going to continue the experiment.

Report No. 138: Hi to all. Started taking *Amanita muscaria* microdoses from1.5–3 g. It was too much for me. After five days of reception, I paused for three days. I felt sluggish and tired. I started to take 0.5 g. In the morning I felt myself **happy and laughing**! All conscious citizens of the ex-USSR big hello!

Report No. 139: My lab blood tests revealed **increased amount of iron**. And since last year I had about a kilogram of dry *Amanita muscaria* fungus; I decided that now is the time to have an experience of treatment with the mushroom. For a month I took 2–3 tablespoons of *Amanita muscaria* in the morning with breakfast. The condition was excellent: sometimes felt slightly high, but it was not reflected at my job, and I smiled constantly like a Cheshire cat. The results of second lab blood test confused the doctor. He said that probably the first test was not made properly. After that I reduced the dose to one coffee spoon; I **felt perfect, irritability and flashes of anger disappeared, lightness in the body appeared**.

Report No. 140: AM microdosing at the moment is pure panacea for me. I am disabled, group three with **chronic polyneuropathy**. There was constant neuralgic **pain** in the legs. I drink AM tea made with one teaspoon of dry powder before bed. For the second week I felt a lot of **positive** things, complete disgust to **cigarettes, alcohol** (that was also main reason to try AM). I react to situations with **calmer and merrier attitude**.

Report No. 141: AM microdosing results: the first few days there were gases, bloats, tingles in the intestines. It passed quickly. The feeling of **hunger decreased** markedly. Food portions became smaller, and I do not eat very often anymore. **Sleep** time has been greatly reduced; I **wake up early, energized**. **Energy increased** greatly during the day. **Emotional-sensual state** is always normal or in plus. Previously, it was often below zero—**anxiety, fears, obsessive expectations of bad events**, etc. Problematic events do not bother me anymore. Looks like I'm getting out of the problem and watching it from the outside. Total **honesty with myself**. Dreams are very bright and realistic, very lively and real. Every dream has a key event, feeling, and emotion that is closely intertwined with real life. Sleep sort of unlocks and shows what requires therapy and healing in the context of relationships and events with these people. For example, fear, shame, guilt, etc. Every morning a new portion for study and healing.

Report No. 142: My AM microdosing report: I picked mushrooms myself, no fermentations, dried at 35°C [95°F], storing over room water heater. I drink AM tea made out of half of small AM cap in the morning. I have **great pleasure** with running on an AM microdose (8 miles), **mood is calm, childlike joy inside, motivation, creativity**.

Report No. 143: Masha, I tested different doses of AM microdoses. The best for me was one teaspoon AM powder at night. It changed my **food preferences**—**meat** does not look appealing anymore.

Report No. 144: Hi! I take one teaspoon of dry powder. AM microdosing results: **Weight reduction. I eat less. I stopped drinking** beer and whisky. **Less being upset**. Stressful situations became easier to solve at work. Staff looks at me with curiosity—what is going on with me? They like my **new attitude**; I did not tell anybody that I'm taking *Amanita muscaria*.

Report No. 145: I take 1 g; AM tea is good for **sleep** vs. the dry form is an **energizer** to me. I took 7 g once; it was not good.

Report No. 146: Ten weeks of AM microdosing. Consumption once a day, in the evening. About 0.6–0.8 g (just over half a teaspoon in thermos with lemon). Immediately affects the arbitrary **concentration of attention in a positive way. Slow down on useless activities**—internet and phone. The **emotional background** is **balanced**. It has become **easier to communicate** with people. **Physical activity** (trainings) generally is simpler, but not fundamentally, coordination does not get better, stretching is markedly deeper, **sensations** from any movement **are richer**.

Report No. 147: The five days of microdoses in the form of dry powder: the first four days up to 3 g and each time a state of mild euphoria and sleepiness. I reduced the dose to 1–1.5 g. Different results, **cheered state**. I noticed that small **wounds healed** very quickly. AM microdosing reduced my **back pain**, and it was gone completely after fifth day. Before AM microdosing, I was limping from that pain.

Report No. 148: Eating AM half cap before bed makes **phlegm** strongly come out of my lungs. My **dreams** are different and surprise me. I ate cooked AM stems once. I experience weak patterns for short time. I think 1 g is enough for microdoses, morning and evening, the **effect is wonderful**.

Report No. 149: Hi, Masha! Three weeks of AM microdosing, 1–2 g a day. At first, there were **migraines, aches** in the body as in influenza, **loss of appetite**, and **intoxication**. They passed quickly, and I think that my parasites are all dead. Now everything is super, no intoxication signs. I had **pain** in the knee joints before AM microdose course; it was painful to walk, now I want to run. Perhaps the rigidity of the effects from the mukhomor depends on the degree of sluggishness of the body and number of parasites. During cleansing it could be difficult due to the mass death of the parasites.

Report No. 150: Microdosing fly agarics for one week. The effect from 1 g is the same as from 2 g. I noticed a change in my **morning wake-up** time. It's around 5 a.m. now. It's very **unusual and pleasing** to me. Also, there was an **unshakable tranquility**. I **don't get annoyed** at people.

Report No. 151: I want to share my several months experience with AM. Mukhomor was in the form of a vodka tincture. Amazing effect. Complete **internal peace, calm attitude** to everything going on around. What might have been out of balance under other circumstances is not even noticed. I gave out a tincture to six of my loved ones and friends to make sure it wasn't a placebo. Everyone had the same result. **Wings behind your back, smiles to your ears, the world is interesting and beautiful**. No nausea or other unpleasant side effects that occur when I microdosed dry AM; no one had these.

Report No. 152: AM microdosing ten days. I brew tea at night with lemon and take before food in the morning. Started from 0.2 g up to 0.5 g. I've had stomach problems for five years. That's why I approach everything with caution. The first thing I noticed was **sight**. The eyes used to itch, tear down, and the picture was fuzzy. Everything passed. Everything became **bright and voluminous**. The **skin on my face** in the area of the nose was peeled before, it became markedly smaller after. I began to get enough **sleep**. The **mood is great, the anxiety is gone**. I began to **eat less. I smoke less**. Overall, the results are **satisfied and pleasant**.

Report No. 153: Six months of AM microdosing, from 1–3 g. The first few days there was nausea and drowsiness, probably the organism had to get used to AM. Then these effects passed and were replaced with **cheerfulness, clarity, and concentration**. Surprisingly after a break, new AM microdose course started right on from the positive previous results.

Report No. 154: One-week AM microdosing: 1–2 times a day, from 0.5 up to 2 g. What happens is inexplicable. Complete **cleaning of the consciousness, the source is open**. (Continued in report no. 164.)

Report No. 155: Experimented with AM microdosing in different ways. I came to the conclusion that the most tangible and effective is AM powder, then drinking water with something sweet on top. AM tea seemed less effective to three people and me. Experiment with AM tincture in progress, four people. Everything is **pleasant, cheer in the body, freshness in the head, easiness in emotional state, dreams bright**.

Report No. 156: I take microdoses of mukhomor about three weeks in a dose of one level tablespoon on average, sometimes a little less, sometimes a little more. My observations: added **energy**, there is **no fatigue**, it became much **easier and earlier to wake up** in the morning, even without an alarm clock. Now I go to bed earlier than before. No euphoria or changed states of consciousness were noticed. It happened when I took a heaping tablespoon—the body became cotton soft, relaxed, the head is clouded and light, as after small shot of vodka. This condition is not a good one for focusing on work. And now that I am a little concerned, my emotional state became vacillated. Before reception it was mainly stable, joyful, confident. Now it can instantly change, from joy to specific apathy and indifference, from boredom to anxiety, from confidence to insensitivity. In general, I would like to hear your opinion, and you may have examples of similar situations. It may be worth trying to take a break, or for doses to increase. But I doubt increasing the dose in the morning—the condition I described above is not suitable for my work. It also seemed to me, the short memory and concentration slightly deteriorated. But it may be because I meditated less. Thanks for attention.

Masha: It was recommended to decrease the dose to 1 g or less.

Report No. 157: Hello to all. I am twenty-seven years old. I want to share my experience of taking mukhomors. Usually, I ate 3 g dry AM every day for two months, and it was all super. Good achievements in a short time frame. I had a lot of **creative ideas** and **thought processes are very easily given**. The **mood** is raised, and there is a **clear understanding** of what you need in life and what you do not need, what you really like, what was imposed on you. My **self-confidence** has very much increased. **Mood is also elevated**. The sense of importance of anything is significantly reduced. My experiment with AM tea: I brewed the same amount of 3 g, intake fifteen minutes after brewing in 80°C [176°F] water. The first thing I felt was that the effect comes very quickly compared to eating a dry mukhomor cap. I didn't like the effect at all. All thoughts disappear, complete silence inside my head, and it becomes difficult to concentrate on anything. Often, I am stuck on a point; working in such a state does not go very well. Productivity decreases, people begin to suspect that I am under the influence of something. My conclusion: If you want to relax and turn off the brain, it is good to take AM tea. If you're looking for productivity, good workability, quick solutions, good creativity, I do not advise you to take AM in the form of a brew. I experienced and realized that the effects are fundamentally different. I intend to microdose for a year without interruptions.

Report No. 158: I want to share my AM microdosing experience. I took an AM microdose for two weeks in the morning, one level teaspoon a day. *Effects:* there is a **cheer and a great mood**. The **inner voice** of an outsider observer is **amplified**, while the **ego becomes quieter**. That allows me to look at any situation from another view. The downside, sometimes at the beginning I became spacy and felt a slight change of mental state.

Masha: Recommended to decrease the dose.

Report No. 159: Chat room conversation:

—Good evening. I suspect the **parasites died** in my body in the beginning of AM microdose course. Because in the chat room it was mentioned before about sugar craving and appetite increase in the first stages. What do you think?

—Yes, I experienced the same. Additionally, I get sour taste in my mouth.

—Confirming the sour taste after AM microdose intake.

Report No. 160: AM microdosing for a month and a half. A third of a tea-spoon in the morning, after breakfast. I tried on an empty stomach, but there was nausea. After breakfast everything is excellent. The actual effects: In the first couple of weeks of consumption there was nausea, light intoxication—all was not pleasant. I was thinking about stopping, but then all these physical aspects just went away. Now, during sports trainings—**endurance and strength are very increased! Great breathing, a beauty around, just running and smiling to surrounding world and myself!** The same words can describe the mental state at this point. **Calm**, **joy** from moments, music brings more **pleasure** than before, I see **beauty in everything** and enjoy it. I began to get great pleasure from **communication and activities** with my child, which was not the case before; there was tenderness to my husband, we micro-dose together. Everything began to bring more joy and pleasure, but such calm joy, quiet euphoria, from which you do not want to jump and yell but simply smile to yourself, freeze, and stop this moment. I also want to note—the effect is really cumulative. Mukhomor opened up for me after 2–3 weeks.

Report No. 161: I tried: AM tea with lemon-ginger-vitamin C; AM tea with salt; AM tea without any additions; dry powder; dry caps not ground. My conclusion: the strongest effect was with dry cap. Next, it was powder. Next, tea with salt. Lemon with AM tea—last on the list. Personally, I prefer dry powder.

Report No. 162: I am taking 1 g AM before food in the morning. Sometimes before bed in the evening. I noticed a **good concentration** on what I need, some ease, a **pleasant internal condition**, and a **dissipation of thoughts**. I personally prefer a tea form to dry powder.

Report No. 163: Mukhomor is very powerful for the good night **sleep**. I use about 0.05 g. I fall asleep quickly, dreams bright, awaken without an alarm clock.

Report No. 164: This is my second week. Previous report was report no. 155—first week. I take once in the evening, brewed tea with lemon infusion from 0.6–0.9 g. I continue to wonder how AM microdosing con-tributes to **concentration and attention**. I am a translator and an editor. The correct words do not come easier, but decisions are made faster and with less brain cost. Everyday decisions are made easier, without much weighing "for and against." **Sense of own importance and guilt trip associated with it losing its grip. Communication** became more situational. **Emotional background** is good, **more control of reactions** than before. Suddenly, AM microdosing gave an **additional dimension to visual perception**—paintings and photographs seem deeper and are perceived intensely. **Perception of music** is changing as well. Body (sports, food) is the same as in the first week. Clearly positive, but without miracles and extremes. Negative—burping and it's not progressing, just stays the same.

Report No. 165: I've taken an AM microdose sporadically for five years, usually before hard work. I cook AM tea in the evening and take it before bed. **Physical endurance** increases many times. **Body agitation** has passed. I used **alcohol** before and it helped. Now I use AM microdosing.

Report No. 166: Recommended AM microdosing to my girlfriend; tea made from half cap of AM with lemon. The result after ten days: her **menstrual cycle** passed easier than usual. She is **eating less** and lost about 3 kg [6.6 pounds].

Report No. 167: My friendship with the mukhomor goes for the fifth month. Morning intake gives tide of **energy**; after night intake I **quickly fall asleep.** I do not take an AM microdose every day, just as needed. In my experience, in the early days AM microdosing made me sleepy all the time. The energy came a week later.

Report No. 168: From Thomas's chat room. I became **kinder** and much **less aggressive**—this is the most important to me. I don't know how it works, but anger and irritability went away on their own, and old resentments went away. That is very pleasing to me. Also, I noticed that my **sleep** is normal.

Report No. 169: From Thomas's chat room. There is no hurry with *Amanita muscaria* microdosing. Be patient, the **effect is cumulative.** I took it for two weeks. First, physical unpleasant moments will pass and pleasant psychological state will come. Do not wait for miracles. *Amanita muscaria* microdoses gave me **calmness.** There are no effects from few intakes. It's not a magic pill. It goes without any signs at first, and in a few days, you realize that you are calm, you smile, and are **cheerful.** And you wonder why so many people are nervous and frowning when there is so much joy around.

Report No. 170: From Thomas's chat room. I became a much **less aggressive** driver, have no aggression behind the wheel. On the contrary, the snotty attitude of other drivers causes a smile. I am using AM tincture. Now, I have two months break from AM microdosing. The irritation doesn't come back. **Life is beautiful, I love everyone.**

Report No. 171: From Thomas's chat room. I have a neighbor, forty-three, a buddy, who had a long period of **heroin addiction**. I gave him a tincture of mukhomor. He did not believe in the success of the treatment at all, but he took it as his last chance for recovery. He used it three weeks, and his addiction went away. For two months he has not consumed a drug and says that he does not want to. He was in shock. We are not sure how long this effect will last, but he is fine for now. He continues to microdose the tincture.

Report No. 172: From Masha's YouTube channel. I am a sixty-two-year-old woman. I picked mushrooms myself; I dried it and prepared the tincture. I used dried *Amanita muscaria* for ten days. I **quit smoking**; it was a thirty-year addiction. I also ate fresh *Amanita* stems, little pieces in the forest, it was good experience, I was tired and it gave me **a lot of energy**. I report a **good night sleep** as well. You are so good, Masha. *Amanita* has long history in our country, and it was all hidden from us. The system lied to us about poison qualities of this mushroom.

Report No. 173: From Masha's YouTube channel. I have **alcohol addition**, daily for about seven years. Three weeks of AM microdosing and no drinking, flight normal, started running, began to **smoke less**. I will know more in the long term.

Report No. 174: From Masha's YouTube channel. Previously: a lot of beer on weekends, although I have problems with the pancreas but could not convince myself to quit and was tormented by this poison. I lived in such a closed circle until I began to microdose the mukhomor. I did not notice how I stopped buying **alcohol**, as if I never drank it. I forgot about smoking cigarettes as well.

Report No. 175: From Masha's YouTube channel. I've microdosed AM for a month. There's no more **alcohol and cigarettes** for me. It's a miracle, a lot of positive effects. I want to slap all zombies and wake them up. Thanks to you BM. You save people.

Report No. 176: From Masha's YouTube channel. Hello, darling! I started microdosing and stopped drinking **alcohol** at all. When I forget to take a microdose for a long while, I get a little alcohol craving. It happened twice already.

Report No. 177: From Masha's YouTube channel. Masha, thanks. Yes, I **quit drinking**, more than a year ago. Also, AM microdosing converted me to **veganism**. Now I feel **chic, cheerful, happy with desire to do things**. There is even no desire [compulsion] to drink alcohol anymore; **marijuana** habit is gone too. Now I can eat increased microdose and feel state of continuous good condition. I plan an AM microdosing break, and I'll check how stable my feelings are.

Report No. 178: Sent to Masha personally via Telegram messenger. Based on my experience of two weeks of AM microdosing, I want to say that mukhomor does not change our consciousness, but simply cleans it up, as well as the whole organism. **All the slag accumulated in a lifetime was gone.** As if AM cleaned a mirror of the pox and dirt. There is no joy, no sadness, no bad, no good, everything becomes what it really is. The pursuit of something is stopped. All our lives we strive for happiness, money, health, spirituality. For example, I chased the knowledge of truth, the supreme self, etc., believing that only my path is correct. But at the same time, I forgot about the most important thing—to live.

We want to live in happiness, live in well-being, live in wealth, live in spirituality. But the root of that is all one—live. In general, I felt this freedom, felt **clarity of mind**, immediately **stepped out of restraints**. I can change the prism of looking at life under different glasses. The first time everything is surprising, fascinating simple things. [. . .] Thank you very much for information!

Report No. 179: From Masha's YouTube channel. Baba Masha, good morning. Everything is right, I confirm, thanks. My husband **quit drinking** beer after AM microdosing; he saw the big difference himself.

Report No. 180: From Masha's YouTube channel. I started AM microdosing with 1.5 g of powder and came to the knowledge that from doses as small as 0.06 g my condition is better and more effective! I recommend starting with a small dose and increase by 0.01 g. I used to make tea, now I just soak *Amanita muscaria* in warm water. The condition is much more interesting!

Report No. 181: From Masha's YouTube channel. Baba Masha, another plus of AM microdosing noticed! The **pigment spot** on my stomach suddenly disappeared after AM microdosing. I had it for a year, and a week ago it was gone. So happy!

Report No. 182: From Masha's YouTube channel. I quit **alcohol** after AM microdosing. I have not drank it for three years now!

Report No. 183: From Masha's YouTube channel. I want to leave an important message to all lovers of freedom and comrades who are looking for changes in life. I have long experience in using red dried *Amanita muscaria* caps. They help a lot to change the point of view to look at the world with real eyes, without prejudice and illusions of mind; a **most powerful and natural antidepressant** in moderate quantities (1–3 caps). More is not necessary because it will be a reverse side for those who are looking for *Amanita muscaria* mushroom high. If the personality is not stable, serious trouble could follow.

Report No. 184: Sent to Masha personally via Telegram messenger (continuation of report no. 155 and no. 164). Third week. Reception is still once a day in the evening between 0.5–1 g. Tea with ground AM in thermos with lemon. In general, the action did not change—**concentration, calm, activity, and fullness of feelings**. Last week there was a lot of **socialization**; I treat it as an experiment, no bad feelings. Important development, I am interested more in entheogens. I want to talk not about symptoms and sensations, but about states of conciseness and energy. AM contributes to fast and situationally correct decisions.

Report No. 185: From Masha's YouTube channel. Thank you. Useful experience. One dry AM cap—**bright colors, calmness, awareness**. Two dry caps—immediately went under the blanket to sleep.

Report No. 186: Sent to Masha personally via Telegram messenger. After taking AM tincture and one dry cap *Amanita muscaria* per day, I refuse **alcohol and cigarettes** now. Light intoxication is present, but it's reenergizing. I "worry" about night erection.

Report No. 187: From Masha's YouTube channel. I am a sixty-year-old man. Last fall I was in a bike accident. Among other injuries—a broken clavicle. The arm mobility did not recover. I couldn't raise my left arm, dressing was very difficult. Practically, the left arm lost its mobility. Examination **revealed**

progressive arthrosis with an adverse prognosis. I used about a quarter liter of AM vodka tincture, rubbing the joints of my arm. The result: the arm is movable with no **pain** and no residual phenomena at all. Now I rub my other leg and arm joints as well. I noticed that the mobility of some joints damaged 10–15 years ago recovered. There is a feeling that I use some potent medicine, purely somatic.

Report No. 188: Sent to Masha personally via Telegram messenger. Baba Masha, thank you for your creativity! I've taken AM microdoses for a month. I want to report to you that seven **warts** on my hands disappeared. I was shocked because I had them for several years and now my fingers are clean like nothing was there at all.

Report No. 189: Sent to Masha personally via Telegram messenger. Hi, Masha! The mukhomor mushroom microdosing experiment, over two months, revealed the following changes. **Awareness**: It is as if you **assess what is happening from the center**, where no one can reach, and all reaction to the surrounding world, all emotions and thought forms are tracked, without identification with them. I catch myself thinking, so to speak. Independence from the opinion of others. It feels great! A **vision of beauty in everything**. The ability to switch itself into a mode of perception without thoughts, without value judgments. Sometimes there is an effect that is difficult to describe, but a scene from movie *The Matrix* comes to mind. When Morpheus told Neo the truth and after "Awakening" and training, they went together to the Matrix, and Neo was surprised and recalled that "here I drank coffee before work, and here such delicious pizza. How can this all be so real and not real at the same time." Physical state: Throughout the experiment it felt that some processes took place in the body. I do not possess knowledge and terms, so I will say only that I trusted these processes, trying not to attach importance to some unpleasant manifestations, such as elevated temperature, severe and mild headache.

It is clear that mukhomor is primarily a tool that is adjusted by the intention to get the desired condition. It's not a magic pill; it's an ally who supports on the way. A wise assistant in achieving awareness. It is interesting, what will be the result of mass rethinking of this mysterious fungus in our country; I believe that the result will be encouraging. I am glad to participate in your good project, happiness of new discoveries and joyful moments to you!

Report No. 190: Sent to Masha personally via Telegram messenger. I've microdosed for two years. I started to take it in a difficult period of my life, sore joints, neurotic states, problems at work, deaths in family. *Amanita muscaria* helped me a lot in everything: **my joints almost do not hurt, I accepted the deaths [of family members], fears went away**.

Report No. 191: Sent to Masha personally via Telegram messenger. Baba Masha, good time. It's been almost a month of taking mukhomors. I used to make a **tea** and later I switched to **dry powder** mixed with tomato juice, as the effect is much better with this method. *Effects*: dreams brighter, **sleep** calmer, I **wake up easily** without harsh thoughts. I am craving more **physical activity**, and regularly as well. I began to monitor very carefully the cleanliness of the house, the body, and clothes. Internal cramps began to be worked out more easily, their reasons begin to open, very interesting discoveries I make for myself in this regard. I work as a programmer. The work was very much optimized with the time of the beginning of the reception of mukhomors: the code became more beautiful and slimmer. I finish easily what I started; earlier there were big problems with it, and unfinished business sucks a lot of energy. Less wasting time. I stopped taking on obligations that I cannot fulfill. I have guts to say "no" more often, where it is necessary. I became **closer to family and friends**. Practically **no more overeating**, I eat less, no more fast food, I cook home more often. And all this in one month.

Report No. 192: From Thomas's chat room. I still feel the effect of the mukhomors, although it's been about half a year since the last reception. Today remembered that he (mukhomor) came in my dream; I think it is time to buy AM again.

Report No. 193: From Thomas's chat room. One morning, as part of a ritual, when you're going to take an AM microdose, you suddenly realize that you don't have to. The organism does not want it. Then after some time, you realize that it is time to use AM help again. I understand that it sounds very subjective, but I experienced that and often heard this from other members of this chat room.

Report No. 194: Sent to Masha personally via Telegram messenger. Baba Masha, I was going to buy some medicine to remove a couple **warts** from my fingers. And here, I read the reviews about warts and AM microdosing,

I looked at my fingers, and warts are absent. I microdosed AM for a month, I am on break now.

Report No. 195: From Masha's YouTube channel. Hi, Baba. What you're doing is great. It was just because of your podcast I tried AM microdosing, and I got rid of many problems with my health. Although I did not expect it to help. I took it for six months. Thanks for information. Respect with all my heart.

Report No. 196: From Thomas's chat room. Masha, I am much older than you. I've taken AM for five years. I regularly use big and small quantities. I introduced all my friends to AM, even my eighty-four-year-old mother.

Report No. 197: From Masha's YouTube channel. I am a fifty-eight-year-old man. Three times I ate mukhomor this autumn. A heaping tablespoon of crushed dry caps with boiled water poured over. Little pinch of salt, and it was excellent mushroom soup. I listen to Baba Masha podcast all the time! And remembered her words: "When you pour that beer in your stomach . . ." There is **no beer** in my life anymore!

Report No. 198: Sent to Thomas personally via Telegram messenger. I do not use AM microdoses by weight. Generally I take half or small whole cap. I definitely noticed that small unopened caps have different effect. A young fungus gives me feeling of **unlimited joy, slight stimulation, and uplifting mood**. Half cap of large opened mukhomor in the morning gave me **contemplation, reflection, mellow**, small waves on the body.

Report No. 199: From Thomas's chat room. When my comrade introduced me to the mukhomor, I responded with anger. So, my friend referred me to a video about fly agarics, and that video triggered me to look for more information. Now I know a lot. I took AM microdoses for two weeks now. I noted only that nothing bothers me anymore, **freedom from anxiety**, no excessive emotions.

Report No. 200: From Thomas's chat room. Thanks to the mukhomor, he returned me to painting again after five years of oblivion. This, by the way, can also be summed up by the last survey about creativity. Mukhomor definitely helped me personally in **creativity**.

Report No. 201: From Thomas's chat room. Review on *Amanita* face oil made by Thomas. My skin is aged and dry. My impressions of oil: I use it with face massage. It removes dryness unambiguously and immediately. The

oil made my skin silky. I repeat, silky and very smooth. Great oil for massage. I used a lot of different expensive creams before. Yeah, they gave me the result. But the result from the oil is more demonstrative. I choose *Amanita* oil. Gratitude to Thomas.

Report No. 202: Sent to Masha personally via Telegram messenger. Dear and adored Baba Masha, I'm sharing my AM microdosing twenty-six-day experience. I started with a coffee spoon, by brewing tea. After day fifteen I switched to dry powder. I like it better this way. The brewed form made me sleepy. The last four days I increased to one teaspoon (3 g). This is my maximum dose that I can take. Someone in the reviews wrote about the feeling of the brain kept in soft palms of God. That's what I feel, too. More effects: **no chatterbox**, no scrolling abstract scenes in my head, this and that pendulum. Before, it used to be constant, and it was exhausting my energy. The **mood** is steadily excellent. Sometimes when longing slips, I accept it. Simultaneously, I'm **building a new positive arch**. It **enhanced my reaction** to events and old destructive reflexes as fuss and **meaningless panic going away** at once. It's a big plus for me. I already have a great relationship with my husband, pleasant and gentle communication. And with AM microdosing it is a honeymoon; he is also microdosing. We've been married for eleven years. My **relations with relatives and friends** are established in positive way now. **Communication** with people who I did not like very much for many years is not annoying to me anymore. I rub *Amanita* oil on my face and neck for a night, the pigmentary light spot gradually leaves. Skin getting softer. Most important aspect for me, I accepted and love myself, unconditionally. I like my reflection in the mirror. Synchronistic events are more and more frequent. I didn't notice the side effects from AM. I will continue microdosing. AM microdosing has no impact on my dreams, but I **sleep** longer. Thanks to the Mukhomorians and Baba Masha! Love, peace, kiss!

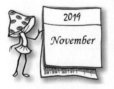

2019
November

Report No. 203: Sent to Masha personally via Telegram messenger. AM microdosing for twelve days, two people—myself and wife. We started with 0.3 g and up to 1.8 gradually through day twelve. At the first reception, 0.3, we both had a mild euphoric effect. My body reactions: from 0.3–1 g—a **sense of muscle relaxation and clear head**. With 1.2 g there was a stimulating effect, similar to a strong cup of coffee. On doses from 1.2–1.5 the stimulating effect lasts six to seven hours; 1.8 g so far, my favorite dose, the effect lasts all day from the beginning of the intake to bedtime. In sports, a significant increase in overall tone, energy, and endurance. For my wife on dose 0.3 g and up, there was **cheer effect**. The effect of higher dose—the extension of the cheer period, light rather than deep sleep. We both have a decrease in **internal dialogue. Brighter senses—smell, vision, hearing**. Increased sensitivity in **sex**. I am experiencing **general positive attitude** and absolutely **different reaction to conflict situations** with humor and positivity.

Report No. 204: From Masha's chat room. This is my second season of AM microdosing. This year I took AM microdoses for one month. I got rid of my severe **depression**. Mukhomor showed me how to work with depression. Usually, I see it as a broken detail on the floor, and I cry. Now I see how to glue details back and fix it. A lot of **internal problems** have been solved. Now just **happiness** in the moment and **harmony**. It's difficult to talk about, it's mysticism. Mukhomor turned out to be my best instrument, and I want to share it.

Report No. 205: From Thomas's chat room. Over one month of AM microdosing. All my life I was the devoted **sweets** lover. After three weeks of *Amanita muscaria* microdosing I lost my **appetite** totally. Then the appetite recovered but sweets were excluded. I do not even look at chocolates at the shop anymore.

Report No. 206: From Thomas's chat room. I use a mukhomor powder, one-third teaspoon, sometimes less. I keep it under my tongue, then swallow. That keeps me in a mocking **mood** most of the time. **Efficiency** slightly increased, **procrastination** slightly decreased. It is easier to **concentrate**. I ate a heaping teaspoon for the night, and I didn't feel the effect.

Report No. 207: Sent to Masha personally via Telegram messenger. I prefer *Amanita* tea, my drink of vital balance, especially at moments of **emotional crisis**. I add vitamin C or lemon to reduce nausea. *Effects:* **emotions** aligned, **anxiety** and darkness retreated. The sincere and active **interest in peace** wakes up. Better **understanding** with others. **Balance and harmony**. Pure consciousness, ready to perceive, listen, maintain **love**. I am in the state of a holistic, balanced person who wants to live, communicate, build, look, understand, and act.

Report No. 208: Sent to Masha personally via Telegram messenger. Three weeks of AM microdosing, one-third teaspoon twice a day. At reception

I noticed a calm **emotional state**, good benevolent **mood**, and **negative thoughts** are **cut out** at the "root." No negative side effects, no pain in kidneys or liver. Few times there were very realistic dreams; it is a separate topic. I will microdose further. So far, everything is good.

Report No. 209: From Thomas's chat room. I was taking *Amanita* raw for two weeks while it was growing in the woods. I quit **smoking**. Less **alcohol** cravings. I eat less **meat**. **Mood** is great.

Report No. 210: From Thomas's chat room. AM microdosing for three weeks, I noted positive support of my nervous system, especially during lots of **stress**. My **sleep** considerably improved. The **digestive system** worked well. There was no need for **alcohol** during the AM microdosing session.

Report No. 211: From Thomas's chat room. After course of AM microdosing **I gave up alcohol**, **meat**, milk, sugar, flour, tea. I mostly eat fruits and seeds, sometimes cereals. But did not help with smoking cigarettes.

Report No. 212: From Thomas's chat room. I started microdosing with 4 g AM. I brewed in thermos for half an hour. I felt nausea and I was too high but it gave me nice **sleep** at night. I decreased the dose to 1–1.5 g, dry, no brew. I feel **comfortable**.

Report No. 213: From Thomas's chat room. First month AM microdosing report. First week I tested doses from 1–7 g at different times—morning, noon, and evening. My resume: big doses do not work—euphoria, no straight thinking, mild headache, lost my sleep. I ended up with my optimal dose of 0.2 g.

Report No. 214: Sent to Masha personally via Telegram messenger. Two months of AM microdosing. I started with 0.3 g and ended up with 1 g. It changed my **diet**—no **alcohol** and no **sweets**. **Antidepressant effects**: much less anxiety, quiet and cozy mood, balanced being with a positive **attitude**. *Amanita* tea also helps my daughter with skin **eczema**. Her hands have cleared; nothing was helping her for the last two years.

Report No. 215: From Thomas's chat room. Thank you for your work. Three months on microdosing, I do everything on your advice. At most 1 g a day. The breaks were done to check the rollback. So far everything is excellent. Total rejection of **alcohol and nicotine**. Initially I was skeptical of the *Amanita muscaria* microdoses. I reviewed all your videos. Read everything I could find. I personally talked to people on AM microdoses. Finally, I began with 0.3 g and raised to 0.5 g in a week. Alcohol and cigarettes are not my friends anymore. Life improved in general. It is hard to explain rationally. I am going to continue microdosing. Now I also have friends on the *Amanita muscaria* microdoses. Some had alcohol problems. Some stopped drinking at all, and some drink much less.

Report No. 216: Sent to Masha personally via Telegram messenger. Four weeks of AM microdosing, tea with 1 g AM with lemon, brewed in thermos in the evening. Good night **sleep**, earlier wake up, great help with **intellectual work**, my **libido** is up, more synchronistic events. I decided to decrease the dose and continue my trial.

Report No. 217: From Masha's YouTube channel. The practice of microdosing for two months turned me away from **alcohol** completely. Fact! Although I did not aim to stop drinking at all. I do not like the taste of alcohol anymore, no pleasure, a turn off, as something alien is entered my body. I don't want any alcohol at all.

Report No. 218: From Masha's YouTube channel. I was heavyweight **alcohol** drinker for seven years. After three weeks of AM microdosing I reduced alcohol and cigarette **smoke**. I started jogging. But I still consider alcohol as a good mental work jumper. We will see in the long run.

Report No. 219: From Masha's YouTube channel. One month of AM microdosing. I quit **alcohol and cigarettes**. It is a miracle, and I am very surprised. I noticed a lot of positive effects.

Report No. 220: From Masha's chat room. I am taking courses of AM microdoses for the fourth year in different combinations of doses and intake time. I want to confirm that there is no dependency to AM, no craving.

Report No. 221: From Thomas's chat room. I offered *Amanita muscaria* alcohol tincture to my heavy-drinker friend. He stopped drinking **alcohol** at first because he was afraid that mukhomor and alcohol could cause undesirable effects. When the tincture ended he did not come back to previous state and now he consumes much less alcohol. We are waiting for the new season and will make more tincture.

Report No. 222: Sent to Masha personally via Telegram messenger. Hello. I'm on AM microdoses for three weeks with weekend breaks. I take a heaping teaspoon for the night. My **sleep** improved; before, I had trouble falling asleep. **Dreams** themselves are colorful and well-remembered. **Alcohol** fell off on its own at once. Given my character and stress, it used to be the surest way to reboot. Stopped following politics and all this "propulsive" arguing and trying to prove anything to anyone. It's just not interesting anymore. Today I noticed that the shoulder joint is not in **pain** (salt deposition). My wife began to take AM microdoses because she watched the change in me. My mother is ready to join us too. Thank you, Baba Masha!

Report No. 223: Sent to Masha personally via Telegram messenger. Good day, Baba Masha. I was taking AM microdoses in 2019, in dry form. It cured my **neurodermatitis** located on my fingers. I suffered from that for nineteen years—monthly I had **painful aggravations** and I used hormonal creams to take it away. It did not come back after the AM microdose course. To the discussion about stability of AM microdosing effects. I am reporting my second day of my pause with AM microdosing. The **mood** is beautiful, the **dream** restored. Thanks to the AM, I have great **sleep** now without taking AM. **Cheer, endurance**, ability to work, **calmness**, and **pacification** are still with me. Today there was a heavy physical workout. Before the course I struggled with exercises; it went away during the course. It stayed with me after the break as well.

Report No. 224: From Thomas's chat room. I used AM in dry form, 2 g. My back **pain** went away.

Report No. 225: From Thomas's chat room. Good evening, I want to report the results of three weeks *Amanita muscaria* microdoses course. As one person has already said in the chat room, it has become **quiet inside my head**, **thoughts** are not jumping, **panic and fears** disappeared, negative thoughts simply bouncing away. Everything is **balanced** and **comfortable**, all is hunky dory. In business this is an optimal solution.

Report No. 226: From Thomas's chat room. My feedback on microdoses and **menstrual cramps**: I want to declare immediately that a miracle happened! For four years I suffered from very painful menstrual periods, and it never went without painkillers, but pills affect my work abilities and the work capacity is lost. **PMS** symptoms bothered me as well. Now I am without any pain and ill being! Well, nothing has ever helped me to achieve that **well-being and balance** during my periods; I remain able to **work, sleep** well, and rejoice in everything and everybody! Microdoses balanced me.

Report No. 227: From Masha's YouTube channel. I am taking AM micro-doses to reach a good and **calm condition**. It works. It took my worries away, I am **tranquil**. I can be comfortable alone or with people around me. My **sleep** improved. For insomnia I recommend to brew a tea with one level teaspoon AM powder with lemon and take it before bedtime.

Report No. 228: From Thomas's chat room. Case of two months of mukho-mor microdoses. First two weeks I ate dry powder, later changed to AM infused tea, 1–2 g. There is the same approximate effect: a changed state of consciousness, a slightly altered state of consciousness but without obvi-ous signs for other people, sometimes fun, small stagnation or vice versa, high activity. I microdose almost every day. I find it is the best to microdose for my work, especially when the job is stressful. I am in a **relaxed state in stressful situations**. I react to it very quietly and don't get angry as usual. I tried bigger doses about 4–7 g. There was no such strong effect, but that amount caused unpleasant nausea. The more I ate, the worse it was for me, so it's better to start from smaller doses.

Report No. 229: From Masha's YouTube channel. I eat one teaspoon of AM powder every day in the morning with glass of water before food. I don't drink, I don't smoke, my food habits are healthy. Mukhomor gave me **a clear head and interesting thoughts and ideas**. It gave me new hobbies, I started reading a lot, I entered a college. I have a positive mood every day. I feel wonderful. Mukhomor works for **well-being**. I tried to eat three tablespoons and became strongly drunk in twenty minutes. In 2–3 hours I experienced light trip with visual distortions, everything was as positive.

Report No. 230: From Thomas's chat room. I did not have healthy lifestyle for fifteen years, active nights and comatose day times, sometimes with no proper **sleep** for several days. AM microdosing right from the start turned me to the correct mode of the **day/night balance**, withdrawal at 10–11 p.m. and very early 5 a.m. rise.

Report No. 231: From Masha's YouTube channel. Actually, when I use AM microdoses, there is no attraction to **alcohol**, especially because I am a big lover of drinking excessively.

Report No. 232: From Masha's YouTube channel. I microdosed mukhomor for three weeks. I experimented with dry and AM tea with lemon. It worked dif-ferently. Dry powder gives me more energy, and tea affects me as alcohol.

Report No. 233: Sent to Masha personally via Telegram messenger. I used AM tincture to alleviate **knee pain** due to my physically heavy job, ten hours plus on my feet. Pain went away in two days; I rubbed it on before bedtime. No discomfort now. I am taking a two-week break; I plan to start again with the intention to quit smoking.

Report No. 234: From Masha's YouTube channel. After taking mukhomor AM microdosing my friend quit everything: **smoking** cigarettes and weed, drinking **alcohol**, and some **drugs**—speed, etc. I witnessed his really scary madness with drugs before.

Report No. 235: Sent to Masha personally via Telegram messenger. I microdosed for two months, 0.5 g twice a day. I have positive effects with my **insomnia**, joint **pain**, **alcohol** cravings, and **diet preferences** (less sugar products). My **mood** is great, a lot of **energy**. I **achieve more** during my work. AM microdosing helped my vision. I am an editor and my eyes are normally very tired at the end of the day.

Report No. 236: From Thomas's chat room. I want to report that only dry form of AM microdose gives me the wanted effects. I do not have effects if I use *Amanita muscaria* infused tea.

Report No. 237: Sent to Masha personally via Telegram messenger. Report: five weeks of AM microdosing. Starting dose was 1 g and reduced to less than 0.5 g. I switched from morning intake to evening due to daytime sleepiness. With microdoses in the form of brewed tea with lemon, I noticed better **sleep**, **better coordination** in my physical activities, **chatterbox** inside my head is not noisy anymore.

Report No. 238: From Thomas's chat room. I suffer with **chronic leg neuropathy**, and pain subsided in second week of AM microdosing.

Report No. 239: From Masha's YouTube channel. I am taking AM microdoses for two months, mostly every day with 1–3 days break sometimes. I use 1 g in a morning and 1 g at night. Very first AM microdose caused very light alcohol-like high effect with a very **cheerful, positive, and humorous condition.** Later it changed to more interesting effects, the degree of **awareness** and **perception** took some other form. What I looked at earlier and did not notice, now I analyze acutely. Past and present information connected in my mind, and the analysis of what's happening is wider now. **Motivation** has grown drastically. I am working on all my previously abandoned ideas! **Self-confidence** has moved to another level: I see that I can, I act, a matrix of earlier settings collapse in front of my eyes. It cured my candidiasis. My dreams now have multidimensional effects; in the morning I wake up as from the cinema, on the positive. Tried to raise the dosage to 5 g, didn't understand much what happened, some set of flashbacks in an hour and then attempts to understand what it was. In general, *Amanita muscaria* microdoses are worth practicing. And with breaks of 2–3 days, the effect of **awareness** does not leave. Reminds me of a stimulant, like putting a layer of bricks under a skewed house that makes the house stand perfectly.

Report No. 240: From Thomas's chat room. I used AM microdosing as supporting tool. After two days of AM microdosing I quit **smoking** cigarettes. I microdosed every day and did not have a craving to smoke. Mukhomor kept me in a good **mood** and I did not have a need to smoke. After a month I stopped thinking about smoking. Before that, I had urges to smoke while I was drinking alcohol. It does not happen anymore. Today is 2.5 months since I quit smoking.

Report No. 241: From Thomas's chat room. Hello everyone. I lost the **sense of smell** due to my smoking habit. In a week after AM microdosing it came back. I smell everything around. I recently smelled freshly cut grass like when I was a kid; it was beautiful.

Report No. 242: From Thomas's chat room. I got **powerful cheer** in the first times of AM microdose receptions; libido was wild. At the moment it seemed that *Amanita muscaria* is a catalyst for that. I didn't notice anything else. *Amanita muscaria* alcohol tincture shows **painkiller** qualities for my wife with back pain and for my mother with back pain caused by a bulged disk. My neighbor's mother uses the same tincture to take away her joint pain.

Report No. 243: From Thomas's chat room. I make AM tea with lemon in thermos overnight and drink it in the morning. Then I do all the morning chores. Breakfast is just about an hour away. And all day I feel like an electric train. The wife has the same effect. The only difference is that her **energy** effect began immediately with minimal doses (0.3 g). I take 1.5 g. My favorite dose is 1.8 g; it charges my all-day vigor. After taking 1.5 g, I have 7–8 hours of energetic effect with a **pleasant relaxation** following.

Report No. 244: From Thomas's chat room. AM microdose course for three weeks. Unfortunately, I had to quit due to my traveling. A miracle continues, it is day four of my break. I feel a certain cumulative effect. If everything around become bleak and ordinary, I stimulate in myself those emotions and patterns that I learned in the course of AM microdosing. I keep my **focus** and accenting attention on important things. All skills remained, feeling of empathy presents, I am in full balance. It did not affect my alcohol, but there was no goal to quit.

Report No. 245: From Thomas's chat room. AM microdosing stimulates my **appetite**. I take AM microdose for a month; I **eat more** and **gain weight**.

Report No. 246: Sent to Masha personally via Telegram messenger. My dad complained a lot while I was preparing AM tincture; he was making fun of me, predicting my horrible death from the mushroom. Until one day he agreed to **use it for aggravating pain** in his leg. The next day he was literally flying with no suffering at all.

Report No. 247: From Masha's YouTube channel. I confirm that AM microdosing **changes thinking**, besides physical health effects. I can say that pretense and hypocrisy are becoming alien. Complexes and internal chains leave. I sprained my ankle. Ice didn't help, I couldn't sleep, the pain was terrible. AM tincture helped me with the **pain** in my twisted ankle, and pain went away really fast. I also use AM tincture as **fever remedy**, massaging it in my soles; it provokes immediate sweating. I feel a lot of trust in this fungus. Thank you, Masha. All thanks to your videos.

Report No. 248: From Thomas's chat room. Very positive two weeks AM microdosing experience of my friend's mom, sixty-four years old. She was very ill after two strokes. First of all, mom could not walk on her own, only with a Socane and her daughter's help. In two weeks the results already visible!!! She was able to walk to the hospital and back with little help. Her **memory improved** as well—where did she put that and this; what did she do yesterday? She also manages to remind us about time for *Amanita muscaria* microdoses intake, and before, she was having real problems with memory.

Report No. 249: From Thomas's chat room. AM microdosing works different for everyone. Only after nine months of AM microdosing I felt changes: the **joints stopped hurting**, the **intestines' work was stabilized, internal mind dialogues left**. It also works for my husband. AM works all over, only for everyone in different ways.

Report No. 250: From Thomas's chat room. It surprised me how AM micro-dosing **turned me away from sweets**. I am even disgusted with them—that never happened before! I do not crave them even though I finished my *Amanita muscaria* microdose course. I ate cakes all the time before, now only a very small piece of dark chocolate.

Report No. 251: Sent to Masha personally via Telegram messenger. Hi: AM microdosing for two months, five days a week in the morning, a heaping spoonful of dry powder. Pronounced effect **of pain relief** on my knee joints. I don't have meniscus, and I suffer with arthrosis. A couple of times there has been blood pressure increase with a panic attack. **Alcohol stopped working for me**. It doesn't produce high effect anymore.

P.S. Recommended to reduce dose to half teaspoon; no negatives came back after reducing the dose.

Report No. 252: From Masha's YouTube channel. I drank alcohol for ten years; the last three years I struggled and felt it drag me to the swamp, to the point that I could not imagine what to do in my spare time, except to drink. Constant thoughts and ideas how to abandon this crap led to no suc-cesses. My life was going down the drain, lack of money, bleak condition, apathy, inability to remember information-consequences caused by alcohol. But this continued until I ate three raw *Amanita muscaria* caps. It appeared to be very heavy on me. That gave me such kick in the butt, I was looking for the fifth corner, **high energy lift**—I was ready to offload the car with sand—while giving me an **awareness** of how to live, what to do for it. The next day I woke up as a new person, as if **alcohol** in my life never hap-pened. The realization of alcohol's futility and absurdness of its consumption became as clear as to eat poop willingly. Even the thought of **smelling alcohol was repulsive**. The consequences of full booze refusal produced all pleasures of life and great feelings.

Report No. 253: Sent to Masha personally via Telegram messenger. Baba, hi! Sharing my experience with AM microdosing. I am thirty-five years old. For thirteen days I consumed mukhomor I collected myself. Dosage is from 0.5–1.0 g twice a day. Changes: **energy rise** from the third day of reception, **improved vision**, **less pain** in the places of intervertebral herniations. I walk for long distances now without pain. Two weeks before AM microdosing I **gave up alcohol**, and during the reception I do not have craving; alcohol smell is not pleasant. My **sleep improved**, body feels rested, healthier food choices, my **mood improved**, became more **balanced, accelerated awareness**. It is easier to track impulses on **internal dialogues. Presence here and now** intensified. Desires such as to prove, punish, guilt were de-energized, and immediately it becomes visible how stupid it was. Thank you!

Report No. 254: From Masha's chat room. I think that one month of AM microdose course is not enough, and mukhomor has a cumulative effect. Regarding dose—it should not be any sensations changed after AM microdosing, and everything should remain normal. Only after a while I realize that **nothing annoys me**, and all I want is to jump and kick without a doubt. And frowning people in the crowd noticed me because I shine as a copper bowl.

Report No. 255: From Masha's chat room. I've microdosed over a month. I take 0.3–0.5 g in the morning and in the evening. The most important thing that a miracle mushroom gives me is **confidence** and that everything is going as it should be. The doubts, unnecessary self-analytical studies, self-digging are all gone. I noticed that this is the first autumn in the last few years when there is **no depressive condition**, so-called autumn blues, **no apathy, no frustration, no reluctance** to get up in the morning and drag to a dull job. My job is hectic and turmoiled, but all this does not cause any negativity anymore, even though earlier I thought about quitting my job.

I was born and raised in a country where there is a lot of sun, and it affected me in a negative way when I moved to Russia where gray days and clouds are common. But now I notice that the mukhomor replaced my sun! I want to tell microdosers who complain about tensions in the liver during AM microdosing—pay attention to the amount of fat and spicy food in your diet. I noticed that this kind of food is not in harmony with this fungus. My **dreams changed**: they became very real and unusual. Once I dreamt that I was the lover of some Russian princess, and she was hiding me from her tsar father. Very real dreams. Maybe these are echoes of past lives? Anyway, I am very glad that this sunny mushroom appeared in my life.

Report No. 256: Sent to Masha personally via Telegram messenger. Two months of AM microdosing, AM infused tea made with 1 g dry. I collected AM myself. The advantages are total rejection of **cigarettes and alcohol** through the realization that I do not need it. **Clear thinking, smiling mood, healthy balance.** Significant decline in neuralgic leg **pain**. There was an internal fear that everything would come back after the AM microdose course. A week without AM microdosing and nothing comes back; I just stopped thinking about it. Before AM microdosing I passed the standard blood and urine test (I've had hepatitis C for twenty years). After two months of AM microdosing, no changes in the tests.

Report No. 257: Sent to Masha personally via Telegram messenger. I've microdosed almost two months. My results are positive and similar to all above here. I persuaded my mother-in-law to microdose; she has problems with mood, sleep, and alcohol. She microdosed two weeks. We noticed improving of her **sleep** and **less alcohol** drinking. Third week all the problems came back. I don't know what to do.

Report No. 258: From Masha's chat room. I eat dry *Amanita muscaria* in the morning and evening. I started with 0.3 g and increased to 0.8 g. My **productivity is maximized**. I have never experienced anything like this in my life; I was lazy and usually ended up with unfinished tasks. Now my life finally is in order.

Report No. 259: Sent to Masha personally via Telegram messenger. Baba Masha, I made AM tincture by your video recipe. Result of using is amazing! My back is singing! I still do not believe, but fact is fact. Thank you for launching this project collecting the information.

Report No. 260: From Masha's chat room. I am taking a heaping teaspoon in the morning and one before bedtime. I slept good without dreams. The feeling is difficult to describe. **Mood beautiful, kindness around, thoughts are clear and in order**. I don't want to fight with anyone, although in the morning before *Amanita muscaria* reception there were a couple of times with tides of anger, but mentally I was able to contain myself. I even washed the dishes far more carefully than I usually do. I am an alcoholic; so far, I successfully **keep myself without alcohol**.

Report No. 261: From Masha's YouTube channel. Reporting my condition after 1.5 months after the *Amanita muscaria* microdose course. The result: **awareness has increased significantly**. It is even a little scary from the high level that I achieved. I read terabytes of literature. I **do not drink alcohol** for three weeks because I love freedom and I want to be free from the system's tricks making me a slave! And according to the books, awakened, visionary, and conscious people are not good for the system. Peace to all!

Report No. 262: Sent to Masha personally via Telegram messenger. I take 0.25 g as a tea; 1 g is too much for me. I think the effect is cumulative. I noticed **enhancements of my mind speed and attention.**

Report No. 263: From Masha's chat room. I was diagnosed with rheumatoid arthritis after the flu two years ago. My knees are in pain. A month ago I started AM microdosing, and I feel much better! AM works as **painkiller**.

Report No. 264: Sent to Masha personally via Telegram messenger. Masha, good evening. AM microdosing for ten days, 0.5 g in the evening before bed. But I suspect that the dose was even smaller than that because I used young AM caps. I found out that the younger mukhomor is, the less active substances in them. I didn't know that, and I was collecting the youngest with unopened caps. My wife took AM microdoses at the same time. She was depressed. At the beginning of the course, her **sleep normalized, depression passed**. But six days later she complained that thoughts began to come into her head about the meaning of life, which was significantly worse than depression for her. It was necessary to interrupt the course. I finished the ten-day course. I didn't feel any special physical changes. There were also interesting, unusual dreams, but not one of them I could remember. After the course **alcohol left my life** completely, although in the last fifteen years I did not actually abuse alcohol, so once every two weeks beer or wine. I didn't stop smoking; it didn't make any difference. Yeah, another unusual effect happened: I stopped masturbating at all; it used to be almost every day before. In normal sex I didn't notice any changes, though perhaps I began to get a little more pleasure. I will wait for next season in August. P.S.: AM has very interesting and strange effects. It looks like there is nothing but there is something. I've never experienced anything like that in my forty-four years.

Report No. 265: From Masha's chat room. Hello, dear readers. I am third day on AM microdosing, and I feel sleepy during the day. At the same time I have very **positive thoughts** directed to self-development, warm and pleasant body vibrations. If I sleep after lunch time, I **wake up rested, in good cheerful condition and mood**. My dose is 1 g per day an hour before eating and 1 g before sleeping. Should I decrease the dose? Everything is good but it is unusual for me to sleep 2–3 hours in the afternoon.

Report No. 266: From Masha's YouTube channel. I microdosed for a month at 0.5 g. I have the same results as I read in the reviews about **good sleep and increased energy**. At the beginning of the course, I experienced light headache and some renal pain. Pain was gone shortly. Mukhomor microdoses definitely work.

Report No. 267: From Masha's chat room. I have a gastric ulcer in remission. During a one-month course of *Amanita muscaria* microdoses, ulcer remains silent; it did not worsen my condition.

Report No. 268: From Thomas's chat room. My *Amanita muscaria* microdose course is ten days with a small coffee spoon of dried powder in the morning. Positive effects: early wake-up, two hours earlier than my regular time. My **energy increased**. My **headaches are gone**! I am surprised, I was twenty years on pills to fight my headache. My **abdominal cramps are gone** as well.

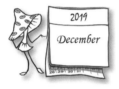

Report No. 269: From Thomas's chat room. Underwater reef/danger. Doses of 5 g AM or more per day for several days in a row lead to **craving**. I mean, feeling like a superhuman who owns his brain in a way many don't dream of. Being able to learn quickly and acquire the right skills. Everything is easily given; tasks resolve without the effort, unlike before. It is difficult for me to deny myself pleasure like this even for one day, and then another day, and so on. To stop becomes more difficult and more difficult every day. If I find strength and stop supplying myself with the necessary fuel, hard depressive days come.

Report No. 270: Today I tried for the first time a brewed teaspoon of AM with honey and lemon. Before, I used to cook AM microdose tea on a water bath. The effect is very different; in 10–15 minutes I literally jumped like I was stung, and I put my place in order in thirty minutes! **Calmness and balance in my head**, **very productive condition**, **full engagement in the moment**, **no nicotine craving**.

Report No. 271: From Thomas's chat room. I take AM once a week, 2–5 g. I do not think that I have to use AM every day. The effect is lasting and good. Everyone is different.

Report No. 272: From Thomas's chat room. The **strength** of mushrooms is also important. I experimented with different AM picked by myself. Mushrooms from the same place and the strength depends on time of the season, ripening of *Amanita muscaria,* drying, soil, and weather. A lot of factors. We are all from different regions, different sexes, different weights, different minds, and individual attitudes. That's why I advise to share only your own experience and report the facts.

Report No. 273: From Thomas's chat room. As my practice shows, yes, I myself passed through it, through such dosages, cancellation, and breakage. For the experiment I stimulated myself for a week with 5–7 g a day, then a **sharp cancellation** and as a consequence of abstinence for almost three days. Not strong, but tangible. The **whole body feels unbalanced**, as if the gear from the tuned mechanism was pulled out and interruptions in work of the whole body begin on all levels—psyche, mental, emotional, and physical.

Report No. 274: From Masha's chat room. General blood test results are good. All indicators in the middle range of the normal, after two courses of 30–40 days with one-week break. Now I can show my results to people who consider mukhomor poison.

Report No. 275: From Thomas's chat room. Mukhomor led me to meditation after two weeks of intake. My **heartache** that I've been carrying from 1.5 years has gone. I just realized why all that past horror happened to me, and it doesn't bother me anymore. I don't know how it works. I trusted in a fly agaric and asked it please to help me, every time at reception—and it does help, the kind and wise mukhomor mushroom.

Report No. 276: Sent to Thomas personally via Telegram messenger. Fourth day of 1 g AM reception. I feel barely **visible tonic, pleasant euphoria, happily aligned mental level, correction of psychosomatics, comfortable and warm feelings, my sleep is fantastic**. My point of assembly clearly turns into **a grateful, creative, efficient, and positive level**, where the dialogue topics are deep and understandable. Dose around 3 g is a torch, 5 g is light trip. I am planning to explore mukhomor's full potential in therapeutic doses. There is something to work on, my mental blocks coming from childhood are serious. Thank you from my heart, Thomas, for investing your soul in this project.

Report No. 277: From Thomas's chat room. I put AM powder in hot water, add little salt, dill, and this saturated broth is tasty. No high, there are **clear mind** and **energy, good-natured humor** and **irony. Kindness** and **awareness** to all.

Report No. 278: From Masha's chat room. From very first reception of 2 g *Amanita muscaria*, I **do not drink alcohol**, although before I was on beer for fifteen years, especially last seven years generally every day. I didn't know what to do with it until a wizard mushroom stopped that, really. And yes, thank you for your work. It makes the world better.

Report No. 279: Sent to Masha personally via Telegram messenger. My wife resisted AM microdosing at first; she was suffering with strong painful menstrual cramps. Apparently, she agreed from hopelessness. From the first intake of half teaspoon AM the **pain went away** in thirty minutes. She's cheerful and merry. She continues for three days, no more complaints about pain. I am on AM microdoses myself; it is a miracle.

Report No. 280: From Thomas's chat room. I have chronic **rhinitis** connected to many nose traumas. I've been on special drops for ten years. I inhaled small pinch of dry *Amanita muscaria* powder with a tube with my nostrils for one week. I noticed great progress, and I have not used the drops since.

Report No. 281: From Thomas's chat room. I was taking AM microdoses for reducing my severe **alcohol dependence** since November. It helps but not much. AM microdosing is better in combination with meditations, jogging, and talking with myself about it.

Report No. 282: Sent to Masha personally via Telegram messenger. I read here a couple of posts about **psoriasis**. My wound became thinner too, looks better. I hope the cumulative effect works. I am waiting.

Report No. 283: From Thomas's chat room. Twelve days AM microdosing. I started taking 0.5 g dry AM as tea in the morning before food. In five days I increased to 1 g, felt some **relaxation and calmness**, sometimes sleepy. Then decided to try in dry powder with drinking water; it seems that acts better. To tenth day the dose increased to 2 g; it gave me **positive thoughts and mood**! Today I took 2.5 g three hours after eating, and an hour later I got euphoria, lightness in the body, energy is beyond imagination, and feeling is not comparable to anything! Not real ease! Perhaps I will stop this dose around 2 g. Kindness to all.

Report No. 284: Sent to Masha personally via Telegram messenger. Hello, Baba Masha. I want to share fourteen days of mukhomor mushroom experience. I am male, twenty-nine years old, 194 cm [6 feet, 3 inches], 90 kg [198 pounds]. I eat 1 g dry powder with drinking water in the morning before breakfast. I feel **very calm**, get up early around 6 a.m., **clear mind**,

inner pure silence, meditative state of mind. No need for coffee in the mornings or cannabis in the evenings. No more "staring at the screens." I am reading a lot. A month ago there were very bad thoughts about myself and life in general, depressive mode. Now I smile thinking about that. [. . .]

Report No. 285: Sent to Masha personally via Telegram messenger. Salute, BM! AM tea brew (70°C–80°C) [158°F–176°F], heaping teaspoon with lemon and honey. This brings me **excellent mood** with the feeling of "halo" behind my head. Only present moment. The **silence and internal rest** come itself, fears go away, acceptance of everything as it comes, **high level of energy, optimistic and positive state, no aggression and demands to others**. I discovered an old habit—internal resistance to humor.

About *Amanita muscaria* alcohol tincture: on fifth drop—feeling of **energy and motivation**; it allows me to set priorities, which are more important at the moment. Calm emotional background feels good. Then bad thoughts and emotions come; they are erased in half a second. Tincture works in the background if you wish to participate in excavations of your own shit. Clear execution of requests in unclear situations or difficult issues, solutions are found easily. It seems like in my mind archives of the past, there is a clerk who, on request, proposes necessary solution.

Report No. 286: From Thomas's chat room. Two months of AM microdosing experiments to find optimum microdose. From 4–1 g dry powder. No more than ten drops of *Amanita muscaria* alcohol tincture, five drops in the morning and evening. Even from 1–2 drops tangible reaction presents. I agree with Baba Masha when she mentioned that **the less the dose, the more it's effective**.

Report No. 287: Sent to Masha personally via Telegram messenger. Hello, Baba Masha. I am practicing AM microdosing, and I have a gentle and pleasant effect. I ate one dry small cap in the beginning; now I like tea with one teaspoon of dry powder. It gives me **good clarity, removes anxiety and worries**. Everything became clear and orderly in my mind.

Report No. 288: From Thomas's chat room. Three months *Amanita muscaria* microdoses course. *Results:* quit thirty-year habit of smoking **cigarettes** and **drinking coffee**.

Report No. 289: From Thomas's chat room. I'm a twenty-seven-year-old male, 65 kg [143 pounds]. I used AM microdoses for a month from 1–3 g on empty stomach in the morning. Breakfast in thirty minutes. It feels like **energy** runs in the body. More energy, **better concentration, good accurate sensibleness, great awareness** here and now. Feels like I am impressed every second! There is **no laziness, no tiredness, no fatigue. Anxiety, fears, doubts disappear**. Five g makes me sleepy.

Report No. 290: From Thomas's chat room. I microdosed from the end of September, as soon as I collected and dried AM. AM microdosing helped me to **quit tobacco**. I have not smoked for two weeks. The tobacco craving went away slowly and the desire does not come anymore. There are many changes in body and thoughts. I want to write an article about *Amanita muscaria* microdoses.

Report No. 291: Sent to Masha personally via Telegram messenger. AM microdosing for 2.5 months; prepare 3 g tea overnight in thermos. After 1.5 months the results became stable. It adjusted my **food addictions**. I hardly eat sweets now, less bread, **alcohol disappeared**. Before, I could drink beer, wine, and strong drinks but not anymore. Today my husband brought some liquor; I took a sip and I immediately had the negative reaction.

Report No. 292: From Thomas's chat room. Forty-five-year-old woman, torn knee ligament over three years causes pain and swelling of legs, all types of treatments were ineffective. Four days of topical use of AM tincture took the **pain and swelling away**.

Report No. 293: From Thomas's chat room. I **tried different AM doses** from 0.5–12 g. At 3 g there was a state of slight high and laziness, could not concentrate. I didn't really like it. One g: apathy and sleepiness. Slept for three hours. I went to gym but could not work out; I left and went home. At 12 g: condition similar to heavily smoked cannabis high, but with mind and drunk body, bad dexterity. My favorite dose is 0.5 g of dry *Amanita muscaria* in the morning and 1 g at night.

Report No. 294: From Thomas's chat room. I had a stomach ulcer, accompanied with bile tract dyskinesia and hepatitis in my past. Now I feel great, and the ulcer is in remission. My tests are better. AM microdosing for four months, 3 g a day. At the beginning it was heartburn; three weeks later everything came back to normal.

Report No. 295: From Thomas's chat room. In summer a small wart appeared on the palm, the size of a match head. I tried some remedies and obviously nothing helped; it appeared again. After ten days of microdosing, the **wart completely disappeared**! This is for me the most obvious indicator of the healthy action of the mukhomor! I started at 0.5 g and smoothly increased the dosage to 2 g per day: 1 g in the morning, and 1 g in the evening.

Report No. 296: Sent to Masha personally via Telegram messenger. One month of microdosing, from 0.5–3 g a day. In general, my microdosing is similar to above comments—everything is fun and wonderful. First few days in the beginning I had light nausea, it quickly passed. I ate 5 g and 10 g on two different occasions, and I fell asleep, nothing much happened. Great results with my **back pain**. I had surgery on my spine; I had chronic pain for years. Pain was gone after a week of AM microdosing. I feel like new! Second achievement, after many years battle with **nail fungus**, I saw effects in two weeks.

Report No. 297: From Thomas's chat room. I made *Amanita* ointment by mixing dry powder with lotion; I keep it in the refrigerator. This ointment took away a **wart** in ten days; I was putting small dabs on the wart and fixed with bandage overnight.

Report No. 298: From Thomas's chat room. Dry AM microdose keeps my stomach **ulcer** in remission. That is *Amanita* healer's known fact.

Report No. 299: From Masha's chat room. Masha, after the week of AM microdosing, the desire to drink **alcohol** completely disappeared, even at the level of psychological dependence. Zero craving. For me this is significant achievement, the ultimate event.

Report No. 300: From Thomas's chat room. AM microdosing affecting physical condition and general well-being very much. For three months of microdosing I got a lot of unexpected bonuses so that it's even somewhat alarming. I'm not used to getting goods at such an easy price. My consciousness starts looking for a catch.

Report No. 301: From Thomas's chat room. Last year I used 50 g of AM for two months microdosing and then took a break. From November 5 of this year, I resumed AM microdosing because I had no need in a single pill since October last year! I use fingernail size of dry AM flake in the morning on empty stomach. Ten minutes later I drink strong tea without sugar. This year AM microdose course was 1.5 month. The result is similar to last year's AM microdose course: **balanced posture, endurance, orderly thoughts, motivation** to exercise, even push-ups and squats feel great! Sometimes in the evening I brew tea from 1 g AM crumbs and I drink without additives. I had no problem with libido before but now it is a fire! Kindness to all!

Report No. 302: From Thomas's chat room. Nothing more could surprise me after the fact that *Amanita muscaria* microdoses took away two years suffering **pain** in the wrist joint. Pain passed in a week. Surprisingly, there is no pain after workload on the wrist. I do not understand how it works.

Report No. 303: Sent to Masha personally via Telegram messenger. About myself: I've smoked cannabis regularly for about fifteen years, the last ten years—daily. I've smoked cigarettes for seven years. AM microdosing from October 2019 with breaks and terminated a week ago (December 5). My body filled with **calm and strong balance**. I don't understand how, but at first, I **quit tobacco** and stopped mixing cannabis with tobacco. About a couple of weeks later, I **stopped smoking cannabis** as well. I've already had three smoke-free weeks, although access to MJ is free 24/7, no desire, I refuse it even with the company of smoking friends. Everything somehow turned around, I began to look at people, things, and relations differently, otherwise. Previously I experienced lack of patience, now it's blossoming. Analysis of errors in progress, with the goal—not to repeat. Health and fun to all.

Report No. 304: From Thomas's chat room. Today on a walk I realized such a thing—that almost all bad and harm comes from fear and the ignorance of truth! I caught myself thinking that inside everything is **calm**; there are no reasons for fuss and stress; there are no conflicts, no need to defend against or to attack someone. There are no reasons to destroy Health. Even for the sake of "pleasure," it's all an illusion. Foolish, knowing the truth and continuing to support lies. The brain calms down as if it's dying; thinking like it used to be has stopped. Deepening in thoughts altogether. I pop to the surface, answers on the surfaces. Simple and clear. I watch stereotypes collapse. It turns out life isn't as bad as I thought before. You can see a lot of things that you usually don't pay attention to. I tried to give up nicotine three times in the last six months. I want to enter the new year without this habit. And all these changes came from AM microdosing.

This time I clearly felt it in my body. Probably concentration level kicked in. My AM microdose now is 0.25 for the night. The bigger amount doesn't let me sleep. Yesterday I decided to check up. I bummed my brain with thoughts about nicotine, experiencing a strong internal fight. In the evening 0.25 AM microdosing changed my inner voice in ten minutes to confident: "Who said it would be easy? Quit once and for all!" This phrase now is my mantra. The world turns out to be not so gray and boring. New interesting reactions developed when people try to manipulate me with guilt or sacrifice—laughter breaks out, nothing I can do. AM is very strong creature. I stopped wanting to prove anything to anyone or turn on "smart me;" I just want to keep quiet and watch what's happening. Thoughts don't bother me anymore; I rely on my own experience; no spam breaks out of me. Finally, my relatives started to use AM tincture. I am happy about that.

Report No. 305: From Thomas's chat room. I smoked cannabis daily for two years. If grass was at home, I couldn't stop smoking until it was gone. A year ago I began to notice that it was hurting me. Anxiety, feeling like I can't handle simple things and planning, that I don't control life. I decided to **stop smoking** about 2.5 months ago combining that with AM microdosing. I have not smoked for over two weeks even though there is grass at home and I don't want to smoke it. And all that comes from AM. In addition, there has come some great **calm and balance**, more **love for myself**, for others, faith in myself, and **more focus in thoughts**. All this seems to compensate for the lack of impressions in life, which I filled with simply meaningless smoking grass. The desire to justify the need for grass in life has disappeared. I feel that it is absolutely not mandatory and does nothing that cannot be found and made sober. Anyway, it's very pleasing. Without cannabis I have much deeper sleep, dreams brighter. If I smoke, I don't see dreams at all.

Report No. 306: From Masha's YouTube channel. Masha, really liked your expression F*** "rocket fuel" toward alcohol! Thank you for opening our eyes. Health, Love, and Good Wishes! I have not got drunk since July, as I started running and began to microdose mukhomors. Now the thought of **drinking alcohol** seems stupid. I am a forty-six-year-old man.

Report No. 307: From Masha's YouTube channel. Four months without **alcohol** in any form! Merci *Amanita muscaria,* a magic thing and a separate thank you, Baba, for the information about AM microdosing. I microdosed three months straight and now I am four months without family scandals, without a sick head and hangovers, etc.

Report No. 308: From Masha's YouTube channel. Three months of AM microdosing. Since June did not take **alcohol**, replaced **food habits**. I tried bigger doses and agree with you that it is better to leave the brain clean. Thanks for your work.

Report No. 309: From Masha's YouTube channel. My mother is a chronic alcoholic. We tried everything and nothing helped. After all it is no longer only on the physical level but also on the mental level. It is very difficult for her to refuse, but for almost three months of AM microdosing the frequency of **alcohol** intake reduced to almost zero. In my opinion, these are incredible results; she was taking alcohol about twenty years. I have not taken alcohol for a year, preferring it to cannabis. After microdosing with magic and *Amanita* mushrooms, I thrill from sobriety. Peace to all and good New Year without booze.

Report No. 310: From Masha's YouTube channel. After AM microdosing, I could not stand **alcohol** and alcoholics.

Report No. 311: Sent to Masha personally via Telegram messenger. I am seventy-two years old, male, suffering from **insomnia** for ages. Three weeks of AM microdosing gave me back my **sleep, rest, and great energized mornings**. My grandson is a big fan. He introduced me to *Amanita*. Of course, I was suspicious at first. God bless you, Masha.

Report No. 312: Sent to Masha personally via Telegram messenger. Hello, Baba Masha! Thank you very much for your education. Two months ago me and my boyfriend started AM microdosing, 2.5 g in the morning. We gave up **meat**. I personally **ceased to be annoyed** by noisy colleagues on public transportation. I meditate rather than going crazy like before. I was pleasantly amazed by how timely my **menstrual cycle** goes now; all my life it has been irregular with terrible **pain**, and here everything is clear, on schedule. There is some discomfort in my abdominals, but I cope with it without painkillers. It became **easier to communicate** with my parents on the phone. I used to be pissed off because they ask the same question about the weather and my answers were dry, as "yes, no, good." Now I ask questions, smile more, look at my mother from a different point, and I feel empathy toward her. I stress much less with my job now. **No more fear** to be fired, no panic, and understanding there are some other jobs around, no one will die. There is only one side effect—I cannot speak about AM microdosing because not many people will understand. I missed a few AM microdoses, and I noticed that my routine irritation comes back sometimes in the evening. Thanks to your channel, we are not alone, and it is pleasing. Happiness to you, and I wish for more fans/subscribers!

Report No. 313: From Thomas's chat room. One month AM tincture. I collected AM myself and prepared tincture. Five drops in the morning and five in the evening. Also, I rub my wrist and knees with it. By the way in external application AM tincture also has a marked change of condition. *Effects:* I feel like I dropped twenty years off my age. There are no signs of intoxication or unnatural euphoria, no side effects. I worked for years with abrasive material, and my right lung was damaged. I could not breathe for many years with full breath and at the same time felt wheezes in this right lung. I was coughing out a lot of weird stuff while microdosing, and my **breath normalized**. I breathe differently and without wheezing; in general, abrasives and silicon dust could not be removed from the lungs. It is a professional disease of miners, and working with abrasive, called silicosis; mine was not in a heavy stage.

Report No. 314: From Thomas's chat room. While microdosing, at one point I realized that I **think more positively, the depressive state disappeared, less negative thoughts, my mood raised**.

Report No. 315: From Thomas's chat room. Male, thirty-seven years old, 95 kg [209 pounds] weight. Came across Baba Masha on YouTube, thank you! I decided to quit taking alcohol, consumed daily with rare breaks, usually couple liters of beer or wine constantly. Boy, I am not a stupid poet and decided to approach it in a comprehensive way. I purchased an anti-stress magnesium calcium cocktail, and I ordered fly agarics. Mushrooms arrived, started microdosing 1–2 g overnight, two hours before sleep. I've been going on for about two months. Now to the essence. **Sleep improved**, bright dreams (but not always). **Increasing energy**, by so much that I slowly engaged in morning gymnastics. I think about more intensive classes. For several years I suffer from **pain in joints** and bones (consequences of trauma). I noticed that the most painful period of the year is the end of autumn and the beginning of winter; it passed without severe exacerbations, but to "miraculous healing" it certainly didn't reach. I don't know because of the fungus or because of the **rejection of alcohol**, and most likely from both—things at work improved, there was excitement, good anger, like a hunter who is chasing prey, which led to me being sent by boss to upgrade school; I was entrusted with a new front of work, I think because they noticed changes in me. At the same time I started to care more about my health. I am planning a visit to dentist. By the way, I noticed that now I want to do more, reach more, as my laziness retreats. I don't know who to say thanks to besides Baba Masha, maybe muk-homor, maybe the universe. Don't despair, guys. Everything is recoverable!

Report No. 316: From Thomas's chat room. I will say—yes, AM pulls away **alcohol** really well, but sometimes there is a momentum in my head and I stand on the verge, in or out! Booze sits deep in my head, and it's scary and very hard.

Report No. 317: Sent to Masha personally via Telegram messenger. After listening to your channel, decided to try microdosing mukhomors—2.2 g in the morning, every day. Today is the thirty-sixth day. I don't recognize myself. In practice, it is difficult to perceive the situation exclusively with the brain. Now without being loaded with self-digging, I remain in **good spirit**, and it is a completely new, incredible experience for me! Before, **panic attacks**, **depression**, **anxiety** were developing on the stress background. The external environment is the same, but my **attitude is different** now. I have clearly become much more optimistic about the future and I say, rejoice in. I recalled all my plans and started meditation again. I think more about good than ever. To be here and now, to love life, to enjoy this temporary but undoubtedly wonderful and very interesting journey. Everything is simple and at the same time we constantly forget about it. I inhale. I exhale. I live. There is something in life on earth; otherwise why did we come here and cherish so much our body, our experience, our life? Thank you, Baba Masha, for your help. For your channel and for blowing my mind three months ago. You pulled me out of my uncomfortable and intense illusion and plunged me into a new, kind, pleasant, and beautiful one. By the way, I brought my girlfriend and brother to your channel, and noticing their changes makes me even happier!

Report No. 318: From Masha's chat room. I sniffed AM powder three times every other day. I liked the effect on consciousness, fifteen minutes of light high and then clarity and a sea of **energy**, but the nose deposits [congestion] remain unchanged.

Report No. 319: Sent to Masha personally via Telegram messenger. I recently learned about the mukhomor. I am a thirty-one-year-old male. I was an **amphetamine addict** for two years and could not do anything about it during those two years. I drank AM as a tea twice a day, and I stopped wanting amphetamine like I never used it. My **sleep** normalized. Next, I bought 100 g of dry AM caps with a goal to totally eliminate my addiction. I ate 10 g at once. Condition was similar to vodka drank, but the head was clear, strong sleepiness, struggle with such euphoria does not compare with anything. My cat joined me, and I understood it as a friend on some different energy level. I woke up next morning feeling reborn. And then I had a month of microdoses combined with work and sports. I am easygoing even after hard work, nothing hurts, dreams bright, thoughts are kind, easy to communicate with people, and everything turned out great. I brewed teas with two teaspoons in 1.5 liter of water; I drank it during the day by small sips, taking 3–4 days break. Now I am on a one-month break, no thought about amphetamine. I understand that only AM helped me to throw out this bad habit.

Report No. 320: From Thomas's chat room. I got rid of the **nail fungus** in half a year with AM microdosing; the nail damage was about 40%. At first the fungus stopped developing, and I just cut fungus off the nail with clippers. Mukhomor mushroom microdoses blocks the growth of the nail fungus, it works.

Report No. 321: Thomas's chat room conversation.

—Yesterday some depression attacked me in the evening; I decided to smoke fly agaric before bed. I **relaxed instantly, great mood appeared**, somehow became easier inside, I calmed down. I also smoked it this morning before work. I got a **positive mood**.

—Smoking mukhomors puts me in dissociative sleep for a couple of hours. I wonder how experiments vary. More research is necessary!

—How much did you smoke?

—A flake fingernail size, crushed with fingers and smoked through a pipe. I do not know the weight exactly.

—And what was the effect?

—Body became very heavy, and I fell asleep for about three hours. The consciousness was cheerful and observed dissociative experience. My dream was very bright and impressive, but nothing similar to our reality; it's impossible to apply the obtained information in our reality and in human language personally for me, any attempts to draw this will be a bleak non-informative smear. I was awake, I was normal.

—I snuffed 0.05 g of AM in each nostril, and I really liked it. First, you're drunk and muddy about 15–20 minutes, and then there was clarity and energy. I've done so much for today that I'm in shock.

—I have a broken nose and I conducted an experiment with AM snuff with a goal to **improve my breathing**. I don't know how much I did by dose. But my nose breathes perfectly. I have a wealth of energy and feel great.

Report No. 322: From Thomas's chat room. Forty-day course AM microdosing, 0.3 g per day. The result is the disappearance of external manifestations of the **candidiasis**. I had these signs since twelve years old, all my life, and mukhomor kicked it out of me.

Report No. 323: Sent to Masha personally via Telegram messenger. Hi, Baba Masha. Can you imagine that AM microdosing cures **eczema**? For seventeen years suffering from eczema, I tried everything from oils to injections, herbs, and nothing helped. Five years ago I had to quit sports because of constant skin trauma affected by eczema areas. Two weeks ago I finally tried the course of mukhomors for general strengthening, but I did not expect that hands will become clean and healthy. It was amazing and nice. I ate [the dose] in the morning, 2–3 g on empty stomach. The problem is, if I miss a daily dose, eczema immediately wakes up. Apparently, I will have to sit on *Amanita muscaria* microdoses, but I will experiment longer with *Amanita* and see how it goes. I am glad it worked!

Report No. 324: From Thomas's chat room. My **gum bleeding** is severe. I put a ground mukhomor on the gums and noticed temporary relief; it started in a week again. So, it only helps for short time. AM microdose intake is not helping at all. Three months microdosing did not have an effect, but topical applications help.

Report No. 325: Sent to Masha personally via Telegram messenger. Hello, I am glad to announce the following changes that have occurred since the beginning of microdosing. I take dry *Amanita muscaria* flake, fingernail size, morning and afternoon.

1. The most striking discovery is the complete disappearance of the **fungus on the toenails**, within 2–3 weeks the toenails became simply perfect, before that it was horrible.
2. I had **chronic back pain** for many years, which was both before and

after surgery on my intervertebral 11 mm hernia. Now no pain, I walk anywhere I want, in any direction, I sit as I want, etc., and nothing hurts! Freedom!

3. **Intercostal neuralgia** also passed.
4. Overall coordination of movements came back; the body easily holds **balance**. Hands small motor skills improved as well, handwriting became clearer, it became easy to tie knots, etc.
5. Excess weight left. Now my body does not take unhealthy products as junk food, alcohol, nicotine, etc.
6. **Alcohol** has simply ceased to exist in my world vs. previous alcoholic me.
7. I am learning to play instruments, which I never even thought about before.
8. The psychological background changed: there **were fears, panic states, depression**. Now everything is gone, **energy** has increased very much. **Sleep**: began to sleep less, better sleep, I stand up with a cheer and immediately want to do something; a lot of thoughts are not crowded. Very strong nootropic exposure. In general, the **mood has improved, nervous disruptions and negative thoughts** almost completely gone. I smile a lot. And this is inexpensive cost, isn't it?! And that's just what I was able to track down.
9. **Marijuana addiction** has gone. Now I can smoke calmly in the morning and forget it for the whole day and continue normal life, rather than as before, then I smoked until I drop down. **Cigarette smoking** has also become much less without fanaticism.

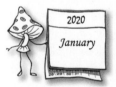

Report No. 326: Sent to Masha personally via Telegram messenger. Three months AM microdosing. I started on October 8, tea with a lemon brewed in the evenings. After six weeks I switched to dry flake in the morning with breaks. Dose is about 1 g. My feeling is that dry AM acts sharply and brings me down at the end. Brewed AM tea with lemon seems to level both the inner background and what happens around, which I need.

In general, the effects are not diminishing with time but became more familiar, and I no longer pay attention to it. Subjectively **concentration** and **"brain capacity"** are higher, the concept's **perception** is panoramic. But in regular routine events, sometimes I am slow and react with a delay of different degrees of criticality. It is **emotionally pleasant** that I do not get immediately involved in any given occasion, like whether I will be offended or someone else will be offended. The **attitude toward my own life** is more instrumental and playable—suspended, but with a plus sign, which suits me. It was always suspended before, but rather with a minus sign and a feeling of discomfort. I am not sure how *Amanita muscaria* microdosing affects my **food preferences**, but there are some changes. **Dreams** changed and became more interesting. I am going to continue AM microdosing.

Report No. 327: From Thomas's chat room. The conditions that AM microdosing gives are the **fearless, fun-filled ease of social communication, endurance, and breadth of thinking**. These states, they remain. After all, it was AM who returned me to the naughty, young, and joyful person of the past. I like it, I keep this condition, the state of vigor of spirit without *Amanita muscaria* microdoses now.

Report No. 328: From Thomas's chat room. I think an AM microdosing course needs an intention to be set up. I started taking a mushroom with a desire to **quit drinking**. I microdosed for a month. At the end AM microdosing completely flipped my consciousness. I became **calm**, there was a desire to think logically, alcoholic psychosis disappeared, no longer irritated the sobriety of consciousness. **Communication** increased and much more. And most importantly, the goal is achieved, I quit drinking! And it does not even pull back into the beer house anymore to drink a cup of another foam. Craving for alcohol is zero. I am pleasantly shocked. I haven't microdosed AM for a month now. Last alcohol drink was two months ago.

Report No. 329: Sent to Masha personally via Telegram messenger. Nine years I was taking Microhydrin **supplements** made for athletes and people engaged in manual labor **for strength and endurance. I quit that** after two weeks of AM microdosing. Now I am free of that for a month. It is a miracle.

Report No. 330: From Thomas's chat room. I noticed that I do not feel good if I smoke **cigarettes** during AM microdosing. I have nausea and uncomfortable head spins, but I still have nicotine craving.

Report No. 331: From Thomas's chat room. My **fears** to be myself went away with *Amanita muscaria* microdoses! I have less boundaries now. I have high work capacity as well.

Report No. 332: From Masha's chat room. Now I'm starting to set a goal during AM microdose course. I am not happy now to drink **alcohol**. Not to say that I was drinking, but on holidays and weekends I was. So, after the first receptions of AM microdose, on New Year's Eve according to the habit I poured a glass of whisky, drank it, and got a headache. I did not connect it yet and next day drank more and got the same result. The next day I got the same result from drinking beer. So, I don't drink now and I don't even want to. Interesting that I even do not go to the liquor department in the store anymore.

Report No. 333: From Masha's chat room. I didn't believe that mukhomor would help me with **alcoholism**. I do not have craving since New Year's Eve. Once I forced myself to drink and felt so bad that I don't want to do it again. Mukhomor takes me out of established trance of repeated events and gives me a chance to act reasonably.

Report No. 334: Sent to Masha personally via Telegram messenger. In five days of AM microdosing, 1 g in the morning on empty stomach in form of infused tea, I had great results. I lost interest in **liquor** and **nicotine** to the point like I never used it in the past. My recipe: In the morning 1 g of ground AM powder added to boiling water, water bath fifteen minutes, then drained, screened, squeezed. Over mushroom body once more I poured boiling water and after twenty minutes combined both decoction to each and drank with adding honey or rosehips syrup.

Report No. 335: From Masha's chat room. I've been eating a bunch of **sweets** for years, by the kilos—candies, pastry, waffles, cookies, etc. After one month of AM microdosing, I stopped eating sugary products. It happened unintended; I did not see it coming. Two months free of my addiction. I ate waffles and some rolls a couple of times during the last two months, and I did not like the taste; I did not want it; I had nausea. Good luck and prosperity! Glory to the fly agaric!

Report No. 336: Conversation from Thomas's chat room.

—Mukhomor ointment from Thomas is a cool thing! I've only applied it in one case so far. My four-year-old daughter often wakes up at night and complains that her legs hurt in the area of calves. I don't know what it is and what causes that, but I remember myself at her age. I had exactly the same until age seven, waking up in the middle of night with similar pulling leg **pain**. Very unpleasant feelings. I went to my mother, complained about this pain, and my mother massaged my legs until the pain passed. Now the same thing is happened with my child. I did the same thing as my mother did in my childhood. I used AM ointment when I got the package, and to my surprise, the pain disappeared right away after applying to the skin of the calves, and my child immediately calms down and falls asleep.

—My husband uses Thomas's ointment to relieve **back pain**; it works, I am wondering if I can eat that too. Did you try to eat the ointment?

Report No. 337: From Thomas's chat room. Yesterday I got a stuffy nose. I decided to sniff AM powder. It irritated my nose mucus a lot. After thirty minutes a lot of goop and slime got out of my nose, and my **breathing normalized**. I jumped with joy.

Report No. 338: From Thomas's chat room. It is pure magic how AM microdosing works with **addictions**. AM lets me take long breaks with my **cannabis and e-cigs** heavy habits. It breaks the addiction trance that I built for many years.

Report No. 339: From Thomas's chat room. Every day for the last two years I have consumed a lot of pastry. Thank god, my figure didn't reflect much. After fifteen days of AM microdoses, I stopped paying attention to **sweets** at all. In general, the goal was to quit smoking. But I did not have enough mushrooms. Effects already seen—the organism was cleaned. I **lost weight**, I feel lighter and more flexible. I am happy.

Report No. 340: From Thomas's chat room. I took a three-week break from forty days AM microdosing by 0.3 g a day. I noticed that my toenails become more healthy and smoother. The most amazing transformation happened with my pinky toe. Due to constant foot stress of wearing tight shoes with a narrowing toe, I had problems with the nail plate. After a close examination I came to the conclusion that my nails were struck by the **fungus**, not particularly visible and interfering, but now, after its destructive effects is clearly obvious. Another manifestation of *Amanita* magic.

Report No. 341: Sent to Masha personally via Telegram messenger. I am going to write full AM microdose report in a month. For now, I can joyfully note that in a week of a microdosing I successfully stop taking the antidepressant Zoloft and also forgot about **depression** at all, which had lasted about nine years!

Report No. 342: Sent to Masha personally via Telegram messenger. I have a very strange situation: For a month I used brewed tea made with one teaspoon AM in the morning with lemon. Then I customized, I increased the dose to two teaspoons and later just dry AM cap with no particular weight, just by eye. The first days are **absolute calm**. As someone wrote in the reviews, it's like a bunch of mini MEs shut up inside my head. There was a feeling of a fresh, clean empty room with a balcony and window. I came to the realization that I do not like my job and decided to quit it. My **sleep** has normalized; I had had some problems with it. Then anxiety came, breakdown, nightmares. Anxiety began to develop into an oppressed state, and "suicidal" thoughts began to climb into the head. I stopped AM microdosing. Despite this experience I want to try it again. The feeling is powerful, the direction is pleasant, but it is strange why I got the opposite result than most on the channel reviews describe. From parallel observations: incredible feeling of sensibleness, great sleep, sharp assessment of situations, and making correct decisions in very difficult in emotional situations.

Masha: You overestimated the dose. According to the data I collected, increasing the dose gives what you described in your own individual version. After conversations with many AM microdose users, it turned out—it is not necessary to exceed the dose more than 1 g. The main thing is the regularity of the intake, not the increase in the dose. One teaspoon of *Amanita muscaria* powder is 3–3.5 g. Two teaspoons are close to 6 g. It's not microdosing anymore, it's minidosing. The minidoses sooner or later lead to negative moments in individual variations, including sleep disorders, apathy, negative thoughts, lack of motivation, anxiety, disgust to the mukhomor, intolerance of its taste or smell, etc.

Report No. 343: Sent to Thomas personally via Telegram messenger. I was addicted to **hashish-alcohol** mix from nineteen years old to twenty-eight. Hashish helped in my struggle with stress and gray weekdays. Then I married, I realized that alcohol and family are not compatible things. Mukhomor showed me the joy of being on this gray rock, understanding of human behavior, gave me empathy. The drinking desire just fell away. Although before, there was a belief that I would never give up drinking. It restored my **memory**, gave me **self-confidence**, eliminated the acquired **allergy** to dust and animal fur, definitely cleaned me of parasites by 1,000-percent, because I do not crave sweets, not at all. It **calmed me** down, I became more **balanced**. Now the absence of THC doesn't bother me as much as before. This is one of the results I expected, it's a miracle!

Report No. 344: From Masha's chat room. I started microdosing around September. My previously stuffy nose cleaned up. Now I **breathe very freely**; the nose is freed from "dirt." My **sleep** was balanced. Before that I could not fall asleep for a long time, and I was getting up early with no rest. Now it's exactly on the contrary. I fall asleep almost immediately, eight hours of great sleep, and I wake up completely rested. Thoughts and psycho feeling [mood] are completely aligned. Before that there was a constant thought of clogged chatter. The psyche was uneven and could blow unexpectedly with no reason. Now I am a lot **calmer**. My stomach was cleaned. There was a lot of "blackness and dirt," if you understand what I am talking about. I dropped approximately 4 kg [9 pounds] in three months, from 59 kg to 55 kg [130 to 121 pounds]. Overall, I am very happy with the results. There's no addiction.

Report No. 345: From Masha's chat room. I admit that at a young age I was fun and laughed constantly. Over time it all went somewhere, and I was sad because of it. That me came back less and less with time and one day did not come back at all. AM microdosing helped me bring him back, a funny guy who was **laughing** over everything and **enjoying simple things** in life. Although my experience with AM is short, only two weeks, I am glad!

Report No. 346: Sent to Masha personally via Telegram messenger. Hi to all. I am writing about my first experience taking an AM microdose. I drank 1 g dry powder stirred in a glass of water in the morning and in the evening. I used 100 g for forty-five days. I finished the AM microdose course a month ago. During the reception and after, I feel physically good. I noted an **increase in physical activity** during reception, and physical heavy work was easier to carry. Very **cheerful morning wake-up**, dreams are beautiful, and **emotions are bright**. **Dreams** almost every night. I am on my first month break now. Only positive impressions. I note similar condition that many wrote already here on **digestion, rejection of unhealthy products** and **dependencies** (coffee and cigarettes). I also use AM oil and ointment from Thomas. I used it with my family. I like AM face oil, cleansing effect. I started to use AM tincture today. I consider AM microdosing completely useful experience for myself.

Report No. 347: Sent to Masha personally via Telegram messenger. Please add a question about **papillomas**. My girlfriend used *Amanita muscaria* ointment five times and a wart on her skin fell off. The result was visible and obvious since day two.

Report No. 348: Sent to Masha personally via Telegram messenger. Hello, Baba Masha. I am a thirty-eight-year-old man. Before AM microdose course I was a **drug addict and alcoholic** for ten years. I also was diagnosed with **Bechterev autoimmune disease**. I took AM microdose by 1 g since last fall, and I felt instant disgust with **alcohol** products. My mother also quit drinking vodka with *Amanita muscaria* microdoses use. Mukhomor cleaned us up and gave us right focus.

Report No. 349: From Thomas's chat room.
—My whole family, my wife, mother, and grandmother, take AM microdose by 1 g in the morning and 1 g before bedtime. Everybody has positive and kind changes except me. Should I increase my dose to 1.5–2 g?
—From Masha: The optimal dose is 0.5 g and should not exeed 1 g. The effect depends also on the reason for taking AM microdose and on the lengh of the course—3 weeks on average—or it might not affect very small group of people at all.
—Taking AM microdose only for 6 days.

Report No. 350: Sent to Masha personally via Telegram messenger. I've microdosed since November. I tried different doses from 1–3–4–6 g. I found out that my ideal dose is 2 g. I am seventy-five days without **alcohol**. I am not irritated like before. I am **relaxed and vigorous**. I continue *Amanita muscaria* microdose course.

Report No. 351: From Thomas's chat room. My wife takes AM microdoses, and she has positive experiences; she got cured from some **fungus** disease on her palms. Skin on her palms became clean and soft. Mukhomor works for her as **sleeping aid** as well.

Report No. 352: From Thomas's chat room. I microdose with 1 g dried *Amanita muscaria* in the mornings, and my **papillomas** disappeared on week two or three. I had these papillomas for ten years.

Report No. 353: From Thomas's chat room. I microdosed *Amanita muscaria* for a month by 2 g and took a blood test. All the numbers of my blood test are normal.

Report No. 354: From Thomas's chat room. I took a blood test twice after two AM microdose courses, one month each. All my tests are normal. I also took abdominal ultrasound examination, and everything is good. I lost 15 kilos [33 pounds] of weight in 2.5 months. My **diet habits** changed, and I do not eat meat anymore.

Report No. 355: From Thomas's chat room. I had to quit *Amanita muscaria* microdoses course because I moved. I was afraid that my condition would become worse because of that. After a couple weeks I realized that I am good and I do not have *Amanita*'s withdrawal symptoms at all; the **effects are stable**.

Report No. 356: From Thomas's chat room. My **depression** was gone after AM microdose course. Before, antidepressants made me a vegetable.

Report No. 357: From Thomas's chat room. In the beginning I took 1 g AM in the morning and 3 g before bed. In three days my condition was not very good. I realized that it was **too much**. I took **two days break**. Now I take 1 g in the morning, and I do not take *Amanita muscaria* at night.

Report No. 358: From Thomas's chat room. I am sure that a lot of people have ideas about mukhomor withdrawal syndrome. I took *Amanita muscaria* microdoses for a month, and now I am on **one week break**. Nothing bad happened to me.

Report No. 359: From Thomas's chat room. After one week of AM microdosing by 1 g, I reduced *Amanita muscaria* dose to 0.3. All negative effects are gone now. I made a mistake like a lot of us here in the chat room. **With mukhomor less is better** as Baba Masha repeats many times for us.

Report No. 360: From Thomas's chat room. Positive effect of AM microdosing. It reduced my **alcohol** consumption, e-cigarettes, and **nicotine** craving. I had **abdominal cramps** for three years after surgery. Now they're gone.

Report No. 361: Sent to Masha personally via Telegram messenger. Masha, first I saw your video about "rocket fuel" and suddenly realized that I am forty years old, I drank **alcohol** since I was eleven, and I am killing myself. Additionally, I was abusing **chemical narcotic substances**. I am eating AM microdose for a month now by 1–2 g a day. I feel great, advised it to most of my addicted friends; they are sending you big thank you. Now I think about alcohol with a smile. I kind of knew about its danger, but I never wanted to admit the truth.

Report No. 362: From Masha's chat room. For twenty days of AM microdosing I have more benefits than for year struggling with **addictions**. Mukhomor works easier and faster.

Report No. 363: From Masha's chat room. I understood all negative effects of **alcohol** and I wanted to quit. It was just beyond me. I took two months AM microdose course, and I did not drink at all for a while. Later on, alcohol came back, much less consumption of course.

Report No. 364: From Masha's chat room. During AM microdose course I have three big positive changes—changing **diet habits**, quitting **alcohol**, and **being present** in the now.

Report No. 365: From Masha's chat room. Baba Masha, to begin with, I want to thank you for the work that you do. Every day I see how many solve their problems through mukhomor. I want to share with you my personal observations regarding mukhomor as well. I am twenty-four years old, male, 170cm/70kg [5 foot, 7 inches; 154 pounds]. Before taking AM, I wrote down the things that bother me in myself and that I would like to change. The main ones are reduce **appetite**, fight **caffeine**, improve my **attention**, self-doubt. My AM microdose course was a month, 0.5 g in the morning on empty stomach. The most obvious for me was the change in taste preferences. I wanted to **give up coffee and tea** for a long time, but the habits were stronger than me. After AM microdosing it was cut off. From **alcohol** too. Yesterday I decided to take a beer; I threw it into the [garbage] urn. I did not like the taste; it does not give any more pleasant feeling; it does not give anything. I eat much less **meat**. Before there was a need for everyday meat consumption; now it does not play such a big role for me. I wake up early now, before an alarm clock with a clear head. Heading to work is now conscious action and not like it was before—"in the fog." **Communication** with customers has become more open; others noticed that. I think I have become more **confident** in myself. I often heard the opinion that the mushroom fills the void with itself. I thought it was nonsense, but the further into the forest . . . although this is possibly a placebo effect, but the most important thing is that it is. **Difficulties pass** easier. I will continue AM microdosing and monitor the changes. Peace to all.

Report No. 366: From Thomas's chat room. Good evening to everyone. I want to talk about my friendship with mukhomor. I've been taking it since October. First, the tincture in a droplet from 1–30 drops, then I began to eat the mushroom in dry form, collected and harvested it by myself. At first, I used 1.5–2 g, and I felt energy and concentration, as many here described. Once tried 4 g and I got euphoria and happiness. But in general, I have no desire to go to Trip. The goal is microdosing only. I haven't set up my comfortable dosage yet. When I took a break, at first everything was fine, and then the days of terrible apathy and physical weakness came back. There was no strength at all for anything; I could not do training or yoga. I started new course with reduced the dosage of 0.5 g. From the visible changes for the entire time of reception: the craving for **sweet** leaves—this is my drug addiction. The real drug addiction is emotional breakdowns. Mukhomor mushroom intake helps me to **cope** with this. I **eat better** now, **training is more effective**, **concentration** is better.

Report No. 367: Sent to Masha personally via Telegram messenger. Good evening. I've used AM tincture for two years and I eat a dry mukhomor between the breaks between tincture intake. In 2013 I was diagnosed with a stage 2 endometriosis ovarian cyst. They prescribed hormone therapy and a bunch of drugs. I refused to take that and looked for alternative methods. A year of vegetarianism did not produce strong results. In 2015 I collected AM with my husband for the first time, and we made a tincture and dried some. The tincture course was incremental, one drop a day, up to fifteen drops and back. Second course, up to thirty drops and back, and then up to sixty. With intermediate breaks of two months. In the breaks between courses, I ate dried mukhomor. I did that treatment on the advice of an experienced herbalist; he said that it is a powerful antiparasitic! And in 2017 there was a medical examination including a gynecologist. To my and gynecologist's surprise, there was no signs of previous condition. **Cysts** disappeared. The doctors asked me, what did I use, and I did not know what to say. After all, during the AM reception, I completely **switched to vegan** style, drinking a lot of juices, sprouted seeds; I stopped consuming white flour, **sugar, black tea**. I took yoga classes and in general I work with my mind to decompress traumatic situations. I revised attitude to people and to life. I can say with confidence that mukhomor is a mystical fungus, for everyone is revealed individually. I treat it with deep respect and love. In our house mukhomor is the family doctor.

Report No. 368: From Thomas's chat room. I took AM microdoses two weeks by 0.3 g, then increased to 0.6, 0.9, 1.2, 1.5, and 1.8.

Results:

1. I started to read books again.
2. I went to dentist (long time due).
3. I became more **communicative**; sense of **humor** became sharper.
4. Some **fears disappeared** after I died in my sleep many times.
5. There was a **desire for physical exercises** again.
6. **Goals** began to appear; before, there was some absolute emptiness and apathy.
7. I became **less dependent** on people; I like my time alone now.
8. I **lost weight** by several kg.
9. **No need to control** myself in some situations; before, aggression showed up.

Report No. 369: From Thomas's chat room. I took AM microdoses for a month, 1.5–2 g daily. I wanted a lightning-fast effect. And it was: **high concentration**, **energy**, great rested six hours **sleep**. In a month my AM supplies ended. After holidays the brutal cancellation syndrome came. Terrible physical weakness, I got up in the morning and couldn't do anything at all, lying like a corpse. Now I'm back to very small dosages—0.3–0.5 g. There are no "effects" physically tangible. But I begin to notice that I became attentive to everything, first of all to my thoughts, and yes, slowly leveling toward high energy resources. It is not necessary to chase the effects; constant stimulation is a load on the nervous system, as a result, the syndrome of cancellation. AM perfectly cures greed.

Report No. 370: From Masha's YouTube channel. I have been taking mukhomor exclusively in microdoses since the beginning of September 2019. I took a break from mid-October to mid-November. Then resumed reception. I've been taking it every day ever since. I found information about AM microdosing from your channel. During AM microdosing time, a lot of positive changes have happened to me. And first of all, I **stopped being nervous and worrying** about any difficult situations. All **fears passed**, which before showed regularly and very strongly. I began to perceive this life as a game, and I have fun with it. Mukhomor gives positive effects on physical health, and it is a very effective psychologist and psychiatrist. Once again, thank you, Baba Masha. Health, happiness, and prosperity.

Report No. 371: From Thomas's chat room. I advise to start small, from 0.2 g AM. No one gives you the right answer. We're all different. There's no right answer for everyone. I have a palpable sensation from tea with 0.2 g AM with lemon and ginger—a lot of energy and fast thinking. So, start small and watch!

Report No. 372: Sent to Masha personally via Telegram messenger. I take 1 g AM microdose in the morning and in the evening, so far, all good. The mushroom balances, makes the mind **concentrate**, takes away **negativity** to some degree, although irritability on some details remains, but my attitude to that has had a positive change—I do not need it and it is not mine. **Dreams** have become more realistic; it feels like I live in other realities on a different frequency.

Report No. 373: Sent to Masha personally via Telegram messenger. I've taken mukhomor microdoses for twelve days, 1 g daily. Steadily **good mood** and armor from negativity. I don't know, write it off for the mukhomor effect, or for the enthusiasm of the neophyte. I think about whether to try mixing AM microdosing with cannabis; sometimes I want more fun. I started microdosing against the background of a long **depression**. Now everything is super, but more thanks to you for putting everything in right direction. Thank you for Telegram and YouTube channels!

Report No. 374: From Masha's YouTube channel. After AM microdose course I got total relief from **pain** in my liver.

Report No. 375: From Masha's YouTube channel. My AM microdosing experience is short. I am reporting sand falling out of my **kidneys** during AM microdose course and urinating with blood. I am not sure if it was the process of purification and it is a positive effect. But I advise to check the disease baggage before taking AM.

Report No. 376: Sent to Masha personally via Telegram messenger. Hi, dear Baba Masha. My AM microdosing I report: I am a forty-nine-year-old man. When I have **pain in the lower back**, I crush 1 g of mukhomor on a cotton disk wetted with vodka and fix it with a patch on a painful spot. I have **relief** in a couple of hours, complete recovery. Dried AM microdose caused depressive states. I switched to 1 g tea with lemon before bedtime; it is the best sleeping pill, and I don't wake up until the morning, which is important for me.

Report No. 377: From Masha's YouTube channel. I took AM microdoses for two months. The dose was regulated experimentally. Too much caused euphoria and a mild headache. I got greater communicability, **excellent mood, good performance, and clear mind**. It became easy to wake up in the morning. Microdosing is really **calming**. Since childhood I lived with **panic attacks. Now they're practically gone**.

Report No. 378: From Masha's YouTube channel. I take a mukhomor tincture in vodka in microdoses. I advise very much to all! It feels incredibly good, and I **sleep** well.

Report No. 379: From Masha's YouTube channel. I had a big **sleep** problem. Microdoses for the night provides a wonderful deep sleep. On breaks I still sleep a lot better. I tried it in the morning instead of coffee; it makes me surprisingly sleepy. Thanks for videos!

Report No. 380: From Masha's YouTube channel. I was diagnosed with bronchial asthma and am taking AM microdoses. The effect is psychosomatics. My worries are gone, and I have less **asthma attacks**!

Report No. 381: From Masha's YouTube channel. Thanks to mukhomor, it turned my life in another direction. Since June 2019 I have completely given up **alcohol, sugar, bread-and-bakery products**, etc. From August to December I used mukhomor to clean my body and reset my brain. By my subjective sensations AM takes all the gimmick and debris out of the body and mentality. The **internal fears** connected with the past and future imposed by society since childhood have **disappeared**, including internal sense of **guilt** (permanent before). Of course, there are some problems in life, but **I look for opportunities**, but not the reasons. I also **lost weight**, 29 kg [64 pounds]. Baba Masha, I adore you and thanks for the world that you opened for many.

Report No. 382: From Masha's YouTube channel. We are colleagues, I am also a doctor. I recently cured my comrade from obsessive **paranoid fear of disease**. It got to the point that he couldn't work. The benzodiazepines he was taking made him sleepy all the time. I brewed four *Amanita muscaria* caps with lemon and honey, and we talked a couple of hours. Then I gave him a few caps and told him to drink one every day. He still doesn't believe how it affected him; he says it's a mind-blowing experience.

Report No. 383: From Thomas's chat room. Good day to everyone. I would like to share a short, but positive experience of AM microdose reception. To be honest, at first, I was aggressive, because I am against all substances that change consciousness. But after studying the benefit of the mukhomor and honoring many reviews here and talking to Baba Masha, I realized that I want to try the wonderful fungus myself. I set up the intentions for AM microdosing and after reception the revelation began. Earlier, I could hardly sleep at night, and sometimes I didn't sleep at all. Sleep was prevented by any small irritants, I often had nightmares. The consequences of **sleep deprivation** were fatigue, negativity, no concentration at work, and in the end of the day I feel like some zombie. Everything changed after I started taking the mukhomor. I fall asleep now easily, dreams bright and saturated, nightmare stopped. I feel that I can keep everything under control, because even in a terrible dream I remain calm. During the day there is no sleepiness, attention increased. Earlier I could get in a negative vortex really easily; now I, to the contrary, became **calmer**. There are no messy thoughts in my head. And I noticed the nuance: I'm a rum lover and I used to have a rum cocktail after work to get some relaxation. Now there is no such desire. I don't want to drink **alcohol** without an excuse at all. The mood is more positive. I take AM microdoses a little over a week. About 0.5 g in the morning and evening.

Report No. 384: From Masha's YouTube channel. Baba Masha, hello, and thank you so much for helping a lot of people. I'm among them. I microdosed this autumn. So many positive emotions, it is hard to conceive. I collected some AM myself; it did not last long. I am waiting for next season. I want to continue AM microdosing. Thank you again from the bottom of my heart.

Report No. 385: From Masha's YouTube channel. It's probably too early for me to talk about any big impact of the mukhomor on my health. Although, I am already observing a **positive effect on the digestive system**. And in three months of not systematic microdosing, I didn't get poisoned and didn't die. Hurrah! But the most unusual thing I find at the moment, is the incredible **ability to wake me up** in the mornings. I can't even believe it! It's a stunner that I experience after every evening tea party.

Report No. 386: From Masha's YouTube channel. The fifth month of AM microdosing without interruption. *Positive feelings:* **Strong positive perception**

of everything. Deep correctness in everything. **Energy** for whole day. Quiet dream. Adapting to the social world, I communicate with relatives, cheers! It used to be difficult. I just want to live with joy and be healthy. *Negative feelings*: Mukhomor kind of builds new mechanisms in the body, which changes consciousness. I eat much less than before and unpleasantly everyone asks why I eat so little. However, I feel that the body no longer requires a lot of food. And **excess weight** . . . I became slender! Therefore, it is hardly negative, although doubts and critical analysis should not leave people.

Report No. 387: Sent to Masha personally via Telegram messenger. Hello. The report on fly agarics: We took a course of AM microdoses for three months. I am a twenty-one-year-old male; my mother is fifty-two. The dosage increased from 0.75–3.5 g. The first two weeks both experienced light nausea and headache, then everything normalized. Immediately noticed an increase in vision brightness. All the colors became very saturated. After each reception a swell of **energy and good mood** began. Mom **quit smoking** cigarettes, switched to vape. Which is a miracle for us, as she smoked thirty-seven years, two packs a day. And before microdosing she didn't think about quitting. Mom finally got herself a vacation for the first time in seven years. She denied herself a vacation before but suddenly realized that life doesn't consist only of a job. **Depressive episodes** almost gone, 90%. Both noticed a fundamental change in thinking. For my part, I noticed an incredible increase in activity. All day I do something and there is strength and desire for it. I reached for the smallest plans that were constantly postponed. I actually forgot the word *lazy*, which is personally very important to me. **Fears and phobias** that prevented our life passed for both of us. It helped us both completely **switch to eating plant food**, which was not possible for three years. Here are such fantastic results.

Report No. 388: From Masha's chat room. My mother is sixty-seven; prior to AM microdosing there were problems connected with high blood pressure for twenty-five years and a lot of different medicines were prescribed. **Blood pressure** was stabilized quickly enough in one month; she is taking much less medicine and not that often. Total AM microdose intake five months. I noticed that her **state of mind, health**, and **mood** has considerably improved also.

Report No. 389: From Masha's YouTube channel. Baba Masha, hello. Thank you so much for helping us. Also microdosed this fall. There are many positive emotions to the mind, it is not comprehensible. I collected mukhomor myself. I was very afraid, so I started with a quarter of the middle-size cap. At the end of the second month at extreme times I steamed two middle caps in a glass of water with a pinch of lemon and drank half in the morning, half in the evening. Once in the evening after the reception I went to the forest with a dog, and I saw a pine tree damaged crying with resin. I hugged it, I cried. How did I feel? Love, sadness, mixed with forgotten children's emotions. I can't explain. My wife looked at me, I didn't tell her a word, and she understood. WITHOUT WORDS. With great gratitude from us, your subscribers.

Report No. 390: From Masha's chat room. And it's like a day of understanding, old bacteria colonies are fighting for a freedom. The whole process is tangible, information with enthusiastic descriptions are many, and negative results are single. I want to know more about the nuances and pitfalls of AM microdosing. For sure it helps with **booze**; I am not easily taken in. This month passed without any mental torment with booze, no craving. I want to continue AM microdosing and not drink.

Report No. 391: From Masha's chat room. There is no information on the side effects because I think thousands of people tried AM microdosing and negative effects in 90% caused by jumping on stimulating big doses. If there was a clear harm to some organs, it would not pass unnoticed with such a great number of people who took AM microdoses.

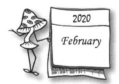

Report No. 392: From Masha's chat room. I rested a month from AM microdosing. I looked back at the results, and realized that it is necessary to continue, a huge number of advantages. I eat much **less bread**, before I ate even pasta or dumplings with bread. The changes were not my personal choice, everything happened itself. It is necessary to introduce it to the masses, but I am not saying it to anyone; I know the reaction in advance.

Report No. 393: From Thomas's chat room. I used *Amanita* tincture with warm water, some honey, and aloe vera gel, mixed in a blender. My recipe: approximately one-third part of the normal teaspoon of alcohol *Amanita* tincture, one tablespoon of honey, half glass of warm water, and a glass of homegrown aloe vera gel diluted with water. My mom also used that. The dose—little baby spoon daily. *Effects:* after the first application slight dizziness before bed, dreams bright, strong sleep, the following days improved well-being, the appetite and food preferences changed (no pasta, etc.). The stool changed, as if it were stagnant in the intestines. Once I saw kind of green porridge came out of me in the toilet. In general, I used that cocktail for a week, now is the third day of the break. I'll start again tonight, before bedtime, I made new portion of cocktail. Mother **stopped taking daily heart pills**. She felt that they were not needed anymore. It turns out that **hypertension** has gone. The first two days I felt a slight tingling in the heart area, and some sensation from the liver, but it passed quick.

Report No. 394: From Thomas's chat room. I microdosed for almost three months, half a teaspoon dried AM in the morning on an empty stomach and after work. Sometimes I prepare 1.2 liters of AM tea in a thermos with 1–2 g of AM dried powder. Me and my sister drink that tea with lemon. **Sleep** improved—it is strong vs. very light sleep before; I used to wake up from every rustle. Stool improved; I was tormented by **constipation** since childhood. No more **sweets**. I became **calmer, no aggression, nervousness** went away. The emotional state elevated significantly. Unusual changes— AM microdosing saved me from craving dependent **relationships**. I tried to increase the dose to 5 g. No good. Loss of coordination, mental chatter, vertigo with my eyes closed, body vibrations—this is not comfortable to me, similar to alcohol intoxication. My choice is a flat teaspoon of dry powder. Shared my experience with a colleague at work. She wanted to put her husband in order. She makes him AM tea with 1 g in the morning, then she eats up the left-over fungus. The effect is present, she feels it. Also, it improved her stool drastically. Peace to everyone!

Report No. 395: From Masha's chat room. I stopped **drinking** beer 100% in five days of microdosing; 1.5 g ground dried AM lasts ten days. It also helped me with **cigarettes and smoking** too much pot. I don't smoke grass as much as I used to. Once a day now vs. six times before. In fact, *Amanita muscaria* microdose intake changes the attitude and interest in all kinds of poisonous habits.

Report No. 396: From Thomas's chat room. My husband has had great success with alcohol tincture to get rid of **knee and back pain**. We tried AM vodka tincture and ointments as well; it did not work very well for him vs. with high alcohol proof.

Report No. 397: From Masha's chat room. I **quit drinking** with the help of a mukhomor; I had a previous coding and course of tricyclic antidepressant. Now, I absolutely have no interest in alcohol, but before, my life was going down the drain.

Report No. 398: From Masha's chat room. I was suffering with **pain from deforming arthrosis** of the joints, one arm totally lost activity, and I could not dress on my own. I used five-year-old AM alcohol tincture, which somehow I found in my dark pantry. Three weeks massaged tincture in my joints—the pain went away for the whole season—winter, spring, and summer, until I collected fresh AM. In the past I was very skeptical about AM tincture storage potency voiced in the public.

Report No. 399: Dialogue from Thomas's chat room.

—I started AM microdosing in October–November to get rid of **alcohol dependency**. I started with 3–6 g dried AM, then found my own dosage: 1–3 g. Now I am three months without any alcohol! There is no craving. I got a tincture from Thomas a week ago. I took it for a week—ten drops morning and evening. Tincture acts stronger. Level of **calm** increased.

—You're right. Dry mushrooms and tincture are very different in effect. I have a pronounced positive effect from tincture. **Activity**, **performance**, **focus** on the task, complete ignoring of bad stimuli. Dry mushroom does not give such obvious advantages. Now I'm experimenting with tincture made from dried AM, so far it is not clear.

Report No. 400: From Masha's chat room. I microdosed for three weeks. Before, I drank a hell of a lot of **booze**, every single day. I drank only three times in the last twenty-one days.

Report No. 401: From Thomas's chat room. I began AM microdosing experience in November last year, and I was amazed by the effect. Some kind of enlightenment happened. The longer I was engaged in the AM microdosing, the clearer and brighter understanding of everything. It is very hard to express in words. In January, after the holidays, I decided to **quit alcohol**; there were some problems that were not particularly terrible, but alcohol interfered with my life. The attraction to alcohol is simply gone, I am very glad and grateful to Grandfather Mukhomor. I can say that **meat** (except chicken) has become somehow not important anymore; I am pleased with that. Mukhomor was taken in the form of brewing tea in a thermos for the night in the amount of 1–2 g. I take it on an empty stomach with lemon juice in the morning. The mind began to work much clearer and in the right direction. Peace to everyone!

Report No. 402: From Thomas's chat room. At the beginning of the AM microdose intake, I had discomfort in my abdomen for two days, then it passed and has not bothered me since October. I am inclined to think that it was fly agaric **cleansing and settling in my guts**. I suffered from gastritis since the army over twenty years now. I could not eat garlic due to immediate pain in the stomach. I did not check my gastritis lately, but after AM microdosing, it is absolutely **painless** to eat a garlic clove at lunch.

Report No. 403: Dialogue from Masha's chat room.

—Masha hello, I took AM microdoses for a week and it's clear that the desire for **harmful habits decreased**; I began to think differently. But now I feel it's all gone, and I'm afraid that maybe the fungus is not working; somehow all of it disappeared. I worry about this very much. I had a head injury. All my life I have had **depression and anxiety**; there was no point in life. But after AM microdosing it seemed I found a way out and I could live without pills. Should I increase the dose or maybe use *Amanita pantherina* instead? Please tell me, if I am in that little percentage of people that AM microdosing does not work. Thank you!

Masha: You are in a group of people who take AM microdoses a few times and think that their problems will immediately disappear from the almighty panacea mukhomor. Unfortunately, this does not happen. I suggest reading the reviews and carefully studying the intake duration, the doses, and how it works for people with similar conditions.

Report No. 404: From Masha's YouTube channel. Fly agaric works miracles! One teaspoon in the morning, after breakfast, daily. I've been taking it for four months. The **emotional background has returned to normal. The brain works like a clock**.

Report No. 405: From Thomas's chat room. After one month of *Amanita muscaria* microdoses, the **alcohol** is down to zero usage. But smoking has become twice as much.

Report No. 406: Dialogue from Masha's chat room:

—I bought AM, and half-opened caps arrived. I milled it in a coffee mill. The first day is 0.5 g, nothing. The second day 0.8 in tea form brewed for fifteen minutes. Half an hour later the wife pulled to the church. We arrived there in the middle of the service. As I entered, stopped and after a couple of minutes I realized how many sounds surrounded me. No hallucinations, just **increased hearing**. I heard rustles in the distance, shuffling feet, etc. I do not like to just stand in the church, so I took my son and went for a walk. As we went outside the bells rang. That day I heard how the vibrations of the bell faded for fifteen seconds, and that never happened before! The **colors escalated**, as if on the television they increased the contrast, but I would not call it hallucinations. The state of a slightly **raised mood** and then for a couple of hours a slight feeling as if the head was a little inflated from the inside. The next day took a pause. Today I tried 1.2 g. Sensations—feel slightly sluggish, sun was bothering my eyes. There is no positive effect as is from 0.8 g. The question is, how to understand what benefits from micro-doses should be? What is the right dose for me? The goal is to reduce red-ness protruding on the skin and reduce pain induced by hard physical work.

Masha: As you indicated the right microdose for you is 0.5. The point is, euphoria is an indicator of effective dosage. The microdose should be incon-clusive in the perception of the surrounding world. The slight sluggishness is the indicator that the dose is too high for you.

Report No. 407: From Thomas's chat room. An interesting observation: the first month, until I figured out the dosage, I took too much—the stimulation effect was strong. My condition was very pleasant, spent time effectively, all **depressant moods and apathy went away**. But due to excessive stimulation, withdrawal syndrome occurred. Further, for the second month I reduced the dosage to 0.5, but in the end, I reached my ideal dosage—1g in the morning only. AM microdosing keeps me awake at night. The whole second month nothing happened, everything returned to reverse: apathy, lethargy, old affections and habits. But I stably continued AM microdosing and tried to stay awake: sports, easy nutrition, yoga, self-education. And hallelujah! In recent days I finally began to wake up cheerful. Today I got up and immediately did a good training without persuasion, and managed to do all things and even more than I expected. I feel like I need to take a break for a week and then continue. In short, we need to listen to ourselves and what the mukhomor broadcasts to us.

Report No. 408: Sent to Masha personally via Telegram messenger. Hi! [. . .] I have about a year of microdosing. I make from mukhomor a magnificent healing product that has been tested on myself personally, and then on rela-tives and friends (at the numerous requests of all). The recipe is simple: I fill the three-liter glass jar with mukhomor caps, pour pure alcohol to cover the caps. Bury the jar to at the depth of a meter for forty days, after which the fungus was removed. We perfectly treat neuralgic, back, and joint **pain** with this remedy. In addition, the effect is colossal for the whole body, when taken by drop dosing, increasing daily by one drop, starting from one to forty and continuing from forty to one. Mukhomor mushroom is a miracle presented by Nature! Thank you for your valuable information.

Report No. 409: From Masha's chat room. Consumption of strong **alcohol**— fell off; the AM microdosing timing is short—about a month. I had a couple of cravings at the very beginning, but it pleases me now that there is abso- lutely no desire for alcohol anymore, given that last year and half I was taking three bottles of strong booze a week and beer nonstop. I still drink beer but not much. I take once a day 1 g dried AM on empty stomach in the morning. I liked the taste right away, even though I was afraid of that mushroom since childhood. Additional features—for the first time, the knee began to bend fully, I do not know what the diagnosis was, but there was constant pain and it did not fully bend. I am not inclined to endorse fly agaric with panacea properties, especially on the cartilage and ligaments, but nevertheless that is that. Now, I **eat much less**, especially **sweet** stuff. My **dependence on pot** has sharply decreased.

Report No. 410: Sent to Masha personally via Telegram messenger. Hi, Baba Masha. Six days of microdosing. On day four I **quit smoking**. I smoked for sixteen years. There were a lot of attempts to quit, well, I could not spend a single day without a cigarette. There were always thoughts about cigarettes. Now I have not smoked for three days without thinking about it. And more, I am disgusted by the smoke, ashes, and everything related to cigarettes. For me, as an avid smoker who had almost two packs a day, this is unbelievable.

Report No. 411: Thomas's post in his chat room. Gentlemen and ladies, new AM M-dosers! I advise everyone to start diaries before microdosing. The first diary entry of your beginning condition will be a point of reference. Describe your current state, mental and physical well-being, everything from boogers to psychoses. Then your goal—why are you microdosing? After each week of microdosing, sit down in a calm atmosphere and read your recordings. Recall and analyze what happened to you in the past week. What changes occurred or failed with you? Do not forget to write down how much you took. This approach will help you better capture and track the changes. You can analyze every day, then the data will be more accurate. There is an example of a diary in my articles. Very often, I see how people take mukhomor a few times without waiting for the result; they begin to shout in all chats that mukhomor did not help them. Listen to your body carefully, try to notice changes that are definitely there, and only over time you begin to understand all the magic of this mushroom.

Report No. 412: From Masha's chat room. There was a problem with the knee. After taking *Amanita muscaria* microdoses my **knee fully bends**, but there is still pain.

Report No. 413: Sent to Thomas personally via Telegram messenger. It began with **a deforming arthrosis** of the left shoulder joint. On August 18 I was in a bike accident. I broke my collarbone. I got it fixed but it seems that the **mobility of the arm** did not recover. I went to the hospital, took an X-ray, and doctors told me that there were no effective treatments, only painkillers. The arm was immobile; it was painful to dress, not to mention riding the bike. I told my friend about that, who had a jar with an AM vodka tincture about five years old. He poured me 300 g, and I rubbed it into my shoulder. After three weeks the pain passed and mobility was fully restored. Next fall, I used tincture by tablespoons and topical additionally. When AM applied externally the action is quite tangible. There was a tangible stimulating action, feelings of overpowering with a potent medicine and some kind of fatigue accumulated. I took a break and after, I reduced the intake to ten drops. The feeling of stimulation remained. For the sake of the experiment, I switched to dried AM. According to subjective perception the equivalent of ten drops is 1 g dried AM. Later I switched to five drops of tincture for the sake of experiment, not because of negative effects. The effect of stimulation smooths, but it is quite palpable if you take regular breaks. Approaching AM usage I do not aim to gain enlightenment or psychic abilities. AM significantly **increases the quality of life** of older age, it stops the symptoms of chronic diseases, and serves to prevent them. In my experience all this unambiguously happens.

Report No. 414: Sent to Masha personally via Telegram messenger. Hello, Masha. I use a tincture of fly agaric made with vodka. Acts positively. I increased it by one drop up to twenty-five. Then a break. I shared tincture with two friends. Two normalized their **blood pressure**, and they quit taking pills. One **cured pain** from dislocated shoulder in two days. It helped with

back pain also then used externally. In general, only positive results. Next year I am going to make a high proof alcohol AM tincture.

Report No. 415: From Thomas's chat room. Health to all! I often have a problem with my back. Usually takes three weeks to recover after a **pinched nerve**. Last time I was in **tormented pain** without sign of reduction. I decided to take half AM cap (about 1.5 g) in the afternoon. The pain passed quickly and I assumed that I had to repeat AM intake next day. But the pain went away! I appreciated this miracle of nature! Recently, my comrade stumbled on the curb, and he was in awful pain. Doctor diagnosed the severe sprain and prescribed painkiller. It did not help much, and I offered to him the mukhomor. He was very impressed with the effect! He began to walk almost immediately. It took only three days to fully recover. AM microdose was taken in form of tea with 1.5 g of dried mushroom.

Report No. 416: From Masha's chat room. For fifteen years I lived with **back pain** after an injury. After taking AM microdose I forgot what pain was. The back has become **more "elastic."**

Report No. 417: From Thomas's chat room. I took AM microdose for a month, prepared in tea form with one-third teaspoon of AM in the morning, on an empty stomach. Last week I blew out my back, the pain was unbearable, any movement caused acute **pain**. On the second day the pain began to pass very quickly. By the end of the day, I was already very active physically, and on the third day it was just a little touchy. And that's it. In general, the back no longer hurts. Surprisingly it was a quick recovery. According to reviews I thought that only the tincture can help for the **back pain**.

Report No. 418: From Thomas's chat room. Greetings. Microdosing over three months. I am on break now for two months. My previous conditions did not come back. All positive moments seem to continue and intensify.

Report No. 419: From Masha's chat room. During *Amanita muscaria* microdosing I noticed growing rejection to sausages and all **meat** products. Even though it's difficult, due to my hard physical work and a lot of training.

Report No. 420: From Thomas's chat room. AM microdosing helped me to **reduce alcohol** and **pot smoking**, which is incomprehensible. Of course, the desire and some efforts are needed, not just shifting responsibilities to magic fungus. That probably won't work. According to my conclusions, AM microdosing hit in two directions—physically on the microflora, mentally on established repetitive patterns of behavior. That makes it very easy to fight alcohol, reducing the desire and making drinks tasteless and hard to absorb. Such a kick is enough to fly into the stratosphere of sobriety. But a strong addiction usually has a lot of psychological heads like a hydra, new heads constantly popping out to replace the chopped off ones. But the magical fungus gives a strong kick in the butt, dependent people spend a lot of effort, money, and time to achieve what the fly agaric mushroom gives for free.

Report No. 421: From Thomas's chat room. I **lost interest in computer games** during *Amanita muscaria* microdose receptions. It just became uninteresting to play anymore.

Report No. 422: From Masha's YouTube channel. Baba Mash, thanks for your efforts. Since I learned about microdoses and your channel, a lot has changed in my life. Most noticeable changes, I **quit drinking and smoking** and my attitude toward these habits changed. Before, my quitting attempts were painful. With AM microdosing, I just got some kind of awareness of the stupidity of these habits. I almost do not eat **meat** anymore, and **sweets disappeared** completely from my home. In general, the food on the table is healthier.

Report No. 423: From Masha's YouTube channel. Hello, dear Baba Masha, thanks to the knowledge that I received from you about the fly agaric, my **vision is improved** through microdosing! I noticed in eleven days of taking dried fungus that the objects stopped blurring. By the way, I **do not drink alcohol and do not smoke cigarettes** any longer for over a month! I recommend your wonderful channel to all my friends! Be healthy, dear!

Report No. 424: From Masha's YouTube channel. Undoubtedly, at first, I was skeptical of everything related to *Amanita muscaria*. But I read reviews, listened to Masha a lot, and I took short *Amanita muscaria* microdose course. There was very little mushroom collected, but the result is great: I am **sober** for six months, and I **do not have the slightest desire to drink**. I am waiting for the summer. I want to make tincture because my back hurts terribly.

Report No. 425: From Masha's YouTube channel. My first 100 g of AM, I took 2–3 g a day, sometimes in the evening as well in the form of tea with lemon. I did not like the effects. I was irritable, annoyed, and my impatience increased. Along with this were a roller coaster of mood changes. I learned by experience, now I take only 1 g a day.

Report No. 426: From Thomas's chat room. Good health to all. The day before yesterday I received a small **ankle injury** in my boxing training class. In the morning it was **painful** to step on my foot, and a bruise appeared. I put AM ointment (badger fat + dried AM) and elastic bandage over it. Relief came in a few minutes, **acute pain left**. During the day I did not walk very much, the leg was mainly at rest. Upon arrival home after work in the evening, the bandage was removed. The pain remained only in extreme positions (if I rotate the foot), the bruise was noticeably gone. Next morning I woke up with no pain. I was very pleased. In the evening I got back to training.

Report No. 427: From Thomas's chat room. I suffered **knee joint pain** from childhood for twenty-five years. Not every night, but with varying constancy. I never went to the doctors. I began to consume mukhomor in December 2019 in the form of dry caps. So far, the pain doesn't bother me for two months. Sometimes it happens, of course, but this is nothing compared to how it used to be. I take about 1 g in the mornings as a tea.

Report No. 428: From Thomas's chat room. I take an AM microdose in the morning about 1–2 g after breakfast. After the surgery on my fractured elbow, I had constant pain and discomfort in my joint especially with hard physical work. After *Amanita muscaria* microdoses **discomfort and pain are gone**.

Report No. 429: From Masha's YouTube channel. I was tormented with **migraines** after a severe concussion with amnesia. The fly agaric mushroom intake completely restored my thinking processes, and the migraines also left.

Report No. 430: From Thomas's chat room. After a half month of AM microdosing, I turned into a deity, alas, I can't find other words. I can't explain it, I just understood everything, everything became clear. **Life turned upside down in a good way**. I expected much less. In my case it works. I read the chat and was surprised how many specific ailments people cured with AM microdosing.

Report No. 431: Sent to Masha personally via Telegram messenger. Greetings to Baba Masha! The old cat had a swollen cheek. Last time I took him to the veterinarian with this problem. He cut the cat cheek and squeezed out pus. This time I wetted cotton ball with AM tincture and treated outside and inside the mouth on the side of the tumor. The next day the **swelling came**

down. Third day there was almost nothing left and cat's appetite returned. In short, everyone must have a home kit for both people and animals.

Report No. 432: From Masha's YouTube channel. Microdoses pulled me out of the deepest **depression**. I did not want to live; there were nervous break-downs one by one. I was healed with fasting, AM microdosing, and "Brain Illiteracy Liquidation" (Masha's audio program). All of it helped a great deal, and now I am happy.

Report No. 433: From Masha's YouTube channel. Hello! First time I heard about the mukhomor on the "Slavic radio." I immediately ordered AM tinc-ture. They sent me instructions for intake. On the twentieth day of reception, a 30 cm **worm came out**! I was in shock! I never saw such monsters alive in my body. Tests never showed that! Later on, I saw the changes in my body— all the sluggish current conditions went away; there was **pain** in my nose, gums, ears, knee joints, and headache. It's all gone! These symptoms were present over five years. First days of AM tincture course were accompanied by diarrhea, acne, but as the instruction said—it is ok. Tincture gives me a magnificent, gradual healing, and everyone else says that I look younger. Now I also take dried AM 1 g, three times a day. I **sleep** better than I ever have in my life.

Report No. 434: From Masha's YouTube channel. I microdosed a month. The result: after the injury, I was prescribed carbamazepine, and for six months I was just a **depressive vegetable**. I **quit taking pills** and switched to *Amanita muscaria* mushroom. I was just fine after microdosing, even a little better.

Report No. 435: Sent to Masha personally via Telegram messenger. Hello, Masha! Thank you for the super channel! I listen to you so much, and I like you so much that my conscience speaks with your voice. Yesterday I went into the kitchen to eat some junk food, and my conscience said with your voice: "Don't be a fool. Feel sorry for your liver. Go do something better." I want to share the experience of *Amanita muscaria* microdoses intake. The daily course duration was sixty-seven days. On some days I made records of my conditions.

Day 1: 0.33 g on an empty stomach in the morning, I felt nothing.

Day 2: 0.72 g, my **appetite was suppressed**.

Day 3: 1 g, I felt like I was wasting my life. I want to be creative, and instead I spent long hours in Moscow to work and back. It is like being in a hell that I haven't noticed before.

Day 6: 1.6 g, **increased attention, excellent concentration**. A lot of strength has appeared. The laziness is gone. I manage to finish all my work. Sexual sensations increased three times. Empathy intensified. No worries. Time began to flow, as if it slowed down.

Day 11: 1.9 g, I came to work, felt wobbly and sleepy. Everything fell out of my hands. The body was like cotton. Colleagues were scared. I joked that I didn't sleep enough. In fact, after 1 g the mukhomor acts on me like sleeping pills. (Since then, I have defined my ideal measure: 0.6–0.8 g.)

Day 20: 3 g on a hungry stomach in the morning and after forty minutes I was knocked out for five hours, or rather, my body was knocked out, but not consciousness. I was pushed into bed. All this time I watched visions and could not move. There was a feeling that I was shown meaningless nonsense. At the fifth hour I was able to move, but I was like a person with paralysis. Fingers twitched on their own, as if they wanted to jump out of my arms, mumbling speech. After two hours my body calmed down, and I was overwhelmed by **euphoria, cheer**, increased **concentration, love**, as if it were ecstasy. Like they pulled me out of the outlet and plugged me back in.

Day 26: 0.9 g, I was introduced into some kind of **spiritual** jet. I always want to talk to God. I am not a member of any religious dogma; the concept of God is not connected in my mind with religion. In general, I always want to have a connection with something Big and to think deeper and larger.

Day 67: Everything has normalized. The **emotional state** is beautiful. Less garbage inside my head. I get joy from the small things. Fears of other people have disappeared. Greater acceptance of oneself. Unimportance of delusions. No more desire of empty chit-chats. I'm not out of the picture; I'm inside the picture of my life. Today I ate 4 g for the night and saw bright **dreams**. I woke up late. This time without twitching. With a **clear head** and with a **desire to create**. I can stare at the cat's coat and see the universe in there. In conclusion, I want to say that the fungus balances individually. Prosperity to your channel and community!

Report No. 436: From Masha's YouTube channel. Once I got **inflammation in my toe joint** and could not walk because of **pain**. I made a compress with AM tincture for two hours, and the next morning the inflammation went away and I could sense the pain only when I squeezed the toe. After second application everything returned to normal. The tincture was made with 50% homemade moonshine. My experience with drying AM: The first time I did it wrong in the oven. Mushrooms baked, lost juice and blackened later, although they dried with an open door and up to 60°C [140°F]. The second time I laid AM caps on the table for a day and a half, without the sun, until "wrinkles" appeared. Then I dried them in the oven with the same temperature and method as first time. They dried in excellent form, in a consistency like chips. I could break it up with my hand into small pieces. The third method was dried simply on the table until completely dried. They have become similar to very hard crumbs and no longer could be broken with the hand. Therefore, if there is no electric dryer for vegetables, you can dry in the oven, but use the second method to get better results.

Report No. 437: Sent to Masha personally via Telegram messenger. I have been unsuccessfully treated for **alcohol dependence** in the past. Then I discovered the mukhomor. I am in a little shock. I **lost alcohol cravings**. **Quit smoking cigarettes**; it became disgusting. I consume 3–4 g in the evening, every second day. I want to know—is that too much?

Masha: Big doses could bring a mood breakdown. Take less: 1 g will be enough.

—Good! I have been alcohol coded since September. I did not drink, but I was tortured with craving. I went to a psychologist, but had hard breakdown anyway and had to go to the hospital. Three weeks ago, I "met" a fungus. I do not need a psychologist anymore. My **head is clear**, no craving. There were some problems at work, but now everything is fine! I do not experience motivation and life excitement yet, as they write here. Laziness is present.

Report No. 438: Sent to Masha personally via Telegram messenger. Four years ago I accidentally stumbled upon the channel of Baba Masha. At first I rejected the information. But as I studied the podcast and other information, it became clear that I need to try it myself to draw my own conclusion. I got together with a friend, gained fly agarics, dried it, and consumed AM microdoses according to the instructions in the video. The effect was quite good; **we quit smoking**, became more positive, things began to be much better and easier. Six months of microdosing in the morning, and in the evening 1.5 g with some pauses. Baba Masha, well done. She carries about a powerful truth of the psychedelic world. Cheers!

Report No. 439: From Masha's YouTube channel. My **dreams** with fly agaric are funny, colored, and very unusual. I **stopped drinking alcohol**. I have not drunk for more than six months. Thanks to Baba Masha for the information.

Report No. 440: From Thomas's chat room. The other day my hand was very badly bruised. I was in pain all night, and I thought it was a fracture, but then I decided that it was likely just a severe bruise of the soft tissues. In the morning a huge bruise formed, descending on the wrist. Next day I rubbed AM vodka tincture over my hand three times a day. In the next evening the pain decreased significantly even if I pressed on the bruise. The next day there was **no pain**, and I was able to train with weights. The bruise passed in three days. I am very impressed!

Report No. 441: Sent to Masha personally via Telegram messenger. I'm forty years old, a cute man. I'll start with the fact that smart people sooner or later face a depression problem. Previously, I could not have thought that a healthy, young man might encounter this diagnosis. Asthenia, guilt, self-eating, feeling of helplessness. I have gone through a number of tests. I was diagnosed with **depression** and prescribed antidepressant Sertraline. Half of the symptoms disappeared. But I realized that living on pills for the rest of my days was not an option. And as it should be, to the modern citizen, I began to look for answers on the internet. Baba Masha appeared in my life. I was like a sponge absorbing her words. How much work and soul she invests in her work to bring to us all the experience of generations. I ordered 100 g of mukhomor and began to microdose. I abruptly removed the antidepressant. AM gave me **strength, vigor, confidence, clarity of mind**. My **fatigue passed, and sleep improved**. I want to paint again, say nice words, read, communicate with people, and be patient and social. It **shook out all the fears** and childhood blocks from my soul! I'm back. There is happiness, gratitude, and love in my soul. I have a clear and bright mind. I'm just learning. I think that we all need to look for a way out from the saddest moments in our lives; they always can be found. Everything works! Baba Masha, thank you very much! Kindness to all!

Report No. 442: From Masha's YouTube channel. Love and peace. I collected mukhomors myself, dried in an electric dryer at 70°C [158°F]. I kept it in a cool, dark place. I use soma (milk AM drink), and I take 3 g of dried AM with juice and honey at night. **Well-being, positive mood, great sleep presents**. Baba Masha, thank you very much!

Report No. 443: From Thomas's chat room. There was a **beer addiction**. The mukhomor removed it. So far 106 days without alcohol or craving.

Report No. 444: From Thomas's chat room. After *Amanita muscaria* micro-doses, the **flu and cold** are afraid of me. Before, I was sick almost once a month. My **migraines passed**. I feel good.

Report No. 445: From Thomas's chat room. I have very **greasy hair**, and I have to wash it twice a day with a shampoo to get rid of it. After a short course of AM microdosing, it was normalized, even though I did not take AM microdoses for that purpose.

Report No. 446: From Masha's YouTube channel. Mukhomor microdoses helped to **stop hair loss**. Eight years I was unsuccessfully using all possible treatments. I take 1–2 g AM microdose in the evening on empty stomach. I cannot take it during the day because they give me a little buzz. My friends began to microdose in early autumn. They look younger, **quit alcohol and smoking**. One of them noticed that AM microdosing stopped hair loss too. Thanks for everything, again. With respect and kindness to you.

Report No. 447: From Thomas's chat room. I want to share a really proven action of an ointment from mukhomor in the fight against **psoriasis**. I am a person who for twenty years unsuccessfully applied everything that is sold in pharmacies to fight psoriasis. Mukhomor ointment has done its job clearly and confidently; the skin has cleared. I made ointment from dried powdered mukhomor and bear fat. I applied ointment before bed. After first over-whelming success I began to apply it twice a day. It took twenty days to get rid of scales. It's just perfect. Be healthy, bring each other positive things.

Report No. 448: From Masha's chat room. All my life I ate bread, adding it to every dish. Surprisingly, I stopped eating bread after one month's of tak-ing AM microdoses, although there were no thoughts to refuse bread. The effect is stable. I paused using AM microdoses now for three weeks, and I **don't eat bread**, and I don't want to.

Report No. 449: From Masha's YouTube channel. I've used AM microdosing for four years. I have all positive effects. I collect, dry, prepare tincture and lotions myself. The drying temperature in dehydrator is between 40°C and 60°C [104°F–140°F]. Lotion made from dried AM with buckthorn oil. I make tincture with high proof alcohol, and the final product is about 38-degree proof. It is interesting that I harvest mushrooms in the same place for years and the power of *Amanita muscaria* mushrooms is different every year.

Report No. 450: From Thomas's chat room. Mukhomor mushroom removed my long-term **caffeine dependence**.

Report No. 451: Sent to Masha personally via Telegram messenger. Baba Masha, hi! In September I began AM microdosing in order to improve mood and quit alcohol dependence. My **mood improved; confidence appeared very noticeably**. However, I was drinking beer during AM micro-dosing every day and I had an excellent mood and noticed that the better my mood, the more I want to drink. Question: How can I use AM to stop the **alcohol habit**?

Masha: Hello, to quit alcohol, you need to want it and keep yourself in control without hope for a miracle. Obviously, microdosing with beer will not help you.

Report No. 452: From Thomas's chat room. According to my feelings there is no rollback if you do not increase the dosage to minidosing. It's been my fifth month of AM microdosing. I had a two-week break and I'm starting AM microdosing again. It is interesting that during the break, I maintained a sta-ble positive state. Before AM microdosing intake there was severe **depres-sion**. At the beginning I experienced **gastrointestinal aggravation**, and it went away quick. Now I'm flying! After four months I felt the cumulative effect, and it definitely does not disappear if I stop AM microdose intake. The general condition is excellent, the **mood is good**, it turned me away from **sweets**, but not completely. It turned me away from **alcohol** too. I do not drink anymore and I do not have a desire to drink. I am planning another month of mukhomor microdosing.

Report No. 453: From Masha's YouTube channel. All January I could not get out of the anabiosis of the post-holiday time. There was no energy at all, stuck at work, did not want to do anything, my sleep was shitty. I read an article about the mukhomor microdosing. After two weeks of AM micro-dosing, I returned to work. From the very first days of reception my **sleep** became good, **dreams** began to be fantastic movies, colorful and interesting. Before AM microdosing I did not see dreams at all for a very long time. I lost all craving for **alcohol**. Before *Amanita muscaria* microdoses I could drink some beer or whiskey with cola; now I have no thought about drinking.

Report No. 454: Hello, I use AM microdosing, fourth day and I already have positive changes. I started with 1 g and lowered the dosage to 0.3 g. **I became more sociable**. I also noticed that the "ego" had become healthier.

In the mornings my thoughts became optimistic; the world became more friendly.

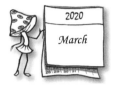

Report No. 455: From Thomas's chat room. My grandmother of eighty-three years, after two weeks of 0.5 g *Amanita muscaria* microdoses in the morning has had great improvement—constant **swelling** on her legs disappeared and **blood pressure** normalized. We did not know the reason for swelling; Grandma refused to go to doctors. We thought that she had problems with her kidneys. She was taking diuretic pills, but they did not help, swelling did not recede. By evening her blood pressure rose to 180 every day; now it's normalized and it is up to 160 only in bad weather. I did not say to grandma the name of the mushroom, so she would not be scared. But I already see that she has confidence in mukhomor.

Report No. 456: From Thomas's chat room. My AM microdosing feedback—I drink less **alcohol** and my **fears** diminished.

Report No. 457: From Masha's chat room. Good day, friends. I want to share my recent six months experience of *Amanita muscaria* microdosing by 1 g per day. In the process of AM microdose course, I **quit smoking** cigarettes, pot, **turned down alcohol** consumption, and many other positive results. It cured **cold, sore throat**, and cough with 4 g AM very quickly. Consciousness is not changed. It lasted about two hours. Then I slept through the night. The next day I felt great. I also signed up for the gym and began to walk. Prior to this, I was engaged in sports about twenty years ago. I continue AM microdose course by 1 g in the morning.

Report No. 458: Dialogue from Thomas's chat room.
—Hello to everyone. For almost two months I take mukhomor from 2–6 g per day, I have constant nausea. What should I do to remove the nausea?
Masha: The dosage gives you the nausea. Microdose is 1 g or less.

Report No. 459: From Thomas's chat room. This is my review of my husband's microdosing. He took AM microdoses for two weeks and quit because he did not see any noticeable effect. But I will describe the facts. In the first days the mukhomor put him to **sleep**, because before he slept usually only for 5–6 hours. He never could sleep for 7–8 hours. There was no stimulating effect. I have a conclusion that if there is no depression, then everything remains as it is and an internal AM microdose reception gave nothing to a healthy and satisfied person. It is interesting that his **skin problems** began to pass. I think he needs to continue working with AM ointment or cream. There was **multicolored chronic fungal infection** in some places of his body. It began to pass during microdosing, but it was not enough because he quit AM microdosing. Also, he could not drink alcohol during AM microdosing; he had a bad reaction on it. It is probably a negative effect for him.

Report No. 460: Sent to Masha personally via Telegram messenger. After the very first AM microdose intake, my seventy-nine-year-old grandma's **skin color** changed from pale to pink. I will continue to observe.

Report No. 461: From Thomas's chat room. Five months of AM microdosing. Obvious changes: several years long-lasting **depression** has completely gone. I still work on my bad habits. It took me awhile to find my ideal dosage. Now I take 0.5–0.7 g once (morning or afternoon). Mukhomor is strict on me. There was no instant enlightenment or miraculous insight, as some described. I am not waiting for an instant miracle from AM microdosing. The first four months I had **mood swings**. Mushroom showed my strengths and weaknesses. Nevertheless, this "training" was accompanied by internal confidence, optimism, and energy. It's like I've grown stronger and older. I saw my mistakes and how I act with people. I began to see the essence of human problems, mine and others. Compassion for people, **empathy has increased**. I have come to understand my call, what I really want to do in life and how to achieve that. I decided to re-learn and master new sciences and to develop my abilities. Creative inspiration appeared. Reality began to manifest itself differently. When I walk around the city (I live in St. Petersburg), I feel some kind of artificiality and absurdity of the metropolis. Like I'm in a matrix. But again, all the observations are high. There's no disappointment. It is very interesting to observe and realize all this. I came to the understanding that microdosing is not for everyone; not everyone is ready to accept their dark side, to change and work on themselves. I think this knowledge should be very carefully distributed, and it is better to be silent in general. I read this chat and understand that many people perceive AM as a magic pill that will do everything for them. It's not. I have such good results and I understand that there is still a lot to be done by myself. My microdosing continues another 1.5 months. Then I will take a long break until the fall. I wonder how the pause will show itself.

Report No. 462: From Masha's YouTube channel. Good day, BM. I wanted to share the effects of one-month AM microdose course. I take a tea made from a teaspoon of powdered AM in the morning. I began sport training. My **internal chatter stopped, fears and worries disappeared**. I feel as a silent **observer** in ringing silence against the background on which all the rest of my being takes place. My words and actions simply arise and occur themselves, both depending on the circumstances and simply on their own, as if a certain impulse gives a kick to my ass. I dealt with my pain and found its cause. After I simply changed to the opposite view. I do not deny anything, and I do not accept, complete neutral view to everything, there is no right or wrong, everything is simply there and everything is fine in nature because it serves something. I wish kindness to everyone and a lot of fly agarics in your home as a first-aid kit.

Report No. 463: From Thomas's chat room. My AM microdose course lasted twenty days. I started with 1.5 g and soon lowered it to 1 g or less. I took it on an empty stomach in the morning, 20–30 minutes before breakfast. I experienced a rush of **energy, positive emotions, empathy** for others. I also want to say on verbal **communication**, it is easy and positive now. I paused AM microdosing, and after ten days, I began to realize many important things that I thought about before as superficial questions with no answers. The main advantage is that I completely lost my **alcohol** craving, and I finally understood what poison it was. I am furious about alcohol's shitty propaganda, describing alcohol as absolutely normal and a cool substance. Alcohol propaganda is absolutely everywhere in our society to young children and adults, designating alcohol superb and great. I also reduced **sugar** consumption after AM microdosing. Only one minus—the thirst for smoking wasn't gone—perhaps became even worse.

Report No. 464: From Thomas's chat room. My experience of "communication" with mukhomor is very positive! Within a month I **became objectively calmer, I stopped having an acute reaction to stimuli**, there is no "offending, criticizing or accusing," etc. I look calmly at worldly fuss and I do not participate in it. I live my life calmly. On the downside—sleep deterioration. But this, as I realized is different for others. I consider microdosing very useful! I don't see any kickbacks yet.

Report No. 465: From Thomas's chat room. I've been microdosing for a month. About 0.5 g in the morning and evening. Sometimes I take a couple days break. During all this time I noticed changes in my behavior. If I waste my time sitting in front of screens, I am getting very angry later, panic arises and the feeling that my life is leaking somewhere. On the contrary, I have huge **clarity** in my head, complete **calm** even in front of the most strenuous deadlines, and a lot of **energy** while working. The laziness still persists, but it is not pleasant anymore.

Report No. 466: From Thomas's chat room. First week of AM microdosing, the energy is like a fountain (I do not have precise scales). I am taking a teaspoon of ground AM in the morning on empty stomach and one hour before bed. Everything leveled out, things are done calmer and precise, without distraction to the surroundings events. **Sleep** without dreams, no problem to wake up in the morning. I am going to finish all 50 g of *Amanita muscaria* and take a break! I expected bright dreams, but they simply are not. I was interested in lucid dreams before and now I lost it.

Report No. 467: From Thomas's chat room. Mukhomor collects all my **energy** into one whole thing; it helps me to **concentrate** on goals, showing me what is not important. I do not worry about the past, the future. I am present in my mind. I fall asleep after eating a gram and plunge into lucid-like dreams. In my sleep the mushroom shows my subconscious fears, which I suppress in myself. **Sleep** is stronger, but sometimes I have too much energy. Sleep time is slightly reduced. Every gram is like a big trip, a lot of awareness when I perform everyday actions like driving or walking down the street. **Sociability, empathy, creativity, attention, concentration.** Perception is increasing, music became brighter, the whole world is perceived differently, the grass is greener, the house is more beautiful. I stick to anything I do; I plunge into it. I have less gloom about the opinion of others about my actions. It is easier to get acquainted with the female gender, less caring when you are refused. It is easy to get away from conflicts; if someone begins to be rude, I look at him with shining eyes, smile, and his desire to fight disappears. I also learned to verbally escape from conflicts. People feel the powerful energy and charm in me, they reach for me, they look at me with some admiration; I attract them to me. The effect is obvious while the mukhomor acts, but here I need to consolidate new habits without a mushroom. If I take a couple of grams, I became an invulnerable fighter who is not afraid of pain, with no doubt about victory, even if there is no chance to win; 2 g give me powerful aggressive energy. If I had known about this mushroom in my younger years, I would've definitely become a fighter champion of something. Mukhomor microdoses are a very useful thing for combat sports.

Report No. 468: Sent to Masha personally via Telegram messenger. First days I took a tea brewed with 0.8–0.9 dried *Amanita muscaria*. Now I am taking it in dry form—0.65 g. At the same time the brewed one acted discreetly and a dried one gave me yucky feeling. AM microdosing returned my former **exuberance and activity**; I can do work again, forgetting about fatigue and food. I get up in the morning without despising the beginning of the day. There is **no more panic and depression**. In the past I had chronic and rapid fatigue, depressing, the state of hopelessness, and lack of opportunity to realize myself. This is no longer. These attacks are most likely associated with nervous overload due to family relationships and subsequent drinking for several weeks. Mukhomor works miracles; just at first I was frightened by the sharp transition to its influence. I will set myself up in the future to meet the Teacher Mukhomor. I want to learn; I've learned so little in this life.

Report No. 469: From Masha's chat room. Hello, Baba Masha. I choose to take this tool seriously and use it only in microdoses. I tried AM trip twice, but it did not happen and I got nausea and flight of thoughts, but happily I did not lose my mind. I learned later on how dangerous AM trips could be. Microdoses helped me cope with deep **depression** after a breakup. My body was also cleaned up, some mucus was coming "out of all holes." After that, I easily rejected **sugar** consumption, although previously I drank about two liters of cola a day and 3.5 spoons of sugar in a cup of tea. Then I refused **flour** and **meat**. I also noticed that I become more aggressive if I eat meat, and my consciousness is lost. Before I ate what different animals (parasites) required inside my body; after mukhomor drove them out, I no longer needed sugar, etc. in such an amount. As to the pros, I **quit playing video games** altogether; it was my problem from childhood, hundreds of thousands of hours of my life spent on this. But now at twenty-three, after I was hit by all the problems—I woke up, my shell split (as you say in one of the videos), and I really **began to notice the signs of the universe**. I feel that I have not noticed before, all these synchronicities and causal consequences in my life. This is so obvious. Thanks to *Amanita* and you, I went headlong into self-development, put myself in order, and there are clear intentions what to do next. Makenna, Leary, Wilson, etc., read out and it all goes straight to cheers. I get such a release of endorphins into the brain by absorbing interesting information. I'm preparing in this way through theory for deeper practices. Sorry for such a huge text, I really wanted to share with you. I respect you very much and thank you for appearing on my way. It means a lot to me.

Report No. 470: From Masha's chat room. AM microdose course about three months. I have been regularly taking half a cap (in the morning and evening). Pros: the **quality of sleep** has improved, I sleep tight, I don't remember dreams. **Nervousness decreased.** There was an appetite. Cons: Drowsiness in the morning. In the early days nervousness increased. What do you advise, continue the appointment or pause?

Masha: Skip morning intake and check if drowsiness goes away.

Report No. 471: From Thomas's chat room. My results of AM microdose intake for four months, 0.5–1 g. I quit **smoking**, I **quit alcohol**, I do **sports**, I eat **healthy food**, I got **inner calm and balance.**

Report No. 472: Sent to Masha personally via Telegram messenger. I am a forty-four-year-old man; my weight is 60 kg [132 pounds]. I began to microdose 2–3 days after I woke up from a month-and-a-half alcoholic binge. Goals: get rid of tobacco and alcohol addiction and cure nail fungus. As a result I don't drink **alcohol** for a month. I read somewhere that there could be a fatal outcome if alcohol is combined with *Amanita.* It is a fact that I do not crave alcohol as before. Smoking, on the contrary, increased. The fungus is still not giving up, but I didn't expect it that quickly. Bonuses: Mukhomor **took away tiredness and chronic fatigue,** which lasted many years. It's like I became 10–15 years younger. I get up early without an alarm clock; this was only in the army, I am amazed! I do not have bad feelings in the beginning of the day! The "energizer bunny" has returned, which was lost many years ago. Before, it was activated only occasionally; now it is easier for me to work. Food preferences have not changed, but I noted that I can eat more spicy food without negative consequences for GI. I experimented with different AM doses from a quarter of the average cap and less. I tried dried and tea form. My optimal dose is from 0.3 to 0.6 of dried AM powder; that keeps me all day in good condition. Mukhomor slowly adjusts and heals me. I wish goodness and health to all! Masha respect!

Report No. 473: From Thomas's chat room. I went through several courses of AM microdosing. It was therapeutic. I got rid of many illusions. Now I **see**

everything with completely different eyes. I also found out that the person closest to me is a manipulator. I was in shock.

Report No. 474: From Thomas's chat room. Hi everyone. I bought mukhomor and just got it. I took half a level teaspoon. There was sweating and mild level of paranoia. I think it could be associated with discomfort in the stomach. Appetite was good. In the evening I went to play football and this perhaps was one of my best games. And I didn't notice it alone; it was a hell of a game. In the evening I drank beer, began to feel the funny taste of beer. I took my usual sleeping pills before bed. I woke up easy in the morning. I have unusual **clarity of thought**. My following studies went easier. Later afternoon I felt a slight sweating and unpleasant light level of paranoia. The dosage was reduced from 0.5 to 0.2 g. In fact, I feel even such a small amount. I use AM microdoses about a month and half. I regain my balance, lot of **energy and concentration** for evening studies, I easily **ignore nonsense**, I **quit computer games**, I have more attention for my family, I **play football better**. I run faster, I make nonstandard decisions in the game, strong movements, much faster shoot, punches, and the reactions are stronger. I consider my mukhomor experience totally positive.

Report No. 475: From Thomas's chat room. *Amanita muscaria* microdoses gave me benefits that I did not expect—**good sleep**, great dreams, and it removed the **nail fungus** (I am in shock, of course). I'm very grateful for the help. My bad **coffee habit** is gone.

Report No. 476: From Thomas's chat room. I take 1 g AM microdose in the morning for two weeks. I have been **energetically** walking to work smiling at all passersby, I am **confident** in myself. At work I do my work much faster now and am way ahead of all my colleagues. This is my fourth AM microdose course. I did not have that effect before. Perhaps the accumulation played an effect; perhaps I bought better mukhomor this time. All four courses were from different sellers, but the last one directly covers all. **No sleepiness** in the morning, I get up charged thirty minutes before the alarm clock.

Report No. 477: Sent to Thomas personally via Telegram messenger. I have an old disturbing **injury to the thoracic spine**. I tried pills, injections, but my condition was going down to the point where I could not always get out of bed. I found Masha's channel in February. On March 16, I started using AM microdose ointment prepared by Thomas twice a day. Today is ten days of use of AM microdose ointment. Pain went away day five, today I managed yoga exercises. I can't believe that it is real; I smile again, I don't have that state of endless **pain**. To be honest it seems to me that this is a fairy tale. I understand that it is emotions, but it is true and it is real. I apologize for the emotions. Thank you very much, Thomas. Health to all.

Report No. 478: Sent to Masha personally via Telegram messenger. I already see the results of AM microdosing in my grandma (seventy-six years old). She takes a tiny pinch only. The quality and awareness of **speech improved, the absence of irritation, elevation of attention and focus** during the conversation without brain freeze and irritations. **Fears gone.** She is feeling younger, vigorous, and much happier than before AM microdose course.

Report No. 479: From Thomas's chat room. I heavily bruised my hand at work. I used an overnight compress made from leftover fungus after tincture preparation for five days. In general, today is the fifth day, I still have the bruise but the **pain** is almost gone, the hypostasis of palm and wrist joint disappeared. It was a quick recovery; I'm already driving and using my hand.

Report No. 480: Sent to Masha personally via Telegram messenger. Masha, hello from the Rostov region. I used AM microdosing for two months with two weeks break, 0.5–1 g a day. **Warts** disappeared. Also, I noticed positive changes in my **mood**. I am planning to introduce AM microdosing to my parents.

Report No. 481: From Thomas's chat room. I took AM microdses by 0.5 g for one month, with one-week break followed with one-month AM microdosing. After completion of reception, I obtained only positive results. There were **no problems with GI or liver**.

Report No. 482: Sent to Masha personally via Telegram messenger. Masha, I'd like to thank you for information about mukhomor. I do not believe in fairy tales, but my grandson slipped me that fungus without telling me what it was. Then he signed me on to your channel. I microdosed over three months, 1 g or less, twice a day, morning and evening. I am seventy-two, so you know it hurts here and there and all other senile gadgets. I feel much easier; I feel younger both internally and externally. I began to walk a lot, just here on the edge of our village, so far without quarantine here. No more **joint pain, the mood is completely positive,** starting right in the morning. I **sleep** so well that you won't wake me up with a gun; before, I used to squirm like an eel until dawn. Bow to you! Peace and happiness to all.

Report No. 483: Sent to Masha personally via Telegram messenger. Hello, Masha. I started AM microdose course with 1 g. It made me sleepy during the day with following **boost of energy**, sometimes aggression. I experimented with the dosage and end up with 0.2 g. This amount gives me the effect of concentrated stimulation on the positive side and raises up my motivation. I feel great, it helps to **eat less** and **move more**. If the doses are slightly exceeded, then I become aggressive and feel that adrenaline rush. I do not drink alcohol and I don't want to smoke anymore. Electronic cigarettes haven't stopped. Now I am permanently in contact with a coronavirus patient, but I am not sick, there are no symptoms. Thank you.

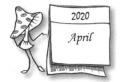 **Report No. 484:** From Thomas's chat room. Good morning, friends. I want to share my month course of AM microdosing, 0.8 g overnight. Additionally, I inhale a little AM powder in each nostril. It fought symptoms of **herpes**, which tormented me for five years. **Sinuses** are actively cleaning. I began to **have fun and laugh** more. I **sleep** well. For me, these are positive results.

Report No. 485: From Masha's chat room. I used alcohol to hide my shy neurotic state, which I especially have while communicating with girls. I switched to AM microdosing. Now I am **relaxed**. If I want to be more active, I take a little bigger amount.

Report No. 486: From Thomas's chat room. I observe different **reaction to different batches of mukhomor**. From some I have slight fever. Today I took 1 g and had some nausea and chills. Earlier, I had eaten another batch and there was no such thing. On the contrary, my father does not feel anything like that at all with the same amount—1 g on empty stomach in the mornings. He did not know what I gave him; he thinks that these are some healing roots. He **lost 4 kg** [9 pounds] in twenty-one days and **feels energetic**. Only this morning I told my father that he's taken AM microdoses for twenty-two days. He laughed. I did not expect such a reaction. He is sixty-nine years old. I love my father. I will send full report after April 13; it will be exactly a month he has been taking *Amanita muscaria* microdoses.

Report No. 487: From Thomas's chat room. My friend treated her mother (eighty-six years) with AM microdosing after a **stroke**. She eventually recovered very quickly, now she walks and speaks well.

Report No. 488: Sent to Masha personally via Telegram messenger. Hello, Masha. I want to share seventeen days of mukhomor reception. In the beginning I did not see any amazing effects except the morning vigor. Later on, I noticed the changes. I **became more balanced**, and it is easier to relate to the surrounding reality. I smile more often and cry less. I plan to take AM microdoses again in the future.

Report No. 489: From Masha's chat room. The effect of *Amanita muscaria* microdosing is not going to be seen immediately. It reveals in a couple of weeks. There will be an understanding that you are already different than before. I do not advise more than 1 g. I personally take 0.5 g before bedtime. I used *Amanita muscaria* microdoses for three weeks; I took a short break and then another month of *Amanita* microdoses.

Report No. 490: From Masha's chat room. The first effect of AM microdosing that I noticed was improved quality of **sleep**, **dreams** became more realistic. The desire to eat **sweets** is gone, although I love it. I began to **get up before the alarm**. I look at the sky and smile; it is a state of **joy** as in childhood. **Worries** are gone, my head is in full order. It is easier to multitask—to solve and find the answers. There's more **energy**. My wife saw my changes and she wanted to try AM microdosing as well, although before she was against it. I also persuaded my parents. My father has **rheumatoid arthritis**; he lost sleep due to the **pain** and now he is sleeping like a child. In general, the quality of our lives has improved many times.

Report No. 491: From Masha's chat room. I took 1 g AM microdose twice a day for a month.
   Results: I do not eat **sugar** (previously I used 3.5 teaspoons in one cup of tea); I quit **alcohol** completely. My mom has changes too; I will write a report later, after she finishes one-month *Amanita muscaria* microdoses course.

Report No. 492: From Thomas's chat room. My father uses AM rubbing alcohol tincture for two months to treat **joint pain**. It works.

Report No. 493: From Masha's chat room. I take up to 1 g AM microdose only once a day. It activates all life systems in absolute harmony, tone, activity, and at the same time there is **relaxation**, **clear thoughts**, I feel and see the **vigor** of my body and spirit. I don't want to eat **sugar** and **flour**. I feel what my body needs. I eat meat, my ancestors ate it, I will not break this system, everything is good with this!

Report No. 494: From Thomas's chat room. I took AM microdose about three months up to 1 g a day. "Red mushroom" works with addictions for sure. I experienced it on myself. I **quit smoking, alcohol, and opium** and I do not have cravings. It is almost six months after I finished the course and my condition is stable. Thomas and Masha, stating that competently and sincerely. Thank you, bless everyone.

Report No. 495: From Masha's chat room. Yesterday, at a training session, I hit my knee with a swing of weights. I came back home with constant **pain** and immediately rubbed an alcohol tincture from the mukhomor extract on my knee. An hour later I noticed that there was no pain at all. Today there is no **swelling**; there is no pain while moving. It is a little painful only if I press hard on the place of impact. It was from just one rubbing!

Report No. 496: From Thomas's chat room. Today I hit my pinky toe, the **pain** was hellish. I had mushrooms in alcohol, last year's crop. I took two mushrooms; they were like a sponge. I wrapped them over the toe in gauze and a plastic bag over. Fifteen minutes later the pain was gone! It is really a miracle painkiller!

Report No. 497: From Thomas's chat room. I take *Amanita muscaria* microdoses for seven months regularly. I take breaks from time to time. **Depression** is gone, no kickbacks.

Report No. 498: From Masha's YouTube channel. I am taking AM microdoses in small doses—a third of a teaspoon in the morning and evening. The effects are soothing, **relaxing, anxious thoughts go away**, I get **calmer** and **kinder**. I start to feel my body; I realize that it needs to be cared for and loved. **Energy raised** and **appetite improved**. I have myopia, my **vision improves** slightly, the colors become juicier. If I take *Amanita muscaria* microdoses in the evening, I have calm and strong sleep with rich dreams. In general, the sensations are positive, I will continue.

Report No. 499: From Masha's chat room. I am a thirty-six-year-old man, 120 kg [264 pounds]. I took AM microdoses for a month. The goal is to bring the inner world into an orderly state, also, as an aid in the fight against alcoholism. I bought 30 g AM on the internet. Beautiful caps came, dry as chips. Started with 1 g in the morning. Vigor and empathy for others in the morning was replaced by sleepiness and deadlock by two o'clock. After 5 p.m. it was gone, and I worked the rest of the day without feeling tired. I reduced the dose to one-third teaspoon in the morning and evening. I stopped feeling anything, but at the same time my sleep normalized and the work ceased to tire, I make furniture from 9 a.m. to 8 p.m. without problems. **Alcohol** craving is gone, but I did not quit smoking. Some powder was used to make the ointment, and mukhomor quickly came to an end. I ordered a second batch, twice cheaper from different person but quality of the product was not good, the caps are darker, not so bright and not so crisp. I continued to take one-third of a spoon (about 0.5–0.6 g) in the morning and evening. I did not experience effects such as an epiphany, awareness, craving for beer came back. I am waiting for the season to collect mukhomor myself.

Report No. 500: From Masha's chat room. Masha, I take a teaspoon and have a negative effect. What it the correct amount?

Masha: It is necessary to reduce quantity until it feels comfortable. The right amount is when the dose does not give an immediate effect—negative or positive.

Report No. 501: Sent to Masha personally via Telegram messenger. Masha, my dose is half a teaspoon, it blasts me with **energy**. Before I used a quarter teaspoon, but it was not enough.

Report No. 502: From Masha's chat room. My husband does not drink **alcohol** anymore after using AM microdoses. His alcohol addiction lasted more than ten years ending up with a stomach ulcer. He was drinking weeks straight from eighteen years old to thirty. He is a strong, thinking, sincere, and kind person; he is free from alcohol now with *Amanita muscaria* microdose's help.

Report No. 503: From Thomas's chat room. I'm a thirty-two-year-old man. There was a **birth injury** and it turned into a shortening of the leg. Up to twenty years old everything was good with mental abilities. After twenty I began to roll into the hole, the brain capacity began to fade. I was in pain caused by many spine protrusions and hernias. At the age of twenty-six, I was diagnosed with **encephalopathy** (there is a cyst from hemorrhage) at the Bekhterev's Research Institute. A violation of venous outflow from the brain was noted. The doctor said that the next stage was already unrecoverable. I quit alcohol flat at that moment, but the snake inside my head continued to seduce me. There were gaps in memory, no ability to concentrate, no desires, speech problems, very fast fatigue, increased uncontrollable salivation, weakness, asthenia. I cried from helplessness. I wanted to live, do business projects, have children, and be happy; those were my inspirations to live. I took prescribed pills, it helped for short while, but then it was a rollback. With time, pills did not have effect on me. In August 2019 I found out about mukhomor. I took 3 g per day for two weeks. I began to blossom, **energy** appeared in the body, wanted to get up in the morning, began to sing at home and at the wheel while driving to work with a smile on my face and in my eyes. I tried 10 g for a trip, and I did not get the desired effect and gave up. Mukhomor brought me to Masha's channel, and after studying all information, I had two courses of AM microdoses using 1 g in the morning on empty stomach.

Results for today: I have a smile on my face. I love my world, and all anger triggers are gone. The level of immersion and empathy during communication is very deep and wise. There is joy within my heart and the soul. Nature, forest, water is my charge. The body is light and clean. I dropped **alcohol**, no more craving. The huge craving for **sweets** has fallen away. I replace it with fruits and honey. I rarely indulge in forbidden chocolate. I have no need to return to pharma pills; earlier, three times per year I had to be on a two-month course of injections and pills. **My spine has become more elastic**, and with the help of physical therapy I manage to remove the blocks, no more bromine use. I **talk freely**, my thoughts easily turn into words. I sing a mantra to a recently born daughter. Fast **fatigue has disappeared** and I can work and live all day from 6 a.m. to 11 p.m. easily. **Cognitive functions** work many times better, allowing me to plan tasks, thinking and consciousness are quite clear. Now I'm learning digital marketing. Of course, I still want to add some brain as in the book *The Wizard of Oz*, since I do not reach super productivity. Once again, I thank Masha and Thomas. Nature and possibilities are magical. Peace and health to all.

Report No. 504: From Thomas's chat room. Before AM microdosing the **pain in spine** was bothering me during my work. Two weeks of AM microdosing fixed it, and the pain comes very rarely and much weaker.

Report No. 505: Sent to Masha personally via Telegram messenger. Hi. I am a thirty-year-old man. I want to leave my feedback on AM microdosing. I started microdosing a month ago and continue now. There is no more

chronic pain in the knee; I also rubbed it with Thomas's ointment. I took *Amanita muscaria* microdoses in different ways; eventually I chose an evening reception, at the tip of a teaspoon. Morning reception caused laziness.

Report No. 506: From Thomas's chat room. I would like to say another big thank you to mukhomor and Thomas! **Psoriasis** appeared on the head. Three weeks of torment, my wife brought some ointment from the pharmacy, I used it for a week with no effect. In connection with coronavirus, doctors were not available. I consulted with Thomas and made my own ointment. I used it a few days, and my skin cleared up.

Report No. 507: Sent to Masha personally via Telegram messenger. Hello, dear Masha. I've taken AM microdoses for fifteen days and there are a lot of positive motives. I watch your AM microdosing questionnaire, very knowledgeable, and most important this is for the greater good and a benefit to all people!

Report No. 508: Sent to Masha personally via Telegram messenger. Good evening. I want to say thank you for what you are doing; I stumbled upon the channel completely accidentally on the recommendations of a friend. I've used AM microdosing for ten days already, and my condition became much better. I have fewer **negative thoughts** in my head. I began to notice little things that I had not noticed before, and I see **more positive** in life. I hope that after a long reception it will be even better.

Report No. 509: From Thomas's chat room. I suffer from **chronic tonsillitis** and fever on an ongoing basis is normal to my condition. Since January I fell ill and could not recover from severely pronounced symptoms. Antibiotics. Two weeks I am ok and then sick leave again. So, I ordered mukhomor. I took 1 g for twenty days. My temperature is normal. I have not seen such numbers for several years, lymph nodes decreased, I feel that I am heading in the right direction. The goal of AM microdosing was physical health, but the bonus is my **panic attacks** and obsessions disappeared. I plan to continue AM microdosing; there is still a lot of work in the body and in the head.

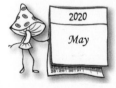

Report No. 510: From Masha's chat. Masha, hi! Thank you for introducing me to mukhomor, and thanks to mukhomor—I **quit smoking** cigarettes, I completely **rejected alcohol**; before, it was the sick topic—beer, every day. The most important, I overcame the **addic-**

tion to marijuana. I didn't admit it before, I smoked a lot and every day and thought it alright, but something clicked in my head, now I do not crave. My wife was shocked about the grass. I thought that I would never have enough willpower to quit, and here I am—clean already for the third month.

Report No. 511: Sent to Masha personally via Telegram messenger. Masha, here's what I want to tell you. I have been taking mukhomor for ten days by 1.2 g in the morning and evening. Microdosing gradually gives me the opportunity to consciously change life and myself like Lego. Yes, the details turned out to be a little plastic quality, but I have learned to rearrange them. I felt a sense of delight, because the game is fascinating, even if it is still a game. Thanks to this feeling, it seems to me that this is the effect of getting out of my **depression**.

Report No. 512: From Thomas's chat room. I have had 200 g of mukhomor in the refrigerator. I eat up to 1 g a day for a month. There was a purge, minor diseases departed, and I did not immediately notice that. Additionally, I am fasting by Islam rules. I like all of it, I began to notice my internal images. I also made a tincture and an ointment from dried mukhomor. The tincture was made with alcohol, and the ointment was mixed with Vaseline. For the time being, my aunt arrived and began to complain about her knees, I offered her to rub the tincture. I made her a compress for the night. In the morning she tells me that her **knees do not hurt** at all. Such a joyful result.

Report No. 513: From Thomas's chat room. My mother is eighty-five years old. She just recovered from coronavirus pneumonia. She has one kidney, pacemaker, esophageal erosion, stomach ulcer, high blood pressure. After ten days on *Amanita muscaria* microdoses and vegetarian nutrition, her condition improved greatly. **She is close to the state in which I remember her** twenty years ago.

Report No. 514: From Thomas's chat room. My feedback on the **dislocated leg** and AM ointment: The first day was difficult to walk. In the evening of the second day, I applied an ointment based on collagen and badger fat. It was 10 p.m. At 4 a.m. I was already walking normally, and a day later there was almost **no inflammation or swelling**. I was skeptical about all the enthusiastic reviews, attributing them more to placebo because I, myself, did not feel any obvious effect from microdosing.

Report No. 515: From Thomas's chat room. Yesterday, my father **hit a toe really hard**. I made him a compress with *Amanita* mushrooms soaked in alcohol. Father said that it is a great **remedy for bruises!** I recommend to everyone! The effect comes almost instantly. My father also used *Amanita muscaria* microdoses for about forty days, 1.2 g in the morning. He is very pleased with the results, irritability disappeared and he is in a **good mood**. He tells everyone at work that mukhomor is a beautiful healing agent! I'll ask him to write his own review at the end of next month.

Report No. 516: Sent to Masha personally via Telegram messenger. Hello, Masha! Thank you for your valuable work! My AM microdosing review: course was for 2.5 months, dosage from 1–5 g, in different ways. The goal is to work out my attitudes, stereotypes, beliefs, etc. The results in physics: a **tick** that I got due to blepharoplasty passed in both eyes. **Hair** began to fall out less, new hedgehogs began to appear. **Periods became easier**. **Constant pain** caused by caesarean surgery that tormented me every morning for several years disappeared. Mental changes: it seems that **depression** is passing. I begin to rejoice in life, allow myself emotions. There were serious troubles that knocked me out of the rut and reversed my life. **Aggression** has been much reduced. There is **hope** for a wonderful future. The other day I had a fight with my husband with a lot of aggression and resentment and desire to divorce him. Later on, I calmed down and came to peace. Also, I can't quit smoking yet.

Masha: Bear in mind that according to information we obtained, an excessive amount of AM leads to spontaneous outbreaks of aggression.

Report No. 517: From Masha's YouTube channel. My comments on AM microdose course breaks: as for the break, I use AM seasonally for 3–5 months after harvest, and I take a break until the next season. **Mukhomor will tell you about your health**; please use without fanaticism.

Report No. 518: From Masha's chat room. Mukhomor microdosing removes addictions, and it seems that the more pronounced the addiction, the better it helps. On the second day I overcame **junk food addiction** and did not want to smoke. After a one week I totally **quit cigarettes** and **coffee**. I am not taking AM microdoses anymore, but I still do not use coffee and cigarettes. No cravings. It's been six months.

Report No. 519: From Masha's YouTube channel. At the age of forty-two, due to health problems after sports and stresses, I **changed my diet** and **quit**

alcohol. Then after two months I found out about Masha and mukhomor, and I took an AM microdose course. Mukhomor and Baba Masha helped a lot to get rid of rubbish in my head and body. I just began to live as I like without accepting dogmas.

Report No. 520: Sent to Thomas personally via Telegram messenger. Good day, Thomas! I want to thank you. I made an ointment based on bear fat with mukhomor by your recipe as you described. When I got **back pain** working in my garden, I rubbed the ointment on my back (May 18). To that point I could not sit or stand because of pain. The pain slowly went away by next day (May 19). I applied the ointment three times and secured it with cellophane wrap. Today is May 23, and I am free of pain! I thank you and the great Power of Mukhomor!

Report No. 521: From Masha's YouTube channel. I realized that I was degraded and began to fall apart from **alcohol addiction**. I began to look for an alternative, and I found the holy mukhomor. I haven't drank booze for almost a year; my wife had more complicated path but managed to quit as well. I recently bought brandy, we drank it, and it we felt awful. Peace.

Report No. 522: From Thomas's chat room. Hi everyone. I **injured my leg** at a football game in the evening. Two hours after the injury, I applied AM cream on my leg and wrapped it with plastic wrap and sock. I prepared cream myself from bear fat and AM that I infused for two months. I got up in the morning, and the pain did not decrease. I reapplied cream + plastic wrap + sock. Additionally, I took a microdose, but this time instead of 0.2 g, I consumed 0.5 g and went to meet my friend. While I was waiting for a man on the street, I discovered that I was walking without limping. About 3–4 hours had passed since the reception. I conclude that the internal intake of the fungus is much more positive than its external use.

Report No. 523: From Thomas's chat room. I want to leave a review of the AM ointment! My husband had major trauma that ended with broken legs and suffers from awful **pain**, especially after physical work. The pain is so strong to the point that he cannot walk. After the very first application of AM ointment, the pain went away very quickly. Such a miracle remedy! We will continue to use the ointment. Great thanks to Thomas!

Report No. 524: Sent to Masha personally via Telegram messenger. Hello, Masha. Thank you, dear, for opening a channel about the mukhomor's medicinal properties. I've used AM microdoses since spring in tea form (0.2 g). It helped with my **sleep and relieves muscle spasm** as well when taken before bedtime. It is also a great tool to energize. I rub AM alcohol tincture in the lumbar region of my back to reduce pain. I noticed that it is better for me to drink AM tea after food, taking it on empty stomach gives me discomfort.

Report No. 525: From Thomas's chat room. The mukhomor normalized my **sleep** duration and its quality. The most important thing is that I began to fall asleep very easily. For five months I have not microdosed, and I am looking forward to a new season.

Report No. 526: Sent to Masha personally via Telegram messenger. Masha, thanks for the book. That's great! So much of your time is invested. I would like to receive a printed copy—the Bible of the Mukhomor. I didn't have time to send my report before the book was published. Although everything coincides with many points described in the book—the disappearance of depression, a decrease in blood pressure, vigor and life joy are present on an ongoing basis. I microdosed for five months with two breaks. I collect AM myself. Waiting for the new season. [. . .]

Report No. 527: Sent to Masha personally via Telegram messenger. Masha, hello, I continue AM microdose course. My problems went away on their own, everything old and unnecessary collapsed without my involvement. The heartburn of many years ago from the **hernia of the esophagus** subsided. Yes, and the appetite weakened. I hope to lose forty pounds. Great! The Mushroom does his job. Thank you, Masha, my bow to you. I heard about the book, and I am going it read with pleasure. I am in L.A. and planning to collect AM in Oregon during new season. We need to make supplies for everyone.

Report No. 528: From Masha's YouTube channel. I do not smoke constantly, but sometimes I experience an awful craving for **nicotine** like an addict. It was erased only with mukhomor. Mukhomor erases the memory of receptors, and you stop reacting and noticing the urge to smoke. It is surprising, especially because I did not take AM microdoses for that purpose.

Report No. 529: From Masha's YouTube channel. Mukhomor microdosing is a great working way to overcome **alcohol** withdrawal syndrome. Masha's opinion is very balanced and causes respect—it is better to motivate for sobriety than for alcoholism.

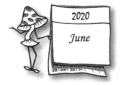

Report No. 530: Sent to Masha personally via Telegram messenger. I'm forty-two, male, weight 78 kg [172 pounds]. I do not have any serious systemic diseases. I used dried AM microdose 1–2 g twice a day. After seven days, I noticed that my vision improved slightly. I **sleep** much better now. The pain in the forehead area caused by frontal sinusitis went away. **Energy** raised, I am **calmer** and more **optimistic** than before. The interesting taste of life appeared. The most significant and the delightful point for me is, of course, a good sleep. Over the past twenty years, I have already forgotten what it is to sleep well and feel awake and active after sleep. Fantastic!

Report No. 531: Sent to Masha personally via Telegram messenger. Thank you, Masha, for the book, very interesting and fascinating, I also participated in surveys about microdosing. Over the year I ate about a kilogram of dried AM with my wife and colleagues from work. I did this because I wanted to collect personal statistics. In general, all participants had their own interests. My personal goal was stimulation in monotonous hard work—processing stone, marble, granite, quartz. My wife is a physician; she finds AM microdosing effects very interesting.

Report No. 532: From Masha's YouTube channel. I use AM microdoses for four days, 0.7–0.8 g every day. I lost desire for social media like Instagram or YouTube that really kill my time. I found out that watching nature and listening to the noise outside the window is much more pleasant. Waking up in the morning from the birds' noise did not cause irritation anymore (as is usually the case), but on the contrary, it is a pleasure and pacification. I began to think less about the actions that I did in the past, who said what about me, what I said, wrote, and have done. I feel the **rise of physical energy**. Now I can easily walk to the fourth floor, before this was accompanied by serious shortness of breath and sweating. I feel that this energy is my internal [self], which always has been inside me but blocked by laziness and apathy.

Report No. 533: Sent to Masha personally via Telegram messenger. Masha, hello, I really want your book in print; as you know our elderly are not computerized and have difficulties trusting the internet. Their heads stuck in TV, full of fears. I really want to drop your book on them so they read and make a choice. About myself: thirty-seven-year-old man, I have been taking mukhomor microdoses since February last year back and forth, after reviewing the results from your first group of sixty-seven people on your YouTube channel. Honestly, I did not believe it myself, but I really wanted a kick against alcohol. The result is striking, not only did **alcohol** leave my life, but also life, thoughts, and health changed in amazing and completely different ways. Thank you, I'm waiting for the printed version.

Report No. 534: Sent to Masha personally via Telegram messenger. They said, "microdosing improves mood." They said, "energy appeared." I almost immediately understood—it is a high! I reduced the daily AM microdosage from 2.5 to 0.9 to 0.4. It is and I understood that there is no boundary between microdose and microtrip! Well, the border is ephemeral. So, today is just a good day, and tomorrow is four hours of energy with waves of intoxication, something similar to ethanol. I am a drug abuser and an alcoholic with more than thirty years of experience. Elephant doses of ethanol and pot, long-term remissions and so on. *Amanita* was a powerful replacement therapy for me. My last affair, mutual, deep passion with pot lasted more than fifteen years daily, with rare short remissions. Five months of AM microdosing and I practically **broke up with grass**. Another thing is **alcohol**. Once in a trip *Amanita* showed me alcohol's true name—"dead." *Amanita* showed me a lot about how alcohol acts, visual 3-D pictures with an effect of experiencing how the living brain shrinks and dries out, emanating an awful stink in front of my eyes. So, on the one hand, small doses of ethanol accelerate the effects of *Amanita*, like energy and psychedelic. On the other hand, I am an alcoholic, and I can't stop at small doses; as a result, I fall into long-term dopamine (this is when I drink a little permanently during the day). Gentlemen, an amazing performance unfolds before your eyes—a battle of psychotropic substances! Place your bet!

About the positive effects of AM microdosing: the **intestine works like a clock**, never worked like that. Mental health is stabilizing, **depression** is relieving, **fears** became empty and unreasonable, **sleep** is recovering, despite the abuse of other substances and numerous stresses. Bonus—bright, detailed fantastic dreams. Things are done easily, strong feeling of open-ness. There is a thrill of doing any job. **Creative uplift, inspiration**—just that pot gave me all these years. Bye my sweet girl, I'll see you after they legal-ize! **Vision has improved** noticeably. And color rendering is amazing! The sky is no longer gray; it is pink, blue, purple. The colors are natural and very soft, it feels like—I just never noticed it before. Psylocibin mushrooms are at rest compared with AM, honestly. Previously, I could not be without sunglasses; now—please, even on a bright sun. The physical condition is improving, yes. Progress in sports. I love everyone!

Report No. 535: From Masha's YouTube channel. Last year I made AM tinc-ture, and I used it to treat myself and my mom's **joint pain**. She calls me a young naturalist. I'm forty-seven. Waiting for this season. I'm going to microdose for the winter. This year I did not have enough AM because I gave it away to friends and family who needed it too. Health to you and long years!

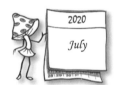

Report No. 536: Discussion from Thomas's chat room.

—I microdose already six days, wildly sick with nau-sea, every day worse and worse, is this normal?

—How many grams do you use?

—Started from 0.3, gradually increased to 3 g. Problems: **depression** and no strength. 0.3–0.5 did not give any energy, so I decided to increase the dose to 3 g and it feels pukey.

—It doesn't work like that. With such dosages, you will only deplete yourself; the dosage is too large for you, and you need to reduce. The meaning of microdoses is not to get high or get immediate results with your diagnosis. AM microdosing has gradual and cumulative effect over time, but not guaranteed. Less expectations, more motivation.

—I agree that mukhomor, like most antidepressants, has a cumulative effect and does not work instantly; this also needs to be taken into account.

—3 g in general can over stimulate emotions and psyche, which then will be rolled back even worse in a depressed state.

—Checked. Proved. I confirm. I ate about 3 g for a week, then for another week I dealt with consequences.

—How much should I take?

—Not more than 1 g or less with no "high" effect. A month or two will pass, and you will see the result.

Report No. 537: Sent to Masha personally via Telegram messenger. Hello. I wanted to share that with the help of AM microdosing I cured **allergy** to fungal dust and mold, which is present in old houses usually. Every year, when I went to my summer vacation house, I choked there. Now it completely passed.

Report No. 538: From Masha's YouTube channel. Masha and mukhomor helped me with **nicotine and alcohol addiction**. Three months of AM microdosing by 2 g, and I do not want to drink any longer. I tried alcohol twice with friends since and I don't like it, I feel stupid, and the taste is unpleasant. Before, I got drunk on weekends, 30% of time totally wasted.

Report No. 539: From Masha's YouTube channel. I made an alcoholic tincture for a friend—three medium caps for 200 g of vodka. He was taking ten drops in the morning on empty stomach. In a month **blood sugar dropped** from 20 to 5, the normal of a healthy person.

Report No. 540: From Masha's YouTube channel. Masha, greetings from Belarus. [I am an] ex-alcoholic, and I have not consumed **alcohol** for ten months, thanks to you and the great and terrible *Amanita muscaria*.

Report No. 541: Sent to Masha personally via Telegram messenger. Masha, I want to tell you how mushrooms changed my life, and I can confidently say that it changed. I am thirty-two years old. I have a family—my wife, children, dog, two cats, and ferrets. I had AM microdose course last year. The result is a complete rejection of **alcohol**. My wife's effects: although she admitted to me that she did not think that she would give up beer on her day off, surprisingly, it has changed. Masha, thank you so much for what you are doing, eliminating brain illiteracy and education about good things. I wrote this with a smile on my face and a feeling of happiness.

Report No. 542: From Masha's chat room. Masha, I have suffered from a **sore back** for ten years, **spinal damages caused by accident**. After AM microdosing by 0.5–1 g I forgot what it is.

Report No. 543: Sent to Masha personally via Telegram messenger. Thank you so much for the book! I'm a fifty-year-old man. I microdose for the third year, a couple of months per year, as long as mukhomor lasts. It rejuvenates me, at least it gives me such a feeling. I have an **increased pulse, but after microdosing my heart beats normal**. Last year I ran a couple of times in the city for a two-kilometer race with a trolley. I won. It is odd, I don't run, and I even don't like running since I was young. And where does such a desire come from?

Report No. 544: From Masha's YouTube channel. For about a year I binged **mephedrone and alpha (designer drug)**. I understood that it would not take long to damage my health, but I could not jump out of that! The gods sent me the right person who helped me cope with my addictions and introduced me to the mukhomor. Mukhomor goes as part of therapy; I have been microdosing mukhomor for two months. I am going to the gym; my life has changed in front of my eyes!

Report No. 545: From Masha's YouTube channel. I microdose Mukhomor Red for a couple of weeks. The other day I scored a whole bucket, tired of drying. I found out the perfect microdose for me, it is 2 g of dried AM. The cosmic peace comes, and the whole world around for the next 5–6 hours become a little muted, as I am in a dream. Waves of some kind of shivering, very pleasant **energy** begin to spill over the body. Literateness, a sense of joy and mild euphoria, **peace and a positive attitude** toward everything around. All this with **complete sobriety and clarity of mind**—I do business, walk, ride a bike, go to training in the gym. At night (optional). Sometimes there are very interesting and bright dreams where I am in a completely different, magical, and pleasant world. I take mukhomor microdoses every other day only.

Report No. 546: Sent to Masha personally via Telegram messenger. I made **AM extract** using Soxhlet extractor. From five average AM caps (20 g dried), I extracted with alcohol and evaporated to about 20 ml. Extraction could also be achieved using a water solution. This extraction process has a number of advantages. There is no need to follow the AM drying protocol. The extract does not need to be infused and fermented as a tincture, and it is ready for use immediately after production.

These AM had no effect in conventional dosages for microdosing and manifested only in extract. I take this extract by 0.5 ml a day. The first and second day it was a noticeable lift of energy, then this effect was gone. In general, my condition clearly changed. It can be described as "uniform activity." Usually, I'm up and down during the day, extremely active and interested, and then I get into a light form of apathy or doze off. There were problems with motivation. Now my forces seem to be distributed for the whole day. In the evening, I am busy until late doing all kinds of interesting things.

Report No. 547: From Thomas's chat room. After three weeks of taking mukhomor by 0.3–0.7 g, I could not drink whisky, or rather I took it as usual and immediately felt acute pain in the back of the head. Next time I decided to drink beer, I drank a can of light beer, felt ok, began to drink the second, and the pain in the back of the head returned. Then there was the moment that there is no pain when I drink, but there is also no high. After a week, I did not even look at the liquor store, my interest in **alcohol** disappeared. Now I can't even bear the smell of alcohol from people's breath. I microdose for four months now, I'm fine. I think it must be also my intention to give up alcohol. Before I eat an AM microdose, I say to myself what I want to get rid of and what I want to change.

Report No. 548: Sent to Masha personally via Telegram messenger. AM microdosing really works, the dead seasons like winter for me are simply woven from the apathy and unwillingness to get out of bed. Now it has become bright and cheerful. I take about 0.5–0.7 g in the morning and evening. **Cheerfulness, concentration, and confidence have increased**. For the fall I plan to take a break from the reception.

Report No. 549: From Thomas's chat room. Mukhomor mushroom cancelled my **alcohol** addiction, and I am very glad of that.

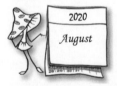

2020
August

Report No. 550: From Thomas's chat room. I'm a forty-year-old man. For fifteen years I was tormented with **back pain**. After an accident my ribs and back were broken and [I had] hernias. There were painkillers, massages, medications without much change. After *Amanita muscaria* microdose 0.5–1 g for a month, the pain passed. After six months the back straightened and began to unbend, hernias decreased + I turned on physical activity. Pain in the internal organs (right underbelly) disappeared. I don't go to the doctors. I continued AM microdosing experience for eleven months. People who knew me before did not recognize me. I feel like I'm seventeen now. There is some kind of **regeneration, rejuvenation** of my body. Alcohol passed away. My life changed: **sports, healthy food**. All that happened during the AM microdose course period. I took a week break during first three months of AM microdosing. Then I went without breaks. In September there will be a year of AM microdosing. My preparation method is drying and vacuum.

Report No. 551: From Thomas's chat room. Mukhomor took away **alcohol** from my life completely. I am very happy about that!

Report No. 552: From Masha's YouTube channel. I am on AM microdoses, my sugar craving went up but my to **alcohol** craving is gone.

Report No. 553: From Masha's YouTube channel. There was no time to wait for the AM "fermentation." I began to eat AM microdose the morning after drying. There is no nausea or discomfort. After the evening reception I **fall asleep almost immediately**; after the morning intake, I am **invigorated** all day.

Report No. 554: From Masha's YouTube channel. Thank you very much for your work and selfless help to people! I am sixty-five, I am cheerful, there are no diseases, but I have bad sleep with frequent awakenings. I started AM microdosing. I ate a piece immediately after drying, no nausea! **Sleep has improved**! The mood has become even better! I keep going. We have a lot of mukhomors in Norway.

Report No. 555: From Masha's YouTube channel. Mukhomor is a good thing. I am taking AM microdoses for a second year. **I don't get sick anymore**, and before I often suffered a cold.

Report No. 556: From Masha's YouTube channel. Two months of *Amanita muscaria* microdoses. The quality of my life improved. I am watching everything that happens from the outside as an **observer**, seeing casual relations, having **good energy**, **cool sex**, **gratitude** for everything.

Report No. 557: From Masha's YouTube channel. In September it will be one year since I quit **alcohol** after three-month microdosing. Also, I am clean from **amphetamines**, **methadone**, **tramadol**, **coke**, etc. I completely forgot about all that shit above. Thank you very much to mukhomor and the individual merci to our Masha for bringing me to this miracle and for pushing the train, which in the future will change the whole planet.

Report No. 558: From Masha's YouTube channel. Masha, your podcasts have given me the strength to **quit booze and "bath salt" narcotics**. I bow to you.

Report No. 559: From Masha's YouTube channel. Hi, Masha. I brew *Amanita muscaria* microdose as tea; I enjoy a good, nice **sleep**.

Report No. 560: From Masha's YouTube channel. I eat 1–1.5 g of dried powdered AM at night. **Sleep has improved, there is no craving for alcohol**. There is a situation after which I used to grab a drink of booze, then I eat another gram and it strengthens my will power. I have these situations less and less. It was interesting to me to **switch food preferences**. Surprisingly, I became a fruit eater. Previously, pear, apples, apricots were not attractive, and now I eat them all day long.

Report No. 561: From Masha's YouTube channel. Yesterday for the first time I made AM tea with 1 g. While it is difficult to describe the effect, it definitely **feels like the brain is rebooting**. It feels like unnecessary thoughts and **fears just disappeared**, some kind of blocking of garbage in the head. I did not even expect anything from 1 g, and there is a noticeable effect. I will continue, today I will try 2 g.

Report No. 562: Dialogue from Masha's YouTube channel.
    —Regarding **tobacco** dependence, microdosing is only getting worse. I use even more cigarettes with AM microdosing.
    —[Reply from another person] On the contrary, I was turned away from **tobacco** altogether. After two weeks of AM microdosing, there was a great desire to stop sucking poisons into myself.

Report No. 563: From Masha's YouTube channel. I also do take *Amanita muscaria* microdoses. I quit **alcohol** completely but am still fighting with nicotine addiction.

Report No. 564: From Thomas's chat. I am a sixty-three-year-old woman. I began AM microdosing due to tension of the mind and body. The last year has been very difficult for me in all directions. My course was 2.5 months of AM microdosing, half dry cap daily in the morning. I like chewing AM pieces. I did not like the tea form. It is really relaxing. I found a healthy fidelity and **cheerful mood**. AM microdosing acts well on the psyche and the body. The greatest respect to mukhomor—it pulled me out of **depression**. My *Amanita muscaria* is not fermented. I was in severe stress. The message is—mukhomor mushroom helped to relax my brain. Specifically pulled me out of stress.

Report No. 565: From Masha's chat room. A year ago I microdosed a couple of weeks *Amanita muscaria*. I noted **an increase in efficiency and a calmer state of mind**. That's the time when I got off antidepressants. Pills are rather dubious assistants in the case of depression, with a bunch of side effects.

Report No. 566: From Masha's YouTube channel. I used **cannabis** for twenty-six years all the time. I used about 200 g of mukhomor by 2.2–2.5 g per day. For the first time in my life, I began to abandon marijuana due to a depressive post-effect right after the AM microdose course.

Report No. 567: From Thomas's chat room. To whom it may concern. Today four people ate three average raw AM caps just collected in the forest. In forty minutes everyone got the worst nausea ever. I don't recommend it. The level of nausea is skyrocketing. Significantly higher than 10–15 g dry.

Report No. 568: From Masha's YouTube channel. I confess that I was lying in bed for four months without getting up after losing my job due to **alcohol**. I went outside just once in three months. **Depression** was severe with constant tormenting thoughts of **suicide**. Now I came back to myself, thanks to the mukhomor mushroom, now I even make jokes! It clearly helps.

Report No. 569: From Masha's chat room. I ate fresh dried AM pieces for a week while they lasted. Surprisingly, it was enough to believe that mukhomor helped to defeat the systematic sluggish habit of drinking **alcohol**; it was a great external stimulus.

Report No. 570: Sent to Masha personally via Telegram messenger. After watching Masha's channels, my life began to change gradually. I read all the information from Thomas as well and chats where people were discussing these issues. I read a lot of different literature on topics and when the whole process began. Three months of AM microdosing. I started to take 0.5 g AM microdose, and gradually increased to 1–1.3 g in the morning an hour or two before eating and another 1 g for the night. I fell asleep quickly, slept well. The awaking in the morning was very hard, and that was repetitive. That was the reason that I switched to once a day intake in the morning. There's a seasonal **allergy** in the spring. On the AM microdose course the nose is clean and easy breathing. It turned out that this was the action of AM microdose, because after the course the seasonal allergy came back. While microdosing I **stopped using glasses**. Vision was not perfect, but I could read a small font without glasses, which had not worked before. After AM microdosing, two weeks later, it all returned to previous again. I needed glasses. I am planning to continue *Amanita muscaria* microdose course.

Report No. 571: From Thomas's chat room. I am very anxious, and it has always been hard to sleep alone. I never liked loneliness and all that. After a course of AM microdosing, it's all great, very **nice deep and sweet sleep**. If I wake up at night, I quickly fall asleep again. There is no **anxiety** in the mornings, appeasement, feels like my consciousness purges.

Report No. 572: Sent to Masha personally via Telegram messenger. I am a forty-year-old woman, behind me is a lot of drama—divorce, the deaths of my beloveds. Finally, I started to look for a cure. I studied AM microdosing for a year. Then we collected AM in the forest and dried it in a dehydrator at 70°C [158°F]. We began microdosing together, 1 g fresh dried in the morning. One-week results: **general feeling of happiness, calm**, and understanding of what is happening in my life. The condition is very interesting: general fun and carelessness, but at the same time, **coordination** and **concentration of attention**! According to my emotions it feels like I am five years old again and summer has just begun. I am surrounded only by friends, a whole eternity and fun discoveries ahead. And most importantly, the message: everything will be fine! Changes at work: there is a desire to communicate with customers and joy in communicating with partners. The level of competitive behavior and irritability decreases. I want to help and hug everyone. Peace, love!

Report No. 573: Sent to Masha personally via Telegram messenger. I am a forty-five-year-old man. A year ago I started watching your channel. I took AM microdoses for three months. My life was changing. I broke up with a woman with whom I lived for six years without love and attraction. I could not eat **meat** and completely refused **alcohol**. Soon, I quit my job and also could not understand why I worked there at all. Now I have better job, I am running all summer in the forest, and doing CrossFits according to my own program. Set the goal, hold your breath underwater for up to fifteen minutes. I can hold 4.5 minutes already; before, I could not hold it for one minute. I had **thrombocytopenia**, there were results of 26. Recently I took a test, and I have 73! This progress happened without pills. I also have **chronic bronchitis, tuberculosis, and thrombophlebitis** of the vessels of the lower limbs; hepatitis B and C are chronic. I was an opiate junky in my youth. Now despite all this I am a happy person. Mukhomor somehow fixed a lot of things in my life, took away a bunch of destructive programs in my head, and put everything in order. I am prepared for a long and comfortable being. Thank you, Masha, you're doing a good thing. I made AM ointment for my mom; it takes away her **arthritis pain**; she forgot about suffering at all.

Report No. 574: Sent to Masha personally via Telegram messenger. Hello, Masha! This is my second follow-up review. News: I completely **refused alcohol**; before, there had been an undefeatable craving for many years. Complete abandonment of regular **cigarettes**. Now the smell is even unbearable for me. But I switched to e-cigarettes. Emotionally there have been many years of **depression**. It changed to awareness and insights. Fears, restrictions, negative attitudes are removed. There is a desire to live and create my life. I think there's still a lot to be realized; I'm in the process, on my way. Thank you! Be healthy!

Report No. 575: From Thomas's chat room. When I started the course in the mornings, there were no scales and I took a teaspoon dried AM powder. It made me sleepy all day long, and I switched to night intake. When I acquired scales it turned out that it was more than 2 g. Now I take around 0.5–0.6 g of *Amanita muscaria,* and everything is fine.

Report No. 576: From Masha's chat room. Today I experienced pot withdrawal syndrome—headache. I took 1 g AM microdose, and it literally removed a **headache** and stopped hurting!

Report No. 577: Sent to Masha personally via Telegram messenger. Hi, Masha. I live in Siberia, our mukhomors come in mid-August. After harvesting and preparation I ended up with 100 g dried AM. I ground it into powder, packed in capsules of 0.6 g. The first three days calibrated the dosage. Mainly, I took from 0.6 to 1.8 g at different times. The sensations these days are very vague, the body seems to get used to the substance, light nausea was often. After three days of adaptation, the mukhomor put me on the rails of consciousness: fog weathered from my head, easier mental state, creativity raised at work, it became easier and more pleasant to communicate with people, anxiety went away. The main goal for myself was to abandon **pharmacy drugs**; they acted on the GABA system. I got used to them when I quit **alcohol** three years ago. Alcohol left—the pharmacy pills stayed. Now for five days I have not been using any pills, I did not expect such a result; before, I could not leave the house without pills due to anxiety, I could not sleep. With AM microdosing my **sleep improved**. I **quit smoking tobacco**! I clearly feel what extra cargoes I drag behind me in my thirty-three years: tobacco, pharmacy, **harmful food**—all this goes away. I began to **smoke less pot**. I can compare this condition with how we feel in childhood when everything is interesting. Problems do not bother me and they are solved systematically, without fuss and anxiety. AM microdosing **helped me to look at myself**, my personality from the outside, to analyze my behavior in a particular situation. I discovered a little toxic monster inside myself that sometimes crawls out, and with passive aggression, can put pressure if someone feels weak. It is uncomfortable because I considered myself a kind and responsive person. Because of this monster, my friends began to shy away from me—I only realized this yesterday! Now that I've discovered it, I'll work with it, with the help of AM microdosing. One more positive thing—I **stopped getting annoyed**! Earlier in some situations I could ulcerate, grin, sarcastically make a person feel like an idiot; now I think for a couple of seconds, without any irritation (and even with pleasure) I answer the question . . . probably this can be called empathy. The food habits were changed; before, I did not eat because of pills I was taking and later at night ate sweets like a pig. Now I do not miss a meal and I **eat good food**—fish, eggs, cottage cheese, cereals, fruits, vegetables, less craving for sweets.

Report No. 578: From Masha's YouTube channel. I've microdosed four days with fresh-dried AM. I suffer from **duodenum problems**. From the very first intake, I began to feel better.

Report No. 579: From Thomas's chat room. Last year I collected *Amanita muscaria* and used for **eczema**, results are great.

Report No. 580: Sent to Masha personally via Telegram messenger. Last year I used Wellbutrin, an antidepressant, for half a year after long-term use of **alcohol and opiates**. It helped me, but I developed an addiction to it. Mukhomor is a miracle for me. I took AM microdoses for three months by 1 g a day, and after the course I **did not need an antidepressant** anymore. It was a miracle. This year I am taking AM microdoses for the second month. My condition is wonderful. The main thing for me is that my bad habits disappeared, thanks to mukhomor mushroom.

Report No. 581: Sent to Masha personally via Telegram messenger. I collected mukhomors, dried at 45°C [113°F], and began microdosing every morning by 0.5–0.7 g. I took the same amount for the night, and my sleep became very deep. It was hard to wake up in the morning. After ten days of AM microdosing, I feel an incredible **energy**, inspiration, and a lot of ideas. Despite the stressful circumstances at my new job, I feel that it is unlikely that something can knock me out of a calm state. Problems are solved as they arrive, without fuss and unnecessary thoughts. I also notice that I have lost excessive emotional attachment to loved ones. I still love them, but I clearly understand that I am independent—they live their lives, and I am mine. According to sports indicators, there are also positive effects: **stamina is higher**, **concentration** on the body is higher, **fear is lower** (I ride the board). I began to **eat more correctly**; I began to clearly understand when I am hungry and when I just want to chew something. I still have craving for nicotine. I made an ointment for my grandma, it helped her with **knee pain**. Masha, thank you for what you're doing.

Report No. 582: From Masha's YouTube channel. I ate two legs and half a cap fresh, my hoarse **bronchi cleaned up** in a few hours, and a **lightness** appeared in my back. I **slept** like a baby.

Report No. 583: From Thomas's chat room. I made an ointment from dry mukhomors and coconut oil. It helped with **dermatitis** that runs in our family. It acts like cortisone ointment.

Report No. 584: From Masha's YouTube channel. Hello, Baba Masha! Thank you. With *Amanita muscaria* microdoses I **quit smoking**; it just became nasty. I **quit alcohol** as well, and I switched to kvas [non-alcoholic Russian beverage].

Report No. 585: From Thomas's chat room. I use *Amanita muscaria* infused aftershave lotions; my **skin** responds to that much better than to regular aftershave lotions.

Report No. 586: From Masha's chat room. I suffered from **back pain** for three days and only when I used mukhomor ointment the pain went away in a couple hours. I cannot believe that! It is a fairy tale.

Report No. 587: From Thomas's chat room. I made alcohol mukhomor tincture for my mother-in-law. She got rid of **psoriasis** on her leg that she had for a long time.

Report No. 588: From Masha's YouTube Channel. I have a history **of anxiety disorder**. After AM microdosing anxiety left, complete victory! Prior to this antidepressants and tranquilizers (Paroxetine, Trittico) did not help. Masha, thank you! AM microdosing also helps with **skin diseases, including fungal**, and removes visible manifestations of **psoriasis**.

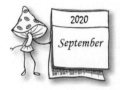

Report No. 589: From Masha's YouTube Channel. Three weeks of AM microdosing in February. Even this short course was enough to feel the potential of the mushroom. Many of the benefits that users write about have manifested to varying degrees. Even the **nail fungus** left. My parents are also pleased with benefits and ask me to prepare more. Overall tone, improved **mood**, optimism, more emotional evenness, **stabilization of blood pressure** (noticeable results), **improved sleep**—these are the main points that they note. They used AM microdosing for several months already.

Report No. 590: From Masha's YouTube channel. I've been eating mukhomor for a long time. I'm a very nervous dude. On this channel I learned about microdoses and just a week ago began an experiment. It seems to me that my condition became better and I am **ready to enjoy life**. In addition, the long-lasting knee **pain** passed. It doesn't hurt anymore. Last year I used vodka AM tincture to cure my back; it helped.

Report No. 591: From Masha's YouTube channel. I am a fifty-year-old male. I prepared AM alcohol tincture myself and used it for old traumas. Old **pain in the shoulder** passed with help of AM tincture compresses overnight. **Minor burns, cuts, bruises successfully treated** with tincture as well. The second effect, seasonal **heartburn**, passed after the first applications. It has purely therapeutic effects.

Report No. 592: From Masha's YouTube channel. With AM microdosing I feel super. It lights in me the **power, wisdom, and inner purity**.

Report No. 593: From Masha's YouTube channel. AM microdosing helped me to **quit alcohol and marijuana**, although I use only 1–1.5 g per day.

Report No. 594: From Masha's YouTube channel. I only learned about AM microdosing this winter. After a course I turned into a talkative, energetic person. My head is clear, I have fantastic dreams. I **quit marijuana**. I began to **eat less**. It's easier to wake up in the morning.

Report No. 595: From Masha's YouTube channel. I started to feel *Amanita muscaria* microdoses effects only after two weeks of consumption. My life became **calmer**. *Amanita* also **works with solutions and stresses**. After microdosing my life has changed to the positive and I have great physical tone.

Report No. 596: From Thomas's chat room. I take 0.5 g for the night as sleeping aid. I fall asleep fast and I have deep **sleep**. Mukhomor taste is nice, no disgust, no nausea.

Report No. 597: From Masha's YouTube channel. I microdosed a month every day, in the morning and in the evening in dried form! **Sleep** has improved, I wake up easily, a lot of **energy** has appeared, the reaction has improved! My body blocks **sugar**! And as Masha said, with mukhomor I grew up mentally!

Report No. 598: From Masha's chat room. I had **chronic cystitis**. It was gone after three months of AM microdosing, although to cure cystitis was not my main goal of microdosing. It's been a year since I've had this disease, and it used to bother me about once a month for sure. Before microdosing I used antibiotics but never had long remission, and it came back again and again.

Report No. 599: Dialogue from Thomas's chat room.

—I want to share my experience in the use of ten-month-old *Amanita* powder. It was stored at 25°C [77°F]. The fourth week of microdosing has gone, and I assure you with confidence that it actually does not work. There are no pure, conscious thoughts, soulful conversations, light spasms in the limbs, and other signs inherent in the reception of AM microdoses. The mushroom powder itself is tasty, clean, and dry. I assume that all the useful substances disappeared. Share your opinion please.

—Yes, I had the same experience. I discovered a stashed bag in the spring. It was stored at room temperature. I tried AM microdosing, and I was disappointed with no action, just like you. I took out another bag from the cold storage room, from the same *Amanita* batch, and tried it. Those were alright. Then I concluded that for long-term storage, the *Amanita* needs coolness.

Report No. 600: From Masha's YouTube channel. I am a fifty-year-old man. I suffered from **joint pain** for a long time and nothing helped me like microdosing dried *Amanita muscaria* and topical application of AM alcohol tincture. Baba Masha, thanks for the information.

Report No. 601: Sent to Masha personally via Telegram messenger. Hello! Feedback on the first experiments in the use of *Amanita*. Previously, I had extensive experience using substances of different classes (psychodisleptics, stimulants, euphoretics, dissociatives).

Over a two-week AM microdose course. Hand-picked mushrooms. Dried in an open oven at a temperature of 40°C [104°F]. Aged in a dark, cool place for about one month. Half a teaspoon of dry ground mushrooms brewed in a thermos for thirty minutes with the addition of lemon and honey: it acted as a stimulator; no intoxication or distortion of perception was noticed. Half a teaspoon dry ground mushrooms consumed after dinner before bedtime: complete absence of dreams, which is opposite my usual condition; a **sharp wake** earlier than usual, similar to the effects of melatonin consumption. Similar to melatonin, early awakening affects subsequent drowsiness during the day. In the morning a slight "hangover" similar to alcohol was felt and the condition worsened by lunch, not critically, but without evening mushroom consumption, **productivity** during the day is higher. With that dosage and regimen, the experience was repeated for several days. The effects are stable and do not change.

Fried stems of fresh *Amanita muscaria:* boiled two times for twenty minutes, washed, and fried. After consumption, a clear psychodisleptic effect. The impact was felt after a short period of time after consumption, a very pronounced manifestation. I do not recommend using mukhomor mushroom as food.

Report No. 602: From Masha's YouTube channel. Recently, I began to microdose with mukhomor, 0.5 g a day, intermittently. There was a feeling that I am **smart, strong, beautiful, successful, and that everything would be fine.**

Report No. 603: From Masha's YouTube channel. Mukhomors are a very interesting tool for creating a positive and not clouded awareness of oneself and the environment. The tool is very powerful. It requires a competent and balanced approach, however, like any other. There is a lot of information about AM, sometimes contradictory, which is understandable. We are all different, with different psych types, metabolism, and life values. Therefore, there can be no universal recipes. The main thing is to start with small quantities. Health and good luck to all! Baba Masha, special thanks to you for the very balanced information and just for the fact that you are with us.

Report No. 604: From Masha's chat room. For fifteen years I have had **pain in my knees**. In June I started an AM microdose course, and in three weeks I suddenly realized that my knees stopped disturbing me. They do not hurt anymore. I am still surprised at this. Although I am not a believer in various miracles, I realized that *Amanita muscaria* helped me.

Report No. 605: From Masha's YouTube channel. I take AM microdoses, I like the condition, **no anxiety, thoughts are bright**.

Report No. 606: From Thomas's chat room. I started AM microdosing because of very strong constant stress over the year. It seemed like my brain would explode. The mukhomor really helped me. I gained a **healthy, calm, balanced state**.

Report No. 607: From Masha's YouTube channel. My **prolonged diarrhea was fixed quickly**; nothing helped before. I used dry *Amanita muscaria* microdoses.

Report No. 608: Dialogue from Masha's chat room.

—Baba Masha, greetings! I brew tea with about 0.7 g of dry AM. Immediately after consumption, I feel some kind of flush of cheer. I want to move. Tell me, is this the norm, or should I reduce the dose so that there is no reaction at all?

—Are you able to do all the normal things in this state?

—Yes, it does not take long and passed.

—Do you feel dizzy? If it bothers you, you can reduce the dosage.

—No dizziness, just immediately energy appears and passes in fifteen minutes. It doesn't bother me. It's just that you said that it is necessary to have no effects at all.

Report No. 609: From Masha's YouTube channel. I only take *Amanita* externally. It removed **back pain** perfectly.

Report No. 610: From Thomas's chat room. There was a **lipoma** on my face for two years, small but not aesthetic. Periodically smeared it with oil with AM and AM ointment of Vaseline. No changes. In October I planned to remove it in the clinic. Three weeks ago I made a paste of 70%–80%

dry AM to 20%–30% lotion. I applied it for a night. Lipoma got inflamed, itched, and popped this morning.

Report No. 611: From Masha's YouTube channel. In several stages I tried micro-AM from 1–2 g. I realized that 2 g is too much. At first, I had a headache and a lower back pain, but then it went away. The world inside me has become **calmer**.

Report No. 612: From Masha's chat room. I microdosed three years on and off. I just passed all [general clinical] tests and underwent a full examination. Everything is normal. Sometimes irritability appears, and then I reduce the AM microdose or take a break.

Report No. 613: From Masha's YouTube channel. I had an experience of 5 g of AM. The condition was disgusting. No cartoons and no other realities. Just a disgusting feeling of intoxication like after alcohol intoxication. No more! Just AM microdosing!

Report No. 614: Sent to Thomas personally via Telegram messenger. I am taking this opportunity to thank you so much from my mother-in-law for AM lotion. It helped with **joint pain**. The painkillers and anti-inflammatory did not help her anymore. She felt the miracle effect of the ointment immediately and the fact was that she did not know about the ointment composition. My sister bows you as well. It turned out that the *Amanita muscaria* ointment is more effective at **rashes of the skin** than official medicine.

Report No. 615: From Thomas's chat room. It's been about three weeks since the start of *Amanita muscaria* microdosing 0.5–1 teaspoon dry powder in the mornings. I noted a **calmer state of mind**. I react less to the negative actions of other people. If misunderstandings happen, I am less involved, not as before, emotional with great dramatic effects. Thanks to Thomas, Baba Masha, and everyone involved in this educational *Amanita muscaria* microdose project and support.

Report No. 616: From Masha's YouTube channel. Taking dried mukhomor during the week, twice a day, morning and evening 0.5–1 g. The results: the **mind is clearer**. I **lost weight**, 4 kg [9 pounds], a feeling of saturation appeared when eating, I became **calmer**. So far, everything is good.

Report No. 617: Sent to Masha personally via Telegram messenger. AM microdosing for a month. 0.5–0.7 in the mornings. Improvements: cognitive functions of the brain increased, I work better, new ideas appeared at work, I received new programming training. There was more **energy** in sports, and I engage in boxing now. **Immunity increased**, seasonal cold passed in three days, usually I am sick for a week with fever. The disadvantages: I became a little more aggressive at the beginning of the course, and then it passed.

Report No. 618: From Masha's chat room. Teaspoons are so different. I took a teaspoon, and then the scales arrived. It turned out that it was 2 g of *Amanita muscaria* powder. That morning dose made me sleepy, and I drank five cups of coffee for the first week to cheer up. With scales I immediately reduced the dose to 0.5 g and everything became okay.

Report No. 619: Sent to Masha personally via Telegram messenger. Hi, Baba Masha! My mom is sixty-five. Three weeks ago she started AM microdosing, half a teaspoon before bedtime. **Sleep** improved, **energy** increased in the morning and during the day. The most important thing—her excessive **alcohol** consumption from boredom and stress is gone. Now there is no traction to drink at all. She is very surprised with the effects. Nausea and altered condition were not observed. Thank you, mukhomor mushroom. Thanks to all.

Report No. 620: From Masha's YouTube channel. I love Baba Masha because I learned about *Amanita muscaria* mushrooms, and I **have not drank** for a month already. I ceased to be dependent on beer and became dependent on her channel. I do not regret.

Report No. 621: From Masha's YouTube channel. I tried a raw *Amanita*. The effect is amazing! I am **in peace** with my husband's relatives. For many years I endured, and now there is silence and peace in the house.

Report No. 622: From Masha's YouTube channel. Over a week of AM microdosing. I take twice a day an average 0.6 g per day. I **sleep** good, dreams are colorful. Before that, I was constantly tormented with insomnia for about three months. In the morning after waking up, I go to work with great pleasure (this has not happened for several years). A day after the receptions, **panic attacks, nervousness, temper began to disappear, the perception of the surrounding world and the people in it changed**. I began to notice the good in people, and not only the bad and what used to be constantly annoying in them. There was an understanding that I very much depend on the opinion of others, and from this I have constant fears and complexes.

I also integrated about my appearance. Now I understand that this is just my perception of me based on some of my fears and invented standards that are imposed on me by this system. It seems that the system constantly keeps people in fear and in a constant race for unfulfilled desires in order to make them easier to manage. I began to understand that I had read a lot of useless books and spent a lot of free time on this. I realized that I used to spend a lot of money on things that I did not need, or on people that were unnecessary to me. I rethought my environment and realized with whom I need to stop communicating (as it seemed to me, listening to people offended by life and injustice, I lose my energy because I absorb all their negativity, and they feed on my positive energy). Previously, I could not be in crowded places for a long time. Now it feels that I and these people of the whole world are one, all people and nature are connected, and all resonate on one wave. I realized that all people are the same and everyone has the same problems.

I rethought the question of religion. I realized that all religions are shit that is imposed by the system and society in which you were born. If you were born in India, you would become a Hindu, in another country another religion, etc., and this would be considered normal. I realized that it is necessary to give a person the freedom to choose a religion and not forcibly baptize in the church when the child is small and does not understand anything. I realized that the repetition of prayers is simply a repetition of words that are invented by an ordinary person, and these repetitions will not lead to anything. I stopped being afraid of everything new. I began to go places that I had not been before.

Pot stepped aside, even the desire to **smoke** disappeared. I don't pay attention to alcohol at all. I don't understand why I used to drink and that this is my greatest stupidity. I run 10 km now three times a week. It is getting easier, **physical endurance**. After the first run (the third day of taking AM microdoses), I felt a very pleasant heat, which somehow spread evenly throughout the body from the heart, and at the end there was some kind of flash in the brain of this warm energy. There was a feeling that I had been sleeping all my life, and now I woke up from some muddy veil in my mind, and now I live as if I have an open cranial box. And it's all just day nine of AM microdosing.

Report No. 623: From Masha's chat room. My *Amanita muscaria* microdoses experience. When the AM reception is over, all the positive qualities achieved from the course are absolutely preserved. Moreover, they continue to grow like a snowball. Then there is no need for intake.

Report No. 624: From Thomas's chat room. I have **protrusions**. I made AM tincture and could not wait forty days because I was in pain. The **pain passed** after the first evening rubbing. There was no pain in the morning as well. It was only the twenty-seventh day of infusion.

Report No. 625: From Thomas's chat room. This year I began AM microdose course with fresh dried AM, no curing. They are effective. I **passed all standard tests** (ALT, AST, bilirubin, etc.) after a week of AM microdosing. I am going to continue AM microdosing and run all tests again in a month.

Report No. 626: From Thomas's chat room. I suffered from **hypertension** for many years. Blood pressure is 160/110. Now is the third week of dry untreated AM microdoses. The numbers are steady 128/83. I am a forty-eight-year-old man.

Report No. 627: From Masha's chat room. Guys, yesterday I accidentally exceeded the dosage of AM. Just now I came to my senses. I would not wish anyone to experience this condition, just horror. I have not experienced anything more terrible in my life.

Report No. 628: Sent to Masha personally via Telegram messenger. Hi, Baba Masha, you are my favorite. Words of love will be in a separate message. I've already microdosed eighteen days. The mukhomors are not cured. I dehydrated it at 50°C–60°C [122°F–140°F] for five hours and milled into powder in a blender. I cool the tea in thermos, boiling water + teaspoon of AM + teaspoon of lemon juice, thirty minutes wait. Took in the morning and evening. First impressions: **deep body relaxation**. The head was tense. So, I saw it as a weakness. Probably should have reduced the dose. I did it, the head felt normal. The state of mind is **calm and balanced**. An adequate picture of the world. I felt positive, in harmony, love, laughter, happiness. All people are different; leave everyone alone, more tolerance to others. The headache bothers me if I take more than a teaspoon. In general, there were no dyspeptic disorders. Psychological condition improved. I have become more tolerant to people, their opinion deserves listening, it's not hard. Why react immediately to the negative? And so forth. I clearly see provocations, and I react to them with laughter, good. Of course, there are ups and downs, but in general, if I had such control, then a maximum of a few hours a day. The body and soul are in a good state, there is no laziness/weakness, everything is fine, I do my favorite things as usual. I am learning German now! My **gastritis** symptoms went away. Prior to this **pain in epigastria** was often accompanied. I will microdose further. Tincture is cooking.

Report No. 629: From Thomas's chat room. Thanks for the advice to **reduce microdose**. I lowered AM microdose from 0.7 to 0.35. **Life played with other colors, irritability left, headache is gone**.

Report No. 630: From Masha's YouTube channel. Baba Masha, hello! I started microdosing a week ago! I took 2–3 g in the morning and 1 g in the evening in powder. At first, there were bright feelings, open shoulders, great, **calm communication with others without neurosis**. Previously, in the conversation I always had to prove my point of view. Under the AM microdose, I did not have that urge. My previously **stuffed nose** got clear, and breathing was good. Everything in my family also became calm. In five days the effect went missing. What does that mean? Weakness appeared, it became again the entire scarecrow, laziness, fatigue as it was before AM microdosing. This morning I decided to take a break 1–2 days. What does it mean? Why so? Please tell me. What's wrong? Thank you!

   Masha: You're taking too much, and this is a perfect example of stimulation followed by decay. Take a break and then decrease the dose to 1 g or less per day. With AM microdosing less means better. Write me back after a couple weeks.

Report No. 631: Sent to Masha personally via Telegram messenger. Good evening, dear Masha. My nose was stuffed for four years. I tried all available meds on the market; I visited a lot of doctors and almost went through surgery. However, after nine days of AM microdosing, I **breathe well** and I am so glad! The reason for AM microdosing was **pain in the hip joint**. The pain is gone and the "side effect"—clearing my nose! I will continue to observe improvements and changes. Baba Masha, I sincerely wish you health, love, and peace.

Report No. 632: From Thomas's chat room. I've taken AM microdoses for four years. This season will be the fifth. My relatives and neighbors take it as well, 2–3 years. We're all in a good shape, alive, and the mushrooms are not growing from our mouths and ears!

Report No. 633: From Masha's chat room. Two days ago, my son cut a piece of the soft part of his finger with vegetable-cutting tool. The flesh was practically cut off, hanging by a piece of skin. I put it together, sprinkled it with mukhomor powder, and bandaged it. The **healing was rapid**. Additionally, was taking AM microdoses 0.5 per day for support. There were no negative reactions.

Report No. 634: From Thomas's chat room. I was on sleeping pills for a long time. My **sleep normalized** after AM microdose course. This is the second year that I did not take sedatives for the night.

Report No. 635: From Thomas's chat room. I've had **hepatitis C** for twenty years. I take *Amanita muscaria* microdoses for the second season. All my medical tests are good.

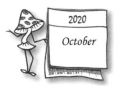

Report No. 636: From Masha's YouTube channel. I've been eating AM microdoses for a week. Condition is **quiet joy** and **clarity**! Thoughts come that this is a natural state of man and in order to come to that without using AM microdoses we need to purify the body and consciousness. In general, everything is super! Thank you for the information, Baba Masha!

Report No. 637: From Masha's YouTube channel. I take *Amanita muscaria* on and off for three years. I was diagnosed with **rheumatoid arthritis** since I was a child. AM microdosing alleviates the symptoms; the most important is that the **pain went away**.

Report No. 638: From Masha's YouTube channel. I microdosed last fall. In a few days I started to feel better. In three weeks the **aversion to alcohol** appeared. I got **good sleep** and **cheer** during the day.

Report No. 639: From Thomas's chat room. I am on my second year of AM microdosing. I tried a tea at 60°C [140°F] and dry form. AM microdosing works either way for me.

Report No. 640: From Thomas's chat room. Greetings to everyone. My wife cured **nail fungus** with AM vodka tincture. She suffers from asthma for ten years, and AM microdosing helps her with **asthma attacks**. That was a really big surprise.

Report No. 641: Sent to Thomas personally via Telegram messenger. My sister has not touched **amphetamines** for seventy days already after AM microdose course. I am sure that she will no longer return to this poison.

Report No. 642: From Thomas's chat room. Before: hellish **pain in my joints**, terrible aggression and rage. Now: the **emotions are stable, good state of mind** during the day, and most importantly, the pain in my back and knees passed, not completely although, but significantly. I am pleased with the results.

Report No. 643: Sent to Masha personally via Telegram messenger. Good afternoon, Baba Masha. My AM microdose course is four weeks, 2 g in the morning, the same dose before bed. The first and most important thing for me is that I stay **calm** in any situation. AM microdosing helps me a lot. The second is my **sleep**. It is gorgeous, strong, and deep. I wake up invigorated with no problems. Third, I **quit boozing** at all. Drugs are all in the furnace, too. **Digestion** is normalized. The only thing that didn't quit is smoking. There may be a lack of desire.

Report No. 644: From Masha's YouTube channel. Greetings to you. I went to the forest, gathered AM, and immediately ate three raw hats. After twenty-five minutes, I puked everything out. After that I started my AM microdose course of dried AM half small cap daily. In two weeks I started to feel better. My **knees and back do not hurt** anymore.

Report No. 645: From Masha's chat room. I have not used mukhomor for more than six months and **the effects remain**. Of course, the effects are not as intense as during the AM microdose course.

Report No. 646: From Masha's chat room. AM microdosing for 2.5 weeks, 2 g per day. I experimented with weight for my own needs. Actually, AM put me on my feet quick. The night **sleep** became magnificent. I calmed down in general. My daily routine is normalized. I go to bed at 8–9 p.m. and wake up at 4:30 a.m. AM is a medicine. Nature knows a lot about medication. Especially cool to see it in contrast to the pharma products that I was selling professionally. After these experiments I realized that *Amanita* is not poison but medicinal. Thank you very much.

Report No. 647: From Masha's chat room. I gave AM tea to my wife; it helps her with **stress** at work. She is not crying anymore. She gets instant relief. I have the same effects, and **pain in my knees** is going away, we are going to continue and observe our AM microdosing trial.

Report No. 648: From Thomas's chat room. AM microdose course is almost two months. I brew a heaping teaspoon with lemon juice in a thermos with a glass of hot water in the morning and night. Of the pros: I became calm as a "tank," a constant **internal dialogue** disappeared, **fear** for the future disappeared, healthy fidelity appeared, everything is given without interruption and effort. There was no interest in unnecessary information (news, information noise, extra people). I began to read classics again and watched many old films. Much more interesting than dumb TV shows. **My eyes opened to many things, a lot became simple and understandable**. There is an understanding of people's problems. Feelings escalated, the world became more colorful, kinder, it reopened for me. I **sleep** perfectly, now I quickly fall asleep. **Dreams** have become an adventure.

Report No. 649: From Masha's chat room. Effects after AM microdose course: **wounds, abrasions began to heal faster**, I cured **psoriasis**, I did not catch cold this year.

Report No. 650: Sent to Masha personally via Telegram messenger. Mukhomor is a wonderful miracle! I take AM caps dried at 40°C [104°F] by 0.5–0.8 g. I brew tea with citric acid and take it before night and in the morning. **Dreams** have become alive and deep; I go to sleep by 10 p.m. now. I also react **calmer** to stimuli since I take AM microdoses. The ass doesn't burn, there's no stress during **communication**. There is great workability of a healthy person. But mukhomor is not omnipotent, it is not a miracle, it cannot force me to wash floors and dishes! The most important thing, after the second week of *Amanita muscaria* microdoses, the symptoms of **prostatitis** went away.

Report No. 651: From Thomas's chat room. I have calm and **balanced sleep**, getting up without alarm clock, and I am in smiling mood in the mornings. Two seasons of AM microdosing three months at a time.

Report No. 652: From Thomas's chat room. I have very stressful job. With AM microdose of 0.6 g, the **calm** comes. Sometimes I feel like a white raven, everything is boiling, the city is rattling, people are furious; well, it is the charms of big city. And I am calmly doing my job. Sometimes I think that I am too calm.

Report No. 653: From Thomas's chat room. I began AM microdose course on September 14, 1 g a day, half in the morning and evening. I collected and dried AM myself. No curing. I noted increase of **energy and endurance**. I have five years of a sleep disorder. On AM microdose I **sleep great**, especially if I take it in the evening. I've eaten much less. More interesting that I lost the "thrill" of a morning cup of **coffee**, now the coffee seems bitter to me. I still drink this cup, but the thrill is gone. I also want to say about my thoughts, in situations where I previously would react hard, there is a clear understanding that this does not have any significance at all. Inner tranquility.

Report No. 654: From Thomas's chat room. I have symptoms of **chronic fatigue and anxiety**. I could no longer sleep. On AM microdose I **sleep** very well, especially if taken in the evening, it turns me off instantly.

Report No. 655: From Thomas's chat room. After two weeks of AM microdosing, I became very **calm**. I'm not angry at all—even yesterday when a big metal piece fell on my foot at work. I sleep like an "elephant" and wake up like an "eagle," invigorated. The most important thing is there are no unnecessary thoughts that were in my head before. **Energy, good mood**, and now instead of beer in the evening I drink kefir or some juice. Doesn't pull on **alcohol** at all, although I drank almost every day for fifteen years. But I can't quit smoking. In general, like many other people in the reports, the rearrangement of life values happened. Thanks to all.

Report No. 656: From Thomas's chat room. The most amazing thing for me is that mukhomor microdose removes **inherited essential tremor** in my hands. It always passed after the mukhomor intake.

Report No. 657: From Thomas's chat room. I could not walk for several months, lying down flat in my bed because of horrible **pain in my back**, and any movement caused pain. And then I found out about AM and began to microdose. This gradually stabilized my spine. Now I fly like a butterfly. I take mukhomor almost constantly. I was scared of upcoming surgery, and I do not need it now.

Report No. 658: From Masha's YouTube channel. Mukhomor generally taught me to LIVE. It saved me from **dependencies**, wasted time, gave the right impetus to thoughts, supplemented the awareness of reality. It came into my life when it was necessary. Thank you very much to universe for that. AM microdosing is an excellent treatment of the soul and body. But be careful. Fools will be punished. I don't particularly advise to get carried away with AM. Two weeks of therapy a year for a couple of teaspoons a day is quite enough. And stop. Too much is not cool.

Report No. 659: Sent to Masha personally via Telegram messenger. Good evening, Baba Masha. I want to inform you that **psoriasis** entered into a wonderful remission after AM microdose intake.

Report No. 660: From Thomas's chat room. Hi. I microdosed *Amanita muscaria* about a month by 1 g per day. What's interesting: **Alcohol** flew off. I just don't want it anymore. The last bottle of cognac is covered with dust. The **pot smoking** also fell away. I realized it wasn't mine. Nicotine didn't leave. I like smoking electronic cigs. Dreams became very cinematic. And more often I began to remember them in the mornings.

Report No. 661: Sent to Masha personally via Telegram messenger. Good morning, Baba Masha. I am taking 1 g in the morning, at lunch, and in the evening. I feel great. There is emotion control. The quality of life went up. I began to run. **I stopped eating bad food**.

Report No. 662: From Masha's YouTube channel. Greetings, Baba Masha, I thank you. This year I began to microdose. I am sure that I have become better, consciousness has become cleaner, there are almost no foreign noises in the head (**negative thoughts**), the head has started to work better, health is normal. There was a **nail fungus** that I treated with AM ointment, it seems to help. Sleep got better. Before, my thoughts just drilled my brain and not all good ones. Now I fall asleep in five minutes after I close my eyes. It is just a miracle.

Report No. 663: From Thomas's chat room. My AM microdosing review. I suffered from **nose bleeding**, especially in the mornings. There was also tightness in my chest and sharp **pain** in the heart area, my left arm was numb. I want to say that I did not check with the doctors, maybe it was not heart problems at all, but banal **neuralgia**. I took AM microdoses for a month; all these symptoms were removed. There is no blood in the nose, the hand was not numb, pain and tightness were gone. I repeat that I did not record these facts with doctors; these are just my personal physical observations. But based on them I can conclude that the mukhomor positively affected my cardiovascular system. Thanks very much to Baba Masha, Thomas, and all the administrators' teamwork! This group has the best content on the entire internet.

Report No. 664: Sent to Masha personally via Telegram messenger. I learned about AM microdosing last year at the end of October, thanks to you, dear Baba Masha. But unfortunately, at this time I could not pick it myself in the Russian Federation. I bought some online and did not have good experience—the zero effects. In 2020 I got my own *Amanita* from the forest, and the effect did not keep me waiting. From the first intake, I felt the very wild **energy**, too much sometimes! But it was really cool! My dose is about 1–1.3 g. I do not miss evening receptions; sometimes in the turmoil of everyday life I miss morning receptions. So, the lyrics are lyrics, and here comes the profile: **Internal dialogue** almost completely stopped. The effect of **alcoholic binges** became sharply bad in the morning, from which the desire to consume alcohol completely disappeared. There was **rationality in actions, pure and systematic thinking. Irritability is gone! Dreams are deep**, most beautiful and long-lasting movie. With my recommendation, ten people switched to the AM microdose, and everyone is delighted. After *Amanita muscaria* microdose course there is a desire to help others with such great knowledge. Thanks again for everything!

Report No. 665: Sent to Masha personally via Telegram messenger. I **sleep** very well after I took four weeks of AM microdose course. I took a break and to my amusement I realized that my sleep is as good as on microdoses. I am ten days off now. The **effects remain**. Thank you, *Amanita*!

Report No. 666: Dialogue from Thomas's chat room.

—I wonder how in general people feel after the cancellation of *Amanita muscaria* microdoses. It seems to me that this is a critical indicator of real success and not temporary. Especially concerning psychological changes, most reviews do not consider that as far as I see. I want specifics. So, you can say about heroin microdoses that they are very cool and help, super, but the main thing after the cancellation—there is nothing to tell.

—I wrote here in the chat room about a hundred times that everything is in order after stopping. But if a person was dependent on drugs, then there will be psychological prejudiced trawls. AM microdosing adjusts, hardens, gives awareness, but we also have to work on ourselves. That's the right life approach.

—I took a six-week AM microdose course in November 2019, and then my wife, father, and mother. The cancellation effect has not been noticed by anyone.

—Are you specifically asking about withdrawal? I did not understand. Withdrawal syndrome is from drugs; it is not present with AM microdosing. But if someone use 5–7 g for five days in a row, from my own experience I realized that I wanted to return to this state but I stopped easily. I took AM microdoses for a year with interruptions of course; all the pros were preserved after cancellation, except for one with marijuana smoke, which was decreased during that year. Later on, I came back to pot, still in smaller amount, I think because I didn't have the desire to quit. Everything else stays—decreased bread consumptions, **alcohol** went to zero, even now no thoughts of pouring it into myself. The family seemed to have been redis-covered during the course. I began to spend time with them and it is inter-esting to me. I am much better with my job. Much less **pain in torn back** than before, **skin sores** are already forgotten about. I bought dumbbells; I do charge in the morning; the last time I did that, it was twenty years ago. Well, a lot more that you notice on a sensation level, not so clearly but very pleasing. I haven't noticed nature for forty years, and now I am in the forest as much as I can. I have all the above, instead of work-house-gadgets-sleep activities in the past. I don't recall anything negative in a year, but a good piggy bank of positive. And the records of my observations helped a lot. I write notes every night: the time of reception, dosage, and sensations.

Report No. 667: From Masha's chat room. I found the best sleeping pills for myself. Five drops of *Amanita muscaria* tincture before bed. I literally **immediately fall asleep** until the morning. I tried that during the day, and I got the same effect.

Report No. 668: Sent to Masha personally via Telegram messenger. Good time of the day! Masha, I really want to hear your opinion. A month and a half ago, I tried AM microdosing. I started with one dry cap to the max-imum dose—2.5 caps morning and night. The effects were **clarity of mind**, **ease**, **high spirits**. **I got a creative rush** to draw, do meditation, go to yoga class, and enjoy music. I maintained a great mood, cheer spirit, energy. Everything was very good. Mukhomor, personally for me, discovered the accumulative effect. After 5–6 days the AM microdose taste became terribly unpleasant with the taste of mushrooms. Right to disgust. Last time I took AM in the forest, it became uncomfortable. I was jagged, a little dizzy, and threw up. What happened? Thanks in advance for the answer!

Masha: You overate the mushrooms. You took too much. Stimulation occurred and then rolled back to negative effects. A gram or less is the microdose, not a few caps a day.

Report No. 669: From Masha's YouTube channel. Mukhomor microdoses are an incredible and accurate tool for **repairing the human body and soul**. We read from Russian classics and the Bible that the meaning of life is love, but under the influence of mukhomor microdoses, this becomes completely obvious. The human language is too poor to describe it. The difference between how you understand it under the influence of AM microdosing is huge, colossal, and completely different level. Do you want to look at the sunset with a child's eyes? Try AM microdosing.

Report No. 670: From Masha's YouTube channel. Symptoms of zombie-putins TV box: dullness, greed, selfishness, envy, anger, alcoholism, immoral behavior, arrogance, and cynicism. Symptoms of AM microdosing: **stable psycho-emotional state**, kindness, love, empathy, healthy **sleep**, body strengthening, world peace, rainbow is beautiful, as well as the dawn. Draw the conclusions yourself.

Report No. 671: From Masha's YouTube channel. Effects of my AM microdose course: complete refusal and desire of **alcohol**; **emotional control**; I became **calmer**; more **concentration** on a problem, an instant decision comes on arisen question; the **internal dialogue** in the head disappeared; **clarity of thoughts**; **focus** on the moment here and now; snots, **nasal congestion** disappeared from both nostrils, like a baby's breathing; extraordinary decisions at work; shoulders flattened, a straight back, ease, posture changed with no effort; people are more willing to communicate with me, before, I did not notice that; strangers with whom for one reason or another I should communicate on the street—there is no fear of communication with strangers on the street. There used to be some kind of panic, avoided communication, now I will willingly explain something if asked; calmer and quieter response to things that annoyed and irritated me before; I **sleep** tight. But it became for some reason difficult to wake up, it is not clear why; the **concentration** behind the wheel increased, I began to drive calmer. My wife notes these facts and confirms! I keep watching my condition.

Report No. 672: Sent to Masha personally via Telegram messenger. Good time of day. I can say, after our last conversation a lot has changed. I **quit cigarettes, alcohol, and drugs**. I run in the mornings, I breathe, and I enjoy it. I created a YouTube channel and share my experience as I come up from the very "bottom" of my nature! Everything is wonderful at home; it has become calmer. My wife smiles. I have great **sleep** rest. Culture of the *Amanita* saved me!

Report No. 673: From Thomas's chat room.

Good evening everyone! I read this chat and see only miraculous healings, and what about **liver damage**, about the **poison effects** on one of the most important organs of our bodies, it's somehow in denial. What do you think, friends?

—That is because there is no harmful effect, so you can't see that in the chat. I took tests for two years in a row after AM microdosing. Everything is exactly correct with the liver; I have been living with hepatitis C for twenty years. I have written about this many times. If there are any negative symptoms, something does not suit or hurts, then stop microdosing, look for other drugs for yourself. But do not write nonsense in the chat! A bunch of people have already tested their liver after AM microdosing, and they're fine!

—If your liver is sensitive, perhaps it's not about the *Amanita muscaria* microdoses, but about your diet, alcohol, vitamins, pills, dietary supplements, and so on.

Report No. 674: Sent to Masha personally via Telegram messenger. Hi, Baba Masha. I regularly microdosed red hats daily for about a month. Before that, I took it irregularly for a couple months. *The effects:* a rooted sense of **self-confidence**. I am out of a toxic relationship. I moved to another town. I started doing what I love. I started singing on stage. I used to be afraid of the scene. Now I feel like a fish in the water. Internal gifts are revealed. In general, a flow of abundance begins to appear. I feel powerful support from the Great Mukhomor.

Report No. 675: From Masha's chat room. Four weeks of AM microdosing. Exposing effects: **Confidence, stress resistance** appeared. **Anxiety and depression** seem to be beginning to release. Heavy emotional moments are easier to endure. I talked to my son, with whom there was a rift. I figured out communication with my mother-in-law without emotional extra involvement (she loves to arrange tantrums).

Report No. 676: From Masha's chat room. I am sharing experience with AM tincture with high-proof alcohol. Absolutely relieves **neurological pain, bruises, and sprains**. I didn't think that such a miracle remedy exists.

Report No. 677: From Thomas's chat room. There is a permanent **hereditary hand tremor**. It goes away with AM microdosing. The higher is the microdose, the more pronounced the effect.

Report No. 678: Sent to Masha personally via Telegram messenger. Hello. I well read reviews in your channel. This is the second week I microdosed together with a friend. Neither I nor him, absolutely no changes or sensations, not to mention those transformations written in the reviews. Well, it can't be like that. I have doubts whether real people write in the chat at all. It hurts everyone and everything is like a copy: energy over the edge, dreams are special, joy, euphoria, thoughts, performance, and much more. And my friend and I have nothing! So far, the only thoughts are that the week is not enough, although they write of the effects in 2–3 days.

Masha: Hello. First, please look at the questionnaire. You will see that there is a percentage of people on whom AM does not work. This is obvious for all available 107 questions. Also, there are votes on negative effects. All the negative effects are subject to discussion in the AM microdosing chat room, and you are welcome to read the chat from the beginning. Second, did you buy your AM online or pick it yourself? Third, what are your reasons to take AM microdoses?

Report No. 679: From Masha's chat room. I started AM microdosing because I got tired of **depression, obsessive conditions, and anxieties**. Four weeks passed, and I can say that I have never felt better than now!

Report No. 680: From Masha's chat room. I have been microdosing for a month. I see the same results: cheer up, **anxiety** down, sleep and rhythm back to normal. It has very interesting and soft action.

Report No. 681: From Thomas's chat room. My own personal example of AM microdosing action on **smoking, alcoholism, and drug addictions**: First, my mother asked for help. I let her read the AM research and reviews. She took AM microdoses for two months, and I can see myself that she **sleeps normally**, finally **quit smoking and alcohol** drinking, she is **calm**. Well done! I've eaten dry AM for three months and tried tinctures externally. Mukhomor pumped me with a sense of measure. I used to sit tight on **opium**. I quit only now, even though I was on substitute replacement therapy for seven years! Everything is even and cool after the end of AM microdose course. This is my second year of taking mukhomor. A close childhood friend of mine, also an **opiates addict**, asked me for AM microdose today. He is very motivated, looking at my success to finish with all this, but is afraid of withdrawal syndrome. Let's see.

Report No. 682: Sent to Masha personally via Telegram messenger. Grandma, hello! I'd like to share a joyful message. After the dialogue with you, I tried to take the smallest dose: a piece of a hat, twice a day. And a miracle! I realized that the mukhomor is precisely for health, not for changing the state of consciousness and not even for an enlightenment. Unpleasant aversion disappeared with AM microdosing. It's such a pleasure. **Sleep** improved, the next day **cheer and creativity**. Everything fell into place. I downloaded your book. I am studying it now; thank you for all the work! Thank you for the dialogue! You are an *Amanita muscaria* mushroom fairy!

Report No. 683: From Masha's chat room. I drank **alcohol** every day! I was not going to quit drinking. I took AM microdose course for different reasons and the craving for alcohol disappeared on microdosing. When I tried to drink, the taste of familiar drinks is still pleasant, but intoxication is not the same and unpleasant. As a result, I don't drink alcohol anymore. I drink tea with lemon instead with great pleasure. Yesterday, the idea came not to return to alcohol after the completion of microdosing.

Report No. 684: From Thomas's chat room. Hello to everyone. I want to leave feedback on AM buckthorn oil. It was a rash (**dermatitis or eczema**) on the ankle of a fifteen-month-old baby. It was itchy and constantly scratched. Nothing helped. The rash was gone after using *Amanita muscaria* buckthorn oil for two weeks, three drops were rubbed without fanaticism in the mornings and in the evenings. Everything has passed. Thanks to this chat; there is really a lot of useful information here.

Report No. 685: From Thomas's chat room. After AM microdosing, I realized that **alcohol** made me dull and stupid. It is more pleasant to be in tone, and the *Amanita* gives it to me.

Report No. 686: From Thomas's chat room. The effect of AM microdosing is individual. I did not want to go to a psychiatrist, and hope for AD, so I have no diagnosis. I am unemployed for more than a year. It was a big problem for me to go outside. I could not **sleep** due to nightmares. It was **suicidal thoughts**. I took *Amanita muscaria* microdoses over twenty days, about 1 g at morning and evening just diluting the *Amanita muscaria* powder in the water. From all possible remedies that I tried, the AM microdose seems the most optimal. The most noticeable effects—normalization of sleep, I have much **less nightmares**. I go outside for a walk; it ceased to be such a problem. I think that twenty days is not enough for the first experience, and I intend to continue. I hope for the best. Although, of course, the mukhomor will not tell me what to do with my life, I do not expect it, but positive changes are already noticeable at this stage.

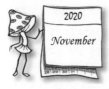

Report No. 687: From Thomas's chat room. During AM microdose reception I clearly improved my health, by all the characteristics. After the reception the direct impact of the mukhomor stops, but the achievements remain! Clearly, with the right approach, it is safe and helps.

Report No. 688: From Masha's YouTube channel. **Depression** down to zero! Yes! And before, I was staying in bed in a dirty house, in pain and sorrow, and complained about everything. After the AM microdose course, I do my home chores with pleasure, I am energetic and optimistic.

Report No. 689: From Thomas's chat room. I also have a **stable effect** after three weeks; the AM microdose probably does not allow me to slip into despondency and apathy, it is easier to act. Other effects: it does not pull on **alcohol** at all, because there is no need anymore.

Report No. 690: From Masha's YouTube channel. I thank you, grandma. Two weeks on the AM microdose, great action, the results are definitely positive.

Report No. 691: From Masha's YouTube channel. I wrote this comment to a zombie commentator, but I want the rest to see my simple arguments: do not rush to draw conclusions under the yoke of fear. For you, this is something new and unfamiliar, plus 100% you watch TV, it immediately reads that TV is your main legislator and authority. People have been hypnotized by TV for many years; they are not able to think clearly themselves, and apply facts to a puzzle. Try to read independent research and look at the benefits and harm from different angles. Here, after the mukhomor, ayahuasca, iboga, and shrooms, people stop addiction to heroin, alcohol, and smoking. But you shout drugs! Danger! My mother and many adult friends are conscious, wealthy, and responsible people and are using mukhomor. And you know what? No one shakes from withdrawal, no high, no trips. It is equal to a full-fledged course of psychotherapy, where you meet with your most potent phobias, which even the most talented psychologist will not be able to excavate. In short, our family results: disconnects **postmenopausal hot flashes**; disables **panic attacks**; **chronic headache** stopped; increased **concentration and attention**; **depression** disappears; calm response to **stressful situations and problems**, it concerns hysterical and frightened women; **insomnia** passes, deep sleep, cheerful morning; new brilliant ideas about business and everyday life appear; infuriation stopped; **alcohol and nicotine** addictions stopped; there is strong craving to play sports. Mukhomor do not kill; Mukhomor has been used for centuries. It is not listed in the classifier of narcotic substances. Pay attention to the poisons in the supermarkets in front of our children with huge sections of alcohol, soy, sugar, and so on.

Report No. 692: From Masha's YouTube channel. Dry *Amanita muscaria* 1.5 g per night knocks out faster and better than any sleeping pills! The quality of **sleep** has improved many times. Plus, a significant decrease in **alcohol** consumption, which also has a beneficial effect on sleep.

Report No. 693: From Masha's YouTube channel. I confirm that on the AM microdose there is an aversion to **alcohol**.

Report No. 694: From Masha's YouTube channel. Hi, Baba Masha! Folks, **do not increase the dosage**, especially for long time. There is a risk of falling back into the "hole." This is not a tool for a high; and taking large doses can knock you down. *Amanita muscaria* microdoses give a thrill, like you won your favorite game, rising mood and motivation. But big doses are fraught with consequences for the body and psyche. I strongly do not recommend big quantities. Thank you! Free body and clean spirit!

Report No. 695: From Masha's YouTube channel. About **alcohol** addiction: I took red mukhomor in a small amount and not regularly. After several receptions I felt a complete lack of desire, craving, and thoughts about buying alcohol, besides catching myself thinking that I don't want or need it at all. Although earlier I had the daily desire to drink in the evening, afternoon, or morning. My wife is in shock. Friends say, well, now there is no one to drink with. I need to get out of anabiosis and learn to live again, fully in real life with real deeds and problems, but again, AM helps to treat this more easily without depleting yourself to a state where only the booze seems to be able to help. True, there is a vacuum associated with the restructuring of consciousness, free from the insurmountable need to run somewhere, buy booze, and F* your own and family time, physical and mental health. There was a time that I killed for booze before, and now I can be devoted to family, business, rest, and sleep. By the way, the quality of sleep improved. My sleep is not an alcoholic coma anymore. Waking up with a hangover is a separate topic, with all that ensues. I never regretted that I quit. I keep working with myself. BM, thanks for your work.

Report No. 696: From Masha's YouTube channel. I **don't drink** for the second year. In many ways, that was influenced by microdoses of the mukhomor. I will not say that I was drinking too much, but enough. My brain returned to factory settings after a year of sobriety, to the state when you stop drinking to communicate with friends and comrades. My surroundings changed by 95%, those who did not accept me sober, they went their way. I responsibly declare that man has to be alcohol free. It kills everything in man. I am talking about the hormone system, the production of dopamine, serotonin, and testosterone is blocked. Add the calorie content of alcohol here, which leads to obesity, including heart problems. Ethanol takes third place on the list of strong active drugs immediately after methadone and heroin.

Report No. 697: From Masha's YouTube channel. I was diagnosed with **flat feet**. I was in **pain** and limping while walking. The doctors said that it could not be cured. I was putting AM tincture compress on my feet for several days, following with AM oil and cream. Two weeks after—no pain, I am not limping. I am also taking *Amanita muscaria* tincture.

Report No. 698: From Masha's YouTube channel. I didn't quit drinking completely after AM microdose, of course. Yesterday, my brother and I succumbed. BUT! The effect is striking and very noticeable. With regular microdosing **alcohol** is simply out. I did not set the goals to quit drinking, but I drink much less! No craving for a strong booze bottle. Sometimes I take a couple bottles of good expensive beer. I wish I could solve the problem with cigarettes.

Report No. 699: From Masha's YouTube channel. I wanted to clean the body with AM microdosing, but did not specifically plan anything. And now, looking back, everything has changed completely in my life. **Alcohol** went away with friends, who were not my friends at all. Instead of alcohol, I prefer silence and the forest, since I left the city. And thanks to grandmother Masha for her videos, everything went much easier and faster, because it's hard for myself to admit that I lived the wrong way.

Report No. 700: From Masha's YouTube channel. Thank you, Baba Masha! After taking *Amanita,* worst habits left. Indifference to **alcohol and porn** appeared.

Report No. 701: From Masha's YouTube channel. **Psoriasis** passed after two months of AM microdosing in the morning and evening. I **quit drinking, smoking, being a druggie**, and signed up for boxing and guitar classes. I've wanted it for a long time. It became easier at work. It may not be AM microdosing at all, but two months ago it was exactly the opposite. I collected AM myself. I take it once a day with a little lemon juice. I feel great.

Report No. 702: From Masha's YouTube channel. I was deprived of my driving license for drinking. Before restoring the license, I was sent for medical examination and blood tests. I was periodically taking *Amanita muscaria* microdoses. Doctors were surprised with my health. All indicators are A+!

Report No. 703: From Thomas's chat room. My neighbor, eighty-year-old grandma, suffered from pain in her arm. It was disabled, and pills were prescribed by doctors; pills did not help. I treated her arm with AM ointment, overnight compress for two weeks. Everything got to normal. She shared AM ointment with her sister. She sent me a box of chocolates. I am a grandma's savior!

Report No. 704: From Thomas's chat room. Good evening. I had **itchy rough spot on my knee**. There was a little help with prescribed ointments. I was smearing raw *Amanita* on the spot while hunting in the forest several times. It took a week for the spot to disappear, only discoloration left.

Report No. 705: From Masha's chat room. In my experience of adopting various means of boosting spirit and cheer, the mukhomors turned out to be the most kind and cool without side effects. I still do not believe that.

Report No. 706: From Masha's YouTube channel. Hi, Baba Masha and her friends. I collected mukhomors myself. I take 1 g in the morning and in the evening. The effects appeared in two weeks. Mukhomor became an alarm clock, at 6:30 a.m. I woke up. I am shaken by **energy**. I microdosed for a month and a half, then there was an aversion to the mushroom. During the course I was craving for missionary work. I began to tell everyone how beautiful the mukhomor is. After that, my friends call me a mukhomor mushroom.

Report No. 707: Sent to Masha personally via Telegram messenger. Hello, Baba Masha! My wife and I read your book and have been taking red mukhomor microdoses for a week (0.5 in the morning, the same in the evening). I feel extremely positive effects, emotionally, psychologically, and physically, even up to the connection with the universe. My spouse gave birth two months ago and is now **breastfeeding** the child. Are there studies on the use of microdoses in breastfeeding?

Masha: Hello. For a child (or fetus), microdose turns into macrodose. I don't recommend it.

—And in the case of psilocybin? Should there be no consequences?

Masha: If you want to experiment with your child, this is your choice. I do not advise or consult on those topics.

Report No. 708: From Masha's YouTube channel. I've microdosed *Amanita muscaria* for one month. I feel super! Childhood colors around. **Mood** is good. In the evening I quickly fall **asleep**. The **depression** is gone.

Report No. 709: Sent to Masha personally via Telegram messenger. I take 0.1 g AM microdose overnight. Mild withdrawal to sleep. The dream is bright. The next day—calm rested state, similar to AD. **Mood** is raised. This is my second course. The first, in December, felt the same. A recognizable internal state of **calm** has arrived. In general, everything is fine.

Report No. 710: From Thomas's chat room. Good morning! I've microdosed for more than two months by 0.3 g. *Effects:* My face cleared from **acne**. I became more observational. I feel people more. I began to feel my body and its reactions to various events. Pleasant **relaxation** after intake. I see my internal fear clearer. I go to work with pleasure now.

Report No. 711: From Masha's YouTube channel. I've used the mukhomor for several years. I think it is the best medicine with wide spectrum of action. Immunity apparently increases. **Herpes**, **colds**, and other shit is cured quick. *Amanita muscaria* defeated my wife's terrible **allergy**. I persuaded her to take AM by showing my results. It worked. I recommend it to everyone, even to "critical individuals."

Report No. 712: From Masha's YouTube channel. Masha, please tell me, is it possible to consume AM during **breastfeeding**?

Masha: Dear Mammas! Come to your senses. Stop experimenting on your newborns. Your microdose is a trip dose for a baby. Isn't that obvious to you?

Report No. 713: From Masha's chat room. I have wild problems with **paranoia** and **physical nervousness** in general. AM microdosing helps, not perfectly, but I feel much better. That's considering I'm getting *Amanita muscaria* microdoses for two weeks.

Report No. 714: Sent to Masha personally via Telegram messenger. For three years I suffered from **pain** under the right underbelly, **bowel cramps** and pain in the solar plexus, especially after stress, and it was hard to breathe from this. Everything went away in five days of receiving the mukhomor.

Report No. 715: From Thomas's chat room. My mother had **heartburn** for years, as it turned out from lifelong prescription drugs and improper nutrition. Pills and other shit from her diet were removed. Mukhomor was added. The word *heartburn* was forgotten.

Report No. 716: Sent to Masha personally via Telegram messenger. Good time of day. Thank you for the work you're doing. I don't want to take a lot of your time, so it's short. In addition to the "standard" results, I wanted to note what I was surprised with after taking AM microdose: **Gum bleeding** went away. "Goose" skin texture decreased on the hands (this a lifetime problem, a hereditary feature of hair follicle's structure, as the dermatologist said; **pimples, acne**, and redness left in the neckline zone and the chin on the face. Neck **spasm left**, and the shoulders flattened. I got normal posture back. If I feel that the "psycho" in me awakens, I take piece of "sedative," after half an hour everything returns to normal. AM works as sleeping pill as well. Also, AM microdosing removed the desire to eat all sorts of shit, even my favorite coffee acquired a disgusting taste. **No more cigarettes and alcohol** in my life. I use fresh dried AM, not cured, for a month at the time. If I use cured, I need bigger dose, 0.3 vs. 1.5 g.

Report No. 717: Sent to Masha personally via Telegram messenger. Hi, I'm a subscriber. I don't remember if there was a questionnaire about the normalization of **digestion and stool regulation**. I'd like to share my observation. I clearly have improvements. Stool became more regular and easier. Previously, there were problems with constipation for two days in a row. Thank you for your work!

Report No. 718: Sent to Masha personally via Telegram messenger. Grandma, hello! My first report arrived. I microdose a red mukhomor for thirty-one days. First, I'll tell you why I came to microdosing. Last summer I had a surgery to remove polyps from the uterus. To prevent their re-growth, I was prescribed an annual course of oral contraceptives. The pills caused a lot of side effects: depression, insomnia, regular headaches, unbalanced libido, acute fear of death. I began to quarrel with people, my character deteriorated, I became plucky. I felt old and lonely. I gained weight. In quarantine I began to eat a lot of sweets, drink a bottle or two of wine a week. No energy, no desire to work. On weekends I stayed in bed, since there was no energy at all to even cook food. All my psychological problems escalated. I've never been so f* up in my life. I did not know that most of my conditions were due to side effects. I just thought that my life had completely turned into a terrible shit and nothing could be done about it. When I **stopped using pills, my mental state improved**. But the doctor offered to continue, and I refused. Somehow, I found your channel and ordered AM. And now about the results of microdosing: For thirty days my craving for **alcohol, sweets, red meat** has disappeared. **Appetite declined. I lost weight. Acne, dark skin spots were gone, skin has become cleaner. Skin papilloma shrank. Libido stabilized.** But the most important and amazing changes occurred with the psyche. I have **physical and mental energy**. I'm happy every day. At the very beginning of AM microdosing, there was generally pure joy as in childhood. Now a stable calm state of the psyche, **self-confidence. Self-sufficiency.** The head began to think better. I feel young, fresh again. I perceive difficulties calmly. I remember my former mental state and understand how bad it was. Now I see some events of my life from the outside. I can analyze them soberly. I began to clearly see toxic people in my environment and smoothly or sharply get rid of their company. The feeling that I am becoming free from stereotypes and can do what I want. Your videos, Grandma, opened up to me in a new way, and in general, I feel that I want to learn new things. Pulled to engage in house plants. I've already bought three. I study how to care for them. I take long walks in the forest next to my house. I really feel the pleasure of the silence of the forest and the nature around.

Report No. 719: From Masha's YouTube channel. Hello. Began to take 1 g AM then to slowly increase and did not feel anything. I reached a dose of 5 g in tea form, and it became nasty. Then I ate 7 g of AM powder with a spoon, felt smashed as the waves shake me badly. Tried 5 g twice a day— not good. What do I do wrong?

Masha: I suggest you download a free book from this channel and read what the AM microdose is.

Report No. 720: From Masha's YouTube channel. I microdosed for about three months, 1.5–2 g per day, morning and night. Currently, I stopped taking morning dose because I became very calm, and I feel that I no longer need it. Thanks to AM for these months, I figured out myself and my life flowed into the right channel, in which everything was great. I still take a night dose because it gives me magical lucid dreams, like second reality. By the way, I used to steadily drink 1–3 bottles of beer a month; since June as I began to microdose, I still haven't drunk anything, only tea or juice. It is difficult to explain, but there was a complete indifference to **alcohol**; it is even an unpleasant memory and the sensations of intoxication. For New Year's Eve I'm going to cook Soma from mukhomor. I think it's somehow more pleasant.

Report No. 721: From Masha's YouTube channel. Many thanks for the work, Masha. Thanks to kind people who share their experience here, in the comments. This summer I also met the mukhomor, very positive impressions remained.

Report No. 722: Sent to Masha personally via Telegram messenger. Hi, Baba Masha! With all due respect thank you for what you are! I want to share my experience with AM. I bought some online from couple of different places, relying on reviews. The first month I took 1 g ground and brewed in warm water with the addition of lemon juice. The **use of beer** was quickly minimized; there was a harmonious state and calm. Sometimes, I even caught some kind of bliss, took breaks in microdosing on average 1–2 days a week. Periodically tried to increase dosages, even reached 7 g. After three months I was taking dry hats, chewing and drinking water. The obvious improvements: I noticed resistance to various seasonal flu and cold. At work everyone gets sick several times, but not me. Now I take 1.5–2 g a day in the morning. It seems that the mental effects are gone. The mood is no longer so elevated. What would you advise to return that first-class action of the AM as it was in the beginning?

Masha: Your AM microdose course got too long. AM is not a stimulant that can be used on a permanent base. It is a medicine. **Overuse** of mukhomor gives a rollback to the previous state or worse. Stop taking it, and enjoy your life without stimulation. You are a healthy young man, and you do not need AM.

Report No. 723: From Thomas's chat room. I'm forty-seven years old. A year ago breast cancer with pleura metastasis was diagnosed. I went through high-dose chemistry, surgery, and radiation. According to doctors my oncology will never go away and we must constantly suppress it. I began taking AM microdoses more than a month ago. I took it in powder 3 g a day. I became more active, more fun, and happier. Tests got better; I feel great. Now I brew 3–5 g in a thermos and drink according to my need. I began not just walking, but I run, I passed 5 km or more. Doctors are very pleased with my results, because they predicted a completely different scenario.

Report No. 724: Sent to Masha personally via Telegram messenger. Yesterday I went to a job interview. I was scared. I took AM microdose two hours before. I was **confident** and there was **no fear**! I passed the interview.

Report No. 725: From Masha's YouTube channel. It's a pity that I did not see this video before. I am ten years on **baklosan [for pain relief]**. Two weeks of AM microdosing and I am free! Life is great!

Report No. 726: From Thomas's chat room. I started *Amanita muscaria* microdosing exactly two weeks ago about 1 g per day. There have been **kidney problems** in the past. All this time (two weeks) I experienced discomfort in the kidneys. This morning I got up and voila . . . nothing hurts!

Report No. 727: Sent to Masha personally via Telegram messenger. My friend has a third week of 1 g AM a day. Says the results are super. **Allergy** on her palms is gone. She's a hairdresser and works in latex gloves. I'll tell her to write a review. She said it was the best thing that ever happened to her. **Panic attacks have disappeared**. **Memory** has improved. In general, she is very pleased. My feedback will be later. I want to drink for a month and then draw conclusions.

Report No. 728: From Masha's chat room. My **appetite has decreased** on AM microdosing. For a month and a half, I lost 2 kg [4.4 pounds]. Yesterday was a stressful situation at work. I passed that with **ease**, not as usual, then I fell into sadness. Good!

Report No. 729: From Thomas's chat room. I want to confirm the statement that **mushrooms from different places are different**. I collected AM from two different places. Until today the microdose was 0.7 g from place number one. Today I decided to try from number two, the usual amount in the morning on empty stomach. Guys, they were stronger, I did not expect that. We need to calibrate AM microdoses for ourselves, because yes, mushrooms are different in strength from different places.

Report No. 730: Sent to Masha personally via Telegram messenger. Greetings to Grandma! I express my great gratitude for your contribution and all the information you bring to the world! I got acquainted with your work from your first channel. I wait for each issue like cartoons in my childhood and digest all the information very carefully. Separately, I want to express gratitude for the information about *Amanita*! The mushroom came to me two years ago. As soon as I heard about it, I immediately ordered from the western part of Ukraine and here I was born again. I steadily take microdose courses and I shine with happiness and warmth!

And now I will tell the story that AM helped me to overcome. In the month of August 2019, I picked up a **tick**, and as it turned out later it was poisonous. At the site of the bite, a red spot appeared that progressed every day; I went to the hospital and turned out to be infected with borreliosis. I was diagnosed with **Lyme disease**. Pills were prescribed and I was pushed to stay in the hospital under observation. I refused all these manipulations and left. By that time I had already read about mukhomor and decided it was time to test it on myself. Since I was told that borreliosis was hard to treat, without much thought I threw away all the pills; I was fasting and drank Soma AM drink. It became noticeably easier for me, the temperature went away, a fever disappeared, and there was a desire to get out of bed. I utilized about twenty AM caps and ran out. After a couple of days, the condition worsened and the pain was even stronger. I realized that I was on the right track; I ordered more AM and started to microdose a tablespoon. I ate it with pleasure as I clearly got better and I felt all the symptoms receded. As a result, in three months I ate 100 g of AM, and by December I forgot that I was bitten by a tick and what it is to be sick. At the request of relatives, in March, I decided to take tests for borreliosis, although I felt completely healthy. The tests showed that my blood was absolutely clean! Doctors could not understand what happened, but my blood was baby-clean. I told them about mukhomor, and they said that I destroyed my liver and pushed me to take tests. The results were 100% clean, and this finally finished off the doctors and our medicine. Today, I collect AM myself, making tincture, ointment, and so on. My mood has no boundaries, always at the highest level, health improved by 200%, as if I changed organs and a skin bag with new sensors. I feel each cell of my body. My nutrition radically became right and healthy. I refused meat for the second year, no desire. I don't want alcohol, I don't want to smoke marijuana as much as before, unless as a microdose, a couple times a month.

I'm surprised myself, but I really like it, I feel great! I'm a twenty-three-year-old man, and I love you, Granny.

Report No. 731: From Thomas's chat room. Good night to everyone! I want to share my experience with mukhomor for **coronavirus**. All family got sick: my husband, two-year-old daughter, and me (I am six months pregnant). Due to the fact that we all smeared the chest and throat with mukhomor ointment, the virus did not descend into the lungs. There was practically no cough. At the beginning I felt congestion in the chest, but as soon as I began to smear with ointment at night, the next morning neither the throat nor the chest were stuffed and irritated. After a week of this treatment, we all recovered. I still have a residual loss of taste and smell. Husband sniffed AM powder in both nostrils and as the result, the next morning sense of smell and taste appeared. Today at night I will also sniff dry mukhomor, just to check if it is a coincidence or not.

Report No. 732: Sent to Masha personally via Telegram messenger. Hello, Baba Masha! Today is about two months as I eat self-picked West Siberian mukhomors. I begin, perhaps, with a description of the "clinical picture" on the way to that event. Last few years I have been haunted by deep, happiness-devouring **depression**. I have abused alcohol for a sufficient number of years to become thoroughly attached to it. In general, I smoked and drank from an early age. The first time I was zero drunk at eleven years old. Periodically threw something "new" to test. Once, seven years ago, I sat on **drug spice** and some **fierce vampire powder** that provoked the aforementioned **depression**. By the age of thirty-two, the body gave unequivocal hints that continuing this course in life will have severe consequences if you continue to ignore it. But the habits were strong. Or rather, I was weak. The body was occupied by parasites that devoured me, and their appetite grew. I did two fasts, tried to change nutrition, to clean myself with other means. And all that seemed barely catchable, on the verge of a placebo.

A year ago I met with the mukhomor, and he declared himself quite vividly. I ordered myself an "eye opener," a source of bliss, a great helper—100 g of hats quickly ended up in my hands. No preparations in the form of fasting or any ascetic at all. I just chew caps and drink water. Somehow his majesty was not in a hurry to please the "master" and ran out of my mouth. Then the hour "X" came, and I managed to eat three to 8–10 cm caps, and mukhomor slightly greeted me. Inside me there was a sense of the presence of another person, a guest who seemed slightly disgusted to enter the temple of my body. I talked with my girlfriend, walked a little, and everything weathered in a couple of hours. The remaining caps were eventually thrown out a year later. To my surprise, the mukhomor itself burst into my life in September this year, when friends—lovers of the forest—began to brag about the harvests. I searched for information again and came across Baba Masha and Epifantsev (BM: Vladimir Epifantsev is a famous Russian actor; he managed 46 g dry AM trip and give an interview to warn the crowd— never, ever repeat that heroic action). Even my parents, whom I wanted to surprise with miraculous knowledge, already found themselves aware of this movement, watched some videos of Baba Masha and many others. After that I harvested and ate raw *Amanita* directly in the forest, mixed dry with raw during the day, making a tasty drink with honey and citric acid. There was a feeling of lightness, sober intoxication, cleansing thoughts, protecting the nervous system, facilitating the perception of reality, depression went away, the hope of leaving the vicious circle of passions and the oppression of invisible managers swept away.

For the first six weeks, I ate 1–2 times a day 3–4 g of dry, crushed mukhomor. About the sixth week, I began to raise dosages to 7–8 g of dry at a time, tried 10 g brewed in boiling water, and nothing. No effects except the tide of strength, which was sharply replaced by exhaustion and **depression**. I paused for several days, digested the lesson, and began to take 1.5 in the morning and evening. Today comes the third day, as my two-month reception course ended. Mukhomor is a wonderful, handsome, wise teacher and good friend. **Alcohol** left me right away, it prodded sharply, it caused me headaches. Several times in two months I drank alcohol, but I did it without the previous pleasure. Even drunkenness is not drunken; I felt the alien nature of this slurry and thought, why? But nicotine, on the contrary, tightened the belts, and I smoked double. The feeling was that the mukhomor wanted this, and he seemed to be guilty of notifying that we were quitting cigarettes a little later.

The cleaning process effects became increasingly pronounced. I lost about 5 kg [11 pounds], although I did not suffer from excess weight. After three sessions of liver tubing in the seventh week, there was a desire to abandon food of animal origin. It stopped pulling the **gallbladder**, and in general I felt my body better, which layer by layer continued to clean. It has become unbearable to listen to people talk with a curse word. I mentally shamed myself if some strong word slips my mouth because of habit. I want to interact with clean people. The understanding has come that the dirt in which we are all flooded here, most may not realize. There was a life model in which the flower of my planetary mission germinates.

Mukhomor helps us, and we in turn must help him. Help the knowledge to regain home. The house is in the minds and hearts of the maximum number of people from our surroundings, of course, those who are ready for this. The masses need mukhomor; it needs to be actively promoted.

Since yesterday I rejected the idea of **smoking cigarettes**, but I continue to blow pot. I hope that the psilocybin shrooms will come soon. I will share my experience with you and the world. Glad to have you, thank you!

Masha: Super! Excellent! Congratulations! At the end, what was the right successful dose for you? 1.5 g twice a day?

—Yes, but sometimes I missed a day or two, and it was a mistake. Mukhomor himself skillfully regulates these moments, makes it clear how much you need to eat and how often! Today, third day, as I stopped the reception, I decided to look around.

Report No. 733: Sent to Masha personally via Telegram messenger. Hello, my father has **multiple hernias** and he suffers from **pain**. Injections and pills do not help. I advised him to try AM tincture. The result—AM tincture helps the best of all medications. Please tell me how often you can use the tincture?

Masha: It should be used when needed, only when pain occurs.

Report No. 734: From Masha's chat room. Grandma, after a six-month AM microdose course I got rid of **skin fungus**, which had been with me all my life. It's probably a coincidence again.

Report No. 735: From Masha's chat room. My friend just reported to me, he lost interest in **alcohol** after a month of AM microdosing.

Report No. 736: From Masha's YouTube channel. After AM microdose course **vascular dystonia, panic attacks, pancreatitis pain** disappeared. Disgust with **alcohol** appeared. It works!

Report No. 737: From Thomas's chat room. AM microdosing is very individual, from 0.3 to 2 g. Above 2 g goes into the category of macrodosing. At first, when there were no scales, I took a heaping teaspoon, the condition was sluggish and sleepy, the head was cloudy, the back of the head was heavy. It turned out to be that my spoon was 2.4 g. Now, I take 0.5 g, and everything is excellent, **clarity** and a lot of **energy**.

Report No. 738: From Thomas's chat room.

—What is **the longest time of AM microdosing** you observed?

—Personally, my record was **six months**, then a break of several days and another six weeks. It's all individual. One day you realize that it's enough. Well, or some side effects appear.

—I've been practicing AM microdosing for about **ten years**. AM microdose courses two weeks.

—I have been with mukhomor since 2013. He helped me a lot.

Report No. 739: From Masha's YouTube channel. I microdosed for two months, 0.3 g twice a day—morning and evening. The goal was to give up **alcohol**. AM microdosing is a good thing, it helped me a lot. After the end of the course, there was no withdrawal syndrome.

Report No. 740: Sent to Masha personally via Telegram messenger. I microdose AM powder since September, 1–1.5 g per day, half for the night, half in the morning, occasionally 2 g, according to feelings. I am not interested in **alcohol**. Unfortunately, this did not work with smoking, although recently I notice that I began to smoke less cigarettes: earlier a pack a day, now one pack is enough for a couple of days, I want to quit altogether. Dreams are bright. I'm glad. **Performance and endurance have increased**. I have new hobby—cycling; I note that indicators are growing. I became calmer, I worry less about problems, it's easier to hold myself my grounds, I look philosophically at everything. Thanks for the educational activities, glad that one day I came across your channel in YouTube.

Report No. 741: Sent to Masha personally via Telegram messenger. Mukhomor cleans so deeply, but it takes two months at least. The environment still manages to bare my nerves, which mukhomor so carefully covers and protects. I am taking about 2 g in the morning and in the evening. My forty-six-year-old girlfriend was also convinced to take the mushroom. Mukhomor in the masses! People should know that there is an alternative to oblivion!

Report No. 742: From Masha's chat room. Two months of *Amanita muscaria* microdose course. I **quit smoking** cigarettes. I did not plan to quit but stopped after 2–3 weeks. Smoking experience, thirty-seven years. After a while **rejection to alcohol** appeared.

Report No. 743: From Masha's chat room. AM microdosing really helps in **sports**. I have great success at kickboxing, mainly on physical and functional level, intuition appears, there is less fear. Thanks to grandma for the information about *Amanita*.

Report No. 744: From Thomas's chat room. I take red for the second month. The first month I took 0.5 twice a day! The second month from 1–2.5 g once a day before bed! There is an increase in energy the next day and a **positive mood**, **easy wake up** even if I fell asleep very late (I work at night and I have broken schedule). **Anxiety and internal anger** passed. I experience a little nausea when taking more than 2 g. In general, I have positive effects! My wife also takes AM microdoses. I picked AM in Kaliningrad region.

Report No. 745: Sent to Masha personally via Telegram messenger. Hey, Baba Masha. I decided to write because I can't be silent. **I am an old druggy**. I used all possible chemicals during my search for happiness. **Alcohol** was daily chore. But all of that stopped with first weeks of AM microdose reception. I took AM microdoses for two months, from 0.3–1 g in powder. Sensations are unbelievable! **Clarity of mind**, **balance**, and **energy**. Thank you so much for being you.

Report No. 746: From Thomas's chat room. Hello to everyone. I want to share my impressions of using AM tincture. It did not suit me internally in the evening; I slept poorly and woke up a lot. But in the morning reception it was **energy** fire! I also had **problems with the scalp**. I rubbed tincture in my scalp after washing my head, while the hair and skin are still wet. The results: itching stopped immediately; greasy skin noticeably returned to normal. I thank *Amanita*.

Report No. 747: From Masha's chat room. I've eaten AM microdoses for a month and drank beer only a couple of times during this time. Although before that I **boozed** every day for five years in a row.

Report No. 748: From Thomas's chat room. Three weeks of dried mukhomor, 1.5 g twice a day gave me ten times more result than a year and a half of expensive **antidepressants**.

Report No. 749: Sent to Masha personally via Telegram messenger. Granny, hello! Today is my fifty-first day of reception. I wrote a month ago that my appetite and libido were reduced. The situation changed now—**appetite and libido** are good, especially libido is at the highest point of my life (BM: report from a woman). Now I am at a comfortable weight. I eat less salt, it is surprising. About AM microdose dosage—different batches of AM affect me differently. Therefore, I advise to carefully test new fungi and track the condition.

Report No. 750: Sent to Masha personally via Telegram messenger. Hello, Baba Masha. My observations on AM microdosing: I took it for twenty-one days, 0.5 in the morning and 1 g at night. I noted that I wake up a lot **more rested** than before after working night shift. My recommendations: do not mix *Amanita muscaria* microdoses with coffee.

Report No. 751: From Masha's chat room. My body has a happy birthday today! It totally refused **ethanol** after a month of AM microdoses. *Amanita* created a miracle!

Report No. 752: Sent to Masha personally via Telegram messenger. Good evening, Baba Masha. At the end of the year, I decided to summarize my success with AM microdosing: **rejection of alcohol, cigarettes, sugar, flour; smooth transition to veganism; completely quit smoking grass; lost 25 kg** [55 pounds]; returned to sports; got rid of **neurosis**; finally realized what I really love and want. This is my result in a year and a half of practice with AM and psi mushrooms, and this is only the beginning of my self-observation. Thank you, Grandma, hugs and kiss on the cheek.

Report No. 753: From Thomas's chat room. I take 0.5 AM microdose in the morning and 0.5 before bed. I **fall asleep** instantly; it was definitely not like that before.

Report No. 754: From Thomas's chat room. Another question about the **combination of mukhomor and psilocybin fungi** together. Separately, both courses work well, but if both are skewed together, then severe fatigue appears. Who has a similar experience?

Report No. 755: From Thomas's chat room. My mother successfully uses AM tincture as **painkiller with varicose veins.**

Report No. 756: From Masha's YouTube channel. Good day! Today is the sixteenth day as I take mukhomor microdoses. On the third day I gave up **cigarettes**. I can't understand why I used these cancer sticks before! The same story with **alcohol**! The world has acquired new colors and become brighter. Energy arrives, mood is great! There is no limit to perfection! Baba Masha, some thanks for the information shared with us.

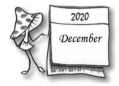

Report No. 757: Sent to Masha personally via Telegram messenger. Baba Masha, hi. I have feedback + question. I've been taking AM for a month. I keep a diary of observations. Here are my results: The **bowel function** was normalized. **Appetite decreased.** I **stopped gnawing my nails**; I've been unconsciously doing this all my life. **Stable, light, permanently positive mood.** Mental lightness. I don't even know how to explain it with words, but inside it's so easy and good, like I was inflated with air and I became a balloon. I am full of energy. All day I feel strength and vigor. And only at 11 o'clock in the evening is it like the battery is discharging and I understand that I want to sleep. Ego! The ego is practically silent! If earlier I achieved this with a lot of practices and meditations and did it forcibly for myself, now this has become my normal state. No emergency situations, I don't want to prove anything to anyone or argue, I became **calm.** I am phlegmatic, however, internally; I have always been inherent in self-esteem and constant internal dialogue with an alarming background. And now I'm still and balanced! It's such a thrill! I became an observer of my emotions and myself. In combination with all the previous results, I was happy for half a month, then it feels like a pullback. Now I feel the same as before AM microdosing. The energy's gone, the inner lightness, too. The only thing that has survived is Ego's silence. Question: Why does it not work for me anymore?

Masha: Please look at the voting post-AM microdosing effects stability. Anonymous poll.

Stable AM microdosing effects: 184 (75%)

Condition returned to its previous state: 54 (22%)

Condition became worse than before AM microdose reception: 7 (3%)

245 people voted so far.

Report No. 758: Sent to Masha personally via Telegram messenger. Hi, Masha! On the last review it would be necessary to note to the author that there are also some recipients of AM microdoses who have not experienced a small part of that wonderful impact described in thousands of reviews. It's all individual. Personally, to me, at a dosage of up to 1 g, I experience the effect of stimulation. More than a gram is a state of intoxication. With 5–6 g, a fever state.

Report No. 759: From Masha's YouTube channel. I dried my AM at 65°C–70°C [149°F–158°F] and ate 1 g before bed. I'm putting my signature under all the words about AM microdosing effects that Masha shared with us. All the effects are positive.

Report No. 760: From Masha's YouTube channel. I've taken AM microdoses since October 15, 2020, **sleep** has normalized. I'm glad, very pleased and alive.

Report No. 761: Sent to Masha personally via Telegram messenger. Good time. I want to share my experience with AM microdosing. In November of this year, I ate AM without understanding up to 7 g, and there were side effects. Now I take 0.2 per day, and that's enough.

Masha: What are your results from 0.2?

—The result is stable, **abdominal pain and stool disorder** have passed.

Masha: What were the goals of AM microdosing?

—Remove asthenia, learn to control my emotions, evaluate myself.

Masha: Is there success?

—**Asthenia** is gone. I am learning to **pay more attention to my actions**.

Report No. 762: From Thomas's chat room. Good morning! I recently read in Masha's AM microdosing reviews that a person began to laugh for no reason during AM microdose course. I started dancing in the morning while I am making breakfast. My AM microdose course is two months.

Report No. 763: From Masha's chat room. Mom is almost sixty. She took AM tincture drops for ten days. Her condition is noticeably changed, the **mood and performance** improved. She was on a pause for two weeks and came back to intake. No complaints.

Report No. 764: From Masha's chat room. I take AM microdose from 1–3 g in the morning. Aggression and fury left, earlier I could explode and curse at relatives easily. No more of that for many weeks. **Depression** is still with me, but I am less involved in it. Watching myself from the outside. No cheer, I am still lazy as before and forcing myself to study. Probably, I didn't get many effects because of the **quality of my mukhomors**. Caps burned while drying and have some black spots.

Report No. 765: From Masha's chat room. I met mukhomor a month ago. The attitude toward life has changed for the best. Finally, I get great **sleep** and do not overeat! I become more active, and everything in business and in relationships is easier. I have a clear understanding of what to do and how do it! Baba Masha, I thank you for information. I constantly watch your videos.

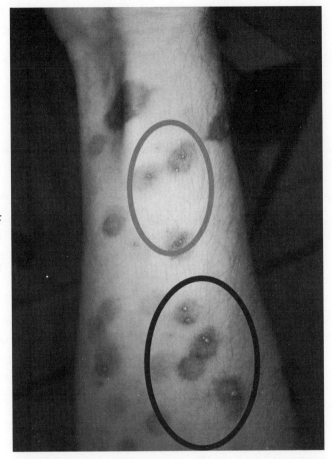

*Photo 4.
Comparison of
rash treated with
AM tincture vs.
nontreated rash*

Report No. 766: Sent to Masha personally via Telegram messenger. Now it is day eight of **chickenpox**. I smear AM tincture on the rashes. On the photo I circled [in grey] those that I smeared and in black those that did not smear. The difference appeared at day five. The same day I began to drink tincture from 5–10 drops. I could sleep well for the first time since I got sick. Also, depression, which turned out to be a companion to smallpox, went away. **Fever** passed; **appetite** came back.

Report No. 767: From Thomas's chat room. My mental state normalized after **depression** because of hormone intake. Cheer and joy appeared. **Papillomas** have diminished. The body was harmonized. Previously, without special drops and tablets, I could not **breathe** through my nose, now it's better, but not 100%, I'm experimenting in this area. I also solved a number of psychological problems, and AM microdosing helps a lot. There was a vision of situations from the outside. By the way, I relate to nature in different ways now, I walk a lot in the woods, I grow plants now.

Report No. 768: From Masha's YouTube channel. Hello to all and Baba Masha! Write it down in your reports for sure! After six months of AM microdosing my liver from fatty **hepatitis**, a stone left the kidney. All blood indicators are like a young girl! I am writing this after checking out of the Yekaterinburg regional hospital. I'm shocked! **Blood sugar** was 9–10, and now it does not rise above 7! I was diagnosed with **giardia and opisthorchis** before *Amanita muscaria* microdoses. It's all gone, and I did not take any meds.

Report No. 769: From Thomas's chat room. My mother was in a vegetable state. As soon as she recovered a bit and it became possible to talk to her, she began to take 0.5 g AM. She still continues with short breaks. She completely refused the pills. **Blood pressure** normalized; all the problems caused by the side effect of "lifelong" drugs passed.

Report No. 770: From Masha's chat room. The constant **chest pain** was gone; it's missing during AM microdose course. I got a great **sleep**; I haven't slept normally in five years. Emotions are in order; it was easier to accept everything as it is. I re-thought a lot. I became more **confident**. It is **easier to talk** to people. Longing disappeared; strength noticeably increased. Since **emotions are in order and under control**, I can make the right decisions in life.

Report No. 771: From Masha's chat room. I like to live in a positive state with confidence in myself and my strength. Thanks to mukhomor, he has safely contributed to that. I became **calmer, less annoyed** at the trifles. I am pleased with the result.

Report No. 772: From Masha's chat room. Hello to everyone. I am not long in this chat but have taken mukhomor already for two months. I started with 0.2 g and now I take around 0.5 g twice a day. There **were problems with the liver, stomach, intestine, and stool**. I am a forty-five-year-old woman. I spent a lot of money on hospitals in three years. And then I was acquainted with mukhomor. The stool got better, all the insides stopped hurting; that was my biggest victory that did not allow me to live. This happened because of *Amanita*. I still have problems with my sleep. I am hypotonic, my blood pressure 110/60, and it felt super. I still have panic attack episodes and headaches, once during this course, and I got better in two days. I stopped eating meat, I lost 2 kg [4.4 pounds]. I've smoked for a long time, I didn't quit, but I didn't mind. However, I began to **smoke less** by 50%. My mom is seventy-one, her joints deformed and in **pain**. The nervous system is not very good. Recently she was hallucinating and seeing people in the house, mice, and spiders. She took AM microdoses for 1.5 months. Mother became calm, not seeing any creatures. People, mice, and spiders left! We ran out of *Amanita,* and it's a disaster for her.

Report No. 773: Sent to Masha personally via Telegram messenger. Dear Baba Masha, Happy New Year! Thank you SO MUCH for all your videos, in particular on the subject of red mukhomor microdosing. Thank to *Amanita,* because I was able to **get out of a sad state** after losing a loved one. I confirm that the best way to use *Amanita muscaria* microdoses is the way Japanese scientists found, and it was described in one of your videos.

Report No. 774: From Thomas's chat room. I am sharing another *Amanita muscaria* microdosing benefit. I suffered from **migraine** all my life since school. I always carried headache pills with me. I rub AM tincture in my scalp during the migraine attack. In an hour, I am fine. The quality of life went up. I used to lie "dead" in bed a few days a month. I take 1 g AM microdose in the morning and in the evening. Wish health to all.

Report No. 775: From Thomas's chat room. AM normalizes **blood pressure**; I regularly check this on my mother. When she takes a break in AM microdose course, the blood pressure jumps up. She got obviously better right in 3–5 days from the beginning of mukhomor microdose course.

Report No. 776: From Masha's YouTube channel. In September was one year that I've been sober after three-month *Amanita muscaria* microdosing course. The reason for AM microdosing was use of **amphetamines, methadone, tramadol, cocaine,** and so on. I am totally clean now. Thank you very much to mukhomor and the individual merci, our Baba Masha for bringing me to this miracle of *Amanita muscaria* and for pushing the train, which in the future will change the whole planet. Thank you.

The following reports are from *Amanita muscaria* users in the United States. I know these people personally and I was witness to the results.

Report No. 777: I am a sixty-four-year-old woman. A dog scratched my leg. I was in **pain** for three days and wound got infected. Redness around the wound expanded and swelling increased. I put on a compress with *Amanita muscaria* alcohol tincture for two hours before I went to bed. The tincture took away the tenderness and pain in 10–15 minutes. In the morning the wound looked totally different—no redness, no discharge, no swelling. It was an amazing difference before and after.

Report No. 778: I am a seventy-year-old man. I got some *Amanita* tincture from a friend and never used it because I was suspicious about that particular mushroom. I started using tincture after experiencing **pain and swelling** in my big toe (spur). As a pain reliever AM tincture is the best. The pain would disappear in minutes. Then after a few days the swelling was gone and has stayed that way for over six months as I write this. I have also used AM for fast healing of cuts and bruises it works wonders. The use of dry *Amanita muscaria* fifteen minutes before bedtime gave me the ability to fall asleep quickly.

Report No. 779: I am a sixty-six-year-old woman. I was picking *Amanita muscaria* on the Pacific Coast and a tick bit me. Thank god it was a "healthy" **tick** with no Lyme disease. The bite was located on my back and I discovered it only at home after four hours. There was **pain and large red swelling** at the bite site. The compress with *Amanita muscaria* alcohol tincture always gives me quick relief from pain, redness, and burning sensation from tick or mosquito bites.

Report No. 780: I am a seventy-six-year-old man and I was diagnosed with prostate cancer. My surgery was scheduled in a month and at that time **my legs got seriously irritated and swollen**. The fluid was building up quick and meds did not help at all. I heard about *Amanita muscaria* from my friends and I decided to give it a chance. *Amanita muscaria* tincture brought my legs to normal condition in seven days, I put it on twice a day to the skin. I did not get much of the tincture and I was afraid that after it was gone, the legs would get swollen again. It did not happen! My surgeon was surprised, he asked me what I used, but I decided that I better keep that a secret.

Report No. 781: Last fall I was experiencing debilitating **pain** in my left foot due to an improperly healed fracture. I had been suffering with painful swelling and it was very painful to walk on. I have also suffered years with painful arthrosis in my knees. I ingested analgesics and used several topical ointments in hope of finding relief but unfortunately with no success. On September 10, I applied *Amanita* tincture to affected areas with an overnight compress. To my surprise, I wake up the next morning free of pain and swelling. I recommended tincture to my friend who also was suffering with a long-term ankle trauma. It helped her instantly after applying. I am a sixty-two-year-old woman and my girlfriend is sixty-six.

Report No. 782: I am a sixty-three-year-old woman who is an experienced mushroom forager. I have encountered **poisonous oak rash** all the time. The allergic reaction I experienced from the poison oak is alleviated by the use of AM tincture. It takes away the swelling, itching, redness, and rash left behind. I have been a consistent patient of chiropractic care because of chronic neck and back pain. When I applied the AM tincture to the affected areas for the first time, I got instant relief, I slept well, I woke up rejuvenated and regenerated. I cancelled three of my chiropractor appointments and finally when I saw him again, (three weeks later) he was so surprised to see such improvement with no adjustments and asked what kind of regimen I was following. I told him about the AM tincture and he was immediately curious to try it, as he has suffered with arthritis in his left shoulder.

Report No. 783: I am a thirty-six-year-old outdoor enthusiast, which includes hiking the forests of Northern California. I am **allergic to poison oak** and if I am not careful, I suffer with hives to my entire body. The only thing that gives me quick relief is the *Amanita muscaria* alcohol tincture. It takes away the pain and irritation as long as I reapply it consistently. I also suffer from constant pain in my neck, which is a long-term trauma from my past surfing activity. Only AM tincture gives me long-lasting relief.

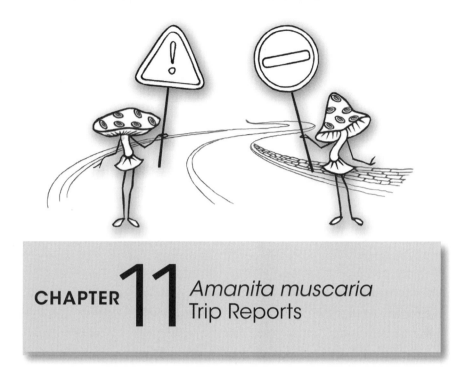

CHAPTER **11** *Amanita muscaria* Trip Reports

The universe is an intelligence test.

TIMOTHY LEARY

I have amassed a large compilation of unsuccessful *Amanita* trips that users sent to me, and I strongly recommend not taking the mushroom in a large amount. Mukhomor is a psychedelic—dissociative. The main psychoactive substances of mukhomor are ibotenic acid and muscimol. When large doses of *Amanita muscaria* are taken, changes are noted in the spheres of consciousness, thinking, perception, attention, self-identification, emotions, motor skills, orientation in space and time, behavior, self-knowledge, speech, memory, and so on.

Changes in the psyche vary individually, depending on the mental warehouse of the host, the quantity, and the potency of the particular fungus. The changes are alternation of activation and inhibition of the central nervous system, euphoria, motor and mental excitation, motor and mental exhaustion, a tide of physical forces, cheer, enthusiasm, intoxication, stupor, comatose state, abundant salivation, vomiting, tremor, drowsiness, kinestic parasthesia, reduction of critical thinking and control over reality, analgesia, hallucinations (visual, sonic, tactile), confusion, anxiety or joy, lack of will regulation, unmotivated aggression, inadequate behavior, getting into mental loop, repeated cyclic hallucinations, distortion of reality, disorientation, delirium, and so forth.

The danger of taking large doses of *Amanita muscaria* is associated with the phenomenon of dissociation (examples of it will given be in subsequent reviews). Dissociation in the *Amanita muscaria* trip is not only mental phenomena such as derealization or depersonalization but also a complete disconnection of thinking and awareness of reality accompanied by amnesia. There is also simultaneous uncontrolled, unrecognized destructive and aggressive body activity.

The trip dosage is undefined and not predictable. There is no guarantee or clear instructions. I ascertained knowledge of several cases of taking *Amanita muscaria* in larger doses without consequences, and then suddenly there was a complete and absolute disconnection from a much smaller amount of the same fungus batch by the same person.

Report No. 784: Hello, Baba Masha. I want to share my experience, perhaps it will be useful to someone. I ate two handfuls of dried AM caps. I definitely can't determine by mass, but my hand is quite large; it was sixteen or eighteen caps for sure. We were in the forest and assembled the tent. At first, there were no sensations, with the exception of abundant salivation. A little later I unexpectedly fell into the state of severe intoxication. Coordination of movement deteriorated, vision blurred, speech become incoherent. My condition was equal to 700–1000 ml of vodka intoxication. Somehow, I got into the tent and laid down. Then my consciousness plunged deep into me; I was very tiny, and there was huge space around. I began to separate— my consciousness remained tiny and my body began to grow and expand. Consciousness was forced to flee the body. I saw my bones, tissues, internal organs grow, and I ran endlessly along them with my internal self. It was continuous, running over and over and over. Each time I died and became small again, continuing to flee the ever-expanding outer self. This endless escape was so terrible that I went crazy, dying over and over again, with which I naturally felt pain from the bones constantly piercing me.

I wake up in a tent, in someone else's clothes, I did not understand why I went to the fire. I drank vodka and sat down. I was covered by the second wave. My vision. With a company of people, I walked through the field on a sunny summer day. Right in the center of the field was a house with bleached walls and a thatched hay roof. On the porch was a man who invited us to drink liquid from a flask. When we drank he said that it was poison and in order not to die, we need to speak some words.

He said the words, we repeated in a circle. Words added up in sentences, speed increased, my inner self screamed in the powerless impossibility to say these words more quickly. They're talking about World War II, about horrors, about pilots, about some night city battle, there was only fire, bursting shells, faces skewed by fear and anger. It was also repeated a number of times, but it was not as terrible as running within oneself. It was much easier to die from explosions than from bones piercing me. It didn't hurt that much. That was my mind.

My body, freed from consciousness at some point, left the tent, came to a cliff and jumped over it into the river fully clothed in sneakers and jacket. The body swam about 5 meters and drowned. My comrades got my breathless body out, and they pumped water out of me. For a while I was aggressive and out of my mind, and finally I fell asleep in the tent.

Report No. 785: Baba Masha, I want to share my experience with large doses to prevent people from mistakes. There are no rules with AM, and it is never sure what it will give and how much. I took 12 g four times, and I did not go further above light fractals. But next time with the same dose, I flew to hell, which I did not remember clearly. I wandered in the forest for a day, woke up in bushes. My clothes were ragged, I was covered in blood and wounds. The severe headache was bombing me for a week. Fingers were twitching for a long time; it was hard to find buttons on my phone. I could sleep at night. One plus—I completely rejected booze after that.

Report No. 786: Masha, two *Amanita pantherina* caps knocked my brain out of me. I was knocked out, smashed, killed, driven out of this reality. It took about ten hours. I was beating my body against the walls, covered with abrasions and cuts. Last five hours I lay down cold in my own blood and urine and without any signs of life. My friend sitter almost pooped in his pants from fear watching me, and thank god, he did not call a mental institution. I still am terrified of what I have done, and I have nightmares. Advise me what I can do to get out of the pit.

Report No. 787: My friend and I discovered mukhomor last year, and we ate 9–12 g dried. I advise—do not abuse it, because the consciousness changes so much that it threatens to disturb the psyche. As a result, my friend has a scattered personality, it's completely decayed. I agree that in small doses it certainly helps, but not in large amounts, as my observations showed a different result.

Report No. 788: I took the mukhomor in large amount and felt nothing; the second time I accepted even more and again almost nothing. For the third time I accepted much less than in the first, and then my brain went off. I woke up naked in the middle of the street with a shovel in my hands.

Report No. 789: A week ago I used mukhomor for the first time. Prior to this there was no experience of using psychedelics. I ate one dried *A. pantherina* cap. When that reality merged with the "other" world, I did not realize. Thanks to my brother and wife for not letting me hurt myself. It was a universal horror and nightmare. I was in an incoherent state, sweating with horror again and again.

Report No. 790: From Thomas's chat. I ate 2 g *A. pantherina* and went for a walk. Four hours I wandered on the streets, and then my consciousness was shut down for five hours, and the body continued to move in the city. I was taken to the hospital about 3 a.m. by some kind people. And another 2.5 hours comatose in intensive care, there I woke up tied to a bed with cuffs on my hands and legs with IVs in my veins. I gave the nurse a signal that I was awake; she looked at me with evil eyes and no longer reacted. The worst thing came to my mind that I killed someone, there was blood on my sheet, and I remembered some flashbacks of blood. Later on, they gave me back my clothes covered in vomit.

Report No. 791: From Masha's chat room. Oh . . . I do not advise anyone to take large doses of mukhomor! Control could be lost completely anytime. In my experience, after 11 g (half of them were *A. pantherina*) I was thrown into such hell with no contact to normal reality. The eternity of hell swept me uncontrollably to the point that I wanted to kill myself with a knife! I was lucky to have people nearby, and they saved me. It took two strong men to hold me down from killing myself, considering that I am a lightweight woman. Don't eat too much mukhomor! This will not turn out to be anything good.

Report No. 792: Masha's chat room. I would also like to warn those who think about "mukhomor trip." You infinitely underestimate the destructive power of what you will feel and what you can do in this state. You might totally lose your mind and get insane. I experienced depreciation of everything; this comprehensive eternity sucked everything itself, and everything that exists was puzzles of the endless cycle of eternity. I was depressed for a long time after that. By some miracle I did not cut off my arms and legs, but I made a mess of my apartment. I was very lucky that my close friend unexpectedly paid me a visit.

Report No. 793: Please be very careful! I ate mukhomor uncontrollably starting from 1 g, next 3 g, and then I ate 2–3 mushrooms at a time. It didn't last long. I ate five or six mushrooms and went to a dark unpleasant trip unprepared. It all ended with the ambulance arriving. Everything would have probably been ok if I had not inadvertently taken this mushroom again in a couple of days, this time only 1.5 g in order to sleep well. This time, I got another horror state, but I managed to escape to this reality. Consequences were much deeper than from the first trip. On the fifth day I went to the hospital because of the effects: vertigo, anxiety, nightmares, tremor, panic attacks, diarrhea. I am in shock.

Report No. 794: The story about what not to do, from me and my wife.

Wife: We ordered 54 g of mukhomor. We both took a quarter, about 12–13 g each, and went for a walk toward the forest. Within an hour there was an effect of light intoxication, gradually changing toward disorientation. I did not want to talk; it was difficult to do. My legs seemed light, as if they carried me themselves. We returned to the city, sat down, and then it began: I see only what is in the center, in front of me, and in the periphery everything flickers white. We went further, reached the traffic light, the euphoria began with hysterical laughter, from the fact that we are here, we are alive.

We were standing at the red light, and a minute stretched like five. For the next ten minutes, everything surprised me: we are alive, we love each other, there are people, there is life. Hysterical laughter did not stop. We reached another traffic light, and I did not want to go—I am afraid of cars, we will die. I became fixated on death, sat on the pavement next to a building, and my mind flew away. My whole life was shown in quick fast scrolls to this moment. And then death. The same place, the same time and dialogue:

"I love you. Love is the universe." "Do you remember Baba Masha?" "We . . . bought . . . fly agarics . . ."

And again: death, life, love, dialogue, over and over, at first slowly, then getting faster. Then the cycle of deaths began. All the bones break at once, and I crumble in the climax of pain, with each cycle increasing. After euphoria with pain, a struggle begins: first, two states slowly change, then faster, as a result, they merge into one single feeling. Then another scroll of my life, the happiest moments, the realization that the whole meaning of my life is in love; as a result, I wake up in the hospital, feeling that I was in a coma for sixty years, calling my husband, doctors say nothing in response. Again, I turn off, again death, again pain in different foci of the body, vicious laughter of doctors in the background. As it turned out later, I really got to the hospital by ambulance. I was tripping unconsciously for five hours. Absolutely all the time I was conscious, but the consciousness itself was not here; I do not remember reality at all. Emotions as a result are only positive, not counting the hospital.

Husband: I will add that yes, we are idiots, violated all the rules that are possible. I was lucky; forty minutes after consumption of fungus I puked it all. I got only light euphoria and slightly changed consciousness. How did my wife's trip look in my eyes? At a certain moment, she began to laugh hysterically in the middle of the street, then she froze, cried, and I could not contact her in any way anymore. Her eyes were wide open, I tried to wake her up. I dragged her in my arms to find some place because it was cold on the street and she had hypothermia. It all ended up with a call to ambulance. In the hospital, outside the emergency room I heard an awful wild wife's screaming. Doctors sent me home in a cab. I picked my wife up from the hospital in couple days. Thanks for the attention, love to all!

Report No. 795: From Masha's YouTube channel. Last year I took 40 g of red dried *Amanita* alone in the forest by a fire. I was out of my brain for three days. That will be enough for my whole life, I am lucky to be alive and sane. People, be more careful.

Report No. 796: From Masha's YouTube channel. My story of "microdosing." There were no psychedelics in my life. I started AM microdosing from 0.5 g and gradually increased 1–1.5 g. Changes went only for the better. Alcohol began to move away, it was a lot of energy, the selectivity of thoughts, food, behavior. But I wanted to try the border condition. I started to use 3 g twice a day until I unexpectable went on a trip with no warnings—change of consciousness and next—I woke up like from a bad sleep. I saw my death. But it turned out that everything is not so simple. The feeling that they threw the settings in my head; there was no feeling of love for my wife, for life, for work. I became a vegetable. The feeling that I would never experience these feelings was frightening. I was saved by my family; they sensed the changes and helped me. Little by little I came back to normal. After a while, I realized that it was NOT microdosing. I overdosed and got punishment for it. Now I pinch just a little piece from dry cap in the morning.

Report No. 797: First of all, I want to say: people, be careful. I drank tea from about 5 g dried *Amanita muscaria* and *pantherina*, 50/50. After an hour, my consciousness was separated, everything was falling out of my hands. There was a complete hell, dreadfulness, and horror. I tried to get to the sofa from the kitchen, fell down, got up, fell again, and passed out. Time stopped, I felt nothing. That terrible thing lasted for four hours. I couldn't feel my legs for a long time after I woke up. I realized I was lucky. Now only AM microdosing and only red mukhomor.

Report No. 798: From Masha's YouTube channel. Do not take the *A. pantherina*. I took it twice and two times overdosed with no high. I died a million times, then I puked for seven hours, so pathetic to the stomach. If you love your family, don't take it! I'm twenty. The cuckoo almost came out. I'm a fool.

Report No. 799: From Masha's YouTube channel. I just arrived from the hospital intensive care after 40 g of dried AM. First couple hours I was running fast like crazy in the apartment supplied with unrealistic energy that fueled me until the ambulance and the police arrived and interrupted my marathon. I ended up in intensive care.

Report No. 800: From Masha's YouTube channel. I ate four caps of *A. muscaria* and 2.5 caps of *A. pantherina*. I got in my car and drove about 5 km [3 miles] in the city rush hour to pay my bills at the office. In twenty minutes I felt that something is changing. I approached the office door, and the door bounced off of me, pushing me back again and again. I called my friend who lived nearby. I could not drive because I began to confuse the car's pedals. I got out of the car and decided to vomit all that I ate. Vomiting is the last that I remember. Two hours I was nowhere, while my friend found me, took me to his place. Then it began to clear up, I could not talk. I saw myself outside my body talking to my friends. Later on, I escaped and I went to the forest at the end of the city. I had a picture superimposed on the picture, a constant feeling that someone invisible was walking next to me. In the morning I woke up at home, like nothing happened. Now everything is normal, but as I remember that, I start shaking.

Report No. 801: From Masha's chat room. My friend ate a bunch of mukhomor raw stems walking through the forest. Soon he got crazy and started running like a furious moose in the forest. After that he completely disappeared somewhere, ran away from us, and we found him two hours later. He fell into the thicket and got knocked out.

Report No. 802: From Masha's chat room. My girlfriend ate a large dose of mukhomor. She was unconscious for hours and woke up bruised in a totally messed up room. She did not remember a thing.

Report No. 803: From Masha's YouTube channel. I want to tell you the story of my AM death trip. I ate *Amanita pantherina,* a quarter cap for a week. I really liked the effect. The energy was a high, mood was raised. Then I ate a medium-sized cap, thinking that it was safe. And everything happened so vaguely. I lost count of time. I passed out on the mattress and it seemed to me that I was a god. I created this world from one sensation and I needed to interrupt the chain in order to find a new embodiment. And I threw myself off the sixth floor. I broke all my ribs, injured my pelvis, broke six vertebrae, and I was ready to die. I woke up in intensive care. God! What a horror that was.

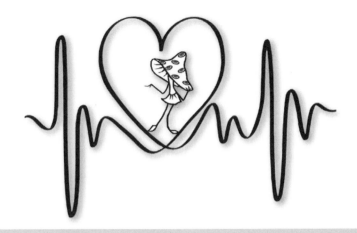

Final Thoughts
on *Amanita muscaria*

Baba Masha and Thomas express great gratitude to all participants of this exciting international project. The new season is not far off, and the study continues. The accumulation of material is taking its course—Telegram channels are open, and feedback arrives. This is a model of the "people's" medicine shared with the whole world. With your help this unique information has been collected for the first time, and many questions are still unanswered. The positive qualities of AM microdose reception are obvious. *Amanita muscaria* (mukhomor) has a long-term positive therapeutic potential with a number of nosological units. It is a promising painkiller and an effective sleep recovery resource. It provides a steady improvement in a person's mental state. *Amanita muscaria* alleviates symptoms of asthenia, depression, and existential agony. It initiates a rethinking of relations with the world, people, and even the user, as well as the destruction of complexes and conceptual stamps of perception of the world, and the ability to stay in balance and interact with others from this point of view. It activates the ability to see the colors of life and feel the value of one's own life and the significance of one's own existence. The importance of *Amanita muscaria* in the treatment of narcotic and drug addictions exceeds all currently known remedies.

We wish our fellow humans health and fun times here on this cozy and beautiful planet!

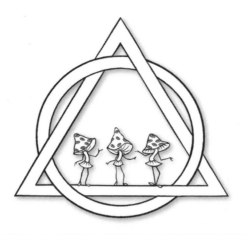

APPENDIX

Similarities in Biosynthetic Pathways in Humans and Fly Agaric

In this book I have provided my data on the effects of AM microdosing. Now I would like to address some interesting parallels between systematized material that I accumulated over a period of two years on AM microdosing effects. By carefully considering the actions and effects of naturally produced neurotransmitters, significant similarities can be found in the effects described below when taking AM microdoses.

Ibotenic acid, muscimol, and muscazone are structurally isoxazoles. Muscarine is structurally related to isoxazoles by a five-member ring in the molecular skeleton. Isoxazoles were reported for their various biological activities. Zhang systematically reviewed the recent researches and developments of the whole range of oxazole compounds as medicinal drugs, including antibacterial, antifungal, antiviral, antitubercular, anticancer, anti-inflammatory and analgesic, antidiabetic, antiparasitic, anti-obesitic, anti-neuropathic, antioxidative, as well as other biological activities.[1] Compounds containing the isoxazole ring serve as an important source of valuable drugs designed to treat infections and diseases of different etiologies.[2] There are reports on the immunoregulatory properties of isoxazole derivatives classified in several categories such as immunosuppressive, anti-inflammatory, immunoregulatory, and immunostimulatory compounds.[3] Among the described compounds, particular attention was paid to the class of immune stimulators with a potential application in chemotherapy patients. Isoxazoles exhibit anti-inflammatory, antimicrobial, antioxidant, and antifungal activities.[4]

The interesting findings are that *Amanita muscaria* fungus contains analogs—chemical compounds structurally similar to another—of three main human neurotransmitters: gamma aminobutyric acid (GABA), glutamate, and acetylcholine. Neurotransmitter receptors transmit the actions of bound neurotransmitters, thus enabling cell-to-cell communication in the nervous system.[5] Neurotransmitter receptors play a vital role in the normal functioning of the nervous system. Controlled modulation of neurotransmitter receptors is critical for proper signaling between nerve cells and effector organs. Factors that disrupt normal neurotransmitter signaling can alter the homeostasis, or balance, of the cells or tissues, leading to adverse effects.[6]

Ibotenic acid resembles and possesses structural similarity to the major stimulatory brain neurotransmitter glutamic acid (glutamate) and acts as a non-selective glutamate receptor agonist. Muscimol is a specific agonist of ionotropic GABA receptors and resembles and possesses structural similarity to the major inhibitory neurotransmitter gamma aminobutyric acid.[7]

Glutamic acid comes under the major group of neurotransmitters. The excitatory neurotransmission is mainly carried out by glutamate receptors in the mammalian nervous system.[8] It is the major workhorse neurotransmitter of the brain. It increases brain function and mental activity. It detoxifies the brain from ammonia by attaching itself to nitrogen atoms in the brain and helps in the transportation of potassium across the blood-brain barrier. It is conjectured that glutamate is involved in cognitive functions such as learning and memory in the brain, although excessive amounts may cause neuronal damage associated with diseases such as amyotrophic lateral sclerosis,

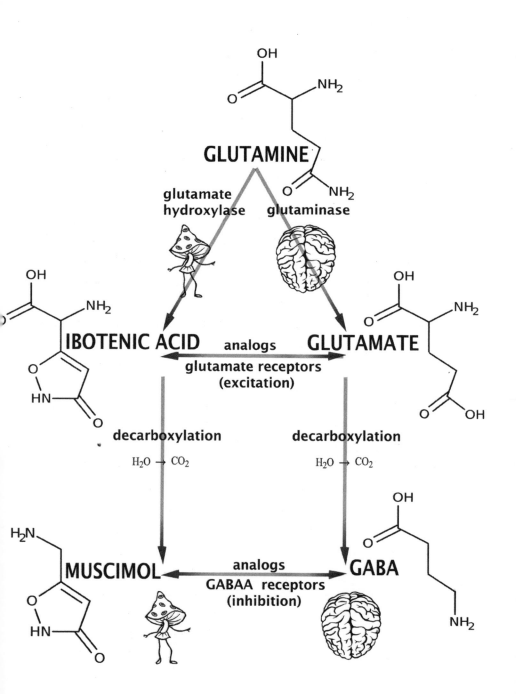

Fig. 80. Biosynthesis in Amanita muscaria and the human body

lathyrism, and Alzheimer's disease.[9] Glutamine is also an energy source for intestinal and immune cells. It helps maintain the barrier between the intestines and the rest of the body and aids with proper growth of intestinal cells. In health and disease the rate of glutamine consumption by immune cells is similar or greater than glucose.[10] Glutamine is an essential nutrient for lymphocyte proliferation and cytokine production, macrophage phagocytic plus secretory activities, and neutrophil bacterial killing.

GABA plays a role in the healthy functioning of the body's immune and endocrine systems, as well as in the regulation of appetite, metabolism, relaxation, pain relief, stress and anxiety, lower blood pressure, improved sleep, balanced mood, and alleviation of pain—a broad range of effects on the body and mind.

GABA is an important contributor to the body's overall mental and physical homeostasis. By inhibiting neural activity GABA facilitates sleep, reduces mental and physical stress, lowers anxiety, and creates a calmness of mood. GABA also plays an important role in regulating muscle tone in combination with glutamate, the body's most important excitatory neurotransmitter. There's also interesting emerging research about GABA's role in gut health and gastrointestinal function where it may work to support motility, control inflammation, support immune system function, and help regulate hormone activity.

Figure 80 (previous page) presents similarities of biosynthesis in *Amanita muscaria* and the human brain. Ibotenic acid biosynthesis in the fly agaric is initiated by glutamate hydroxylation.[11] These findings indicate that the ibo genes are responsible for ibotenic acid production in at least three *Amanita* species. The first committed step is glutamate hydroxylation by IboH, and the last step is decarboxylation of ibotenic acid to muscimol by IboD (tryptophan decarboxylase). This discovery revives the long-dormant research on biosynthesis in the fly agaric. Now it is obvious that the biosynthetic pathways in humans and fly agaric are similar: it reveals the reactions that lead to the isoxazole core in both species—human and *Amanita muscaria*.

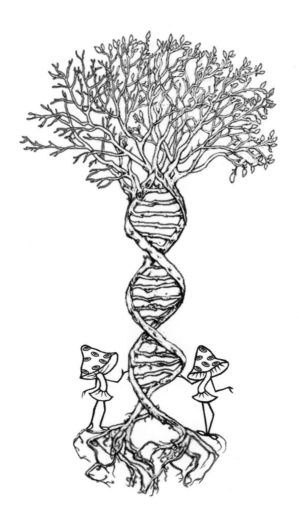

Notes

Foreword

1. Brown and Brown, *The Psychedelic Gospels*.
2. Rose, "The Poisoning of Count Achilles de Vecchj and the Origins of American Amateur Mycology," 37–55.
3. Rubel and Arora, "A Study of Cultural Bias in Field Guide Determinations of Mushroom Edibility Using the Iconic Mushroom, *Amanita muscaria*, as an Example," 223–43.
4. Viess, "Further Reflections on *Amanita muscaria* as an Edible Species," 42–50.

Chapter 1. Introduction to
Amanita muscaria

1. Geml et al., "Evidence for Stronger Inter- and Intracontinental Phylogeographic Structure in *Amanita Muscaria*," 694–701.
2. Geml et al., "Beringian Origins and Cryptic Speciation Events in the Fly Agaric (*Amanita muscaria*)," 225–39.
3. Michelot and Melendez-Howell, "*Amanita muscaria*," 131–46.
4. Spencer and Gillen, *The Native Tribes of Central Australia*.
5. Samorini, "The Oldest Representations of Hallucinogenic Mushrooms in the World," 69–78.
6. Heim, *Les Champignons Toxiques et Hallucinogenes;* Festi, *Funghiallucinogeni* [Hallucinogenic mushrooms].
7. Ruck et al., *Mushrooms, Myth & Mithras*.
8. Wasson, *Soma*.
9. Hoffman, "Entheogens (Psychedelic Drugs) and the Ancient Mystery Religions."

10. Hajicek-Dobberstein, "Soma Siddhas and Alchemical Enlightment," 99–118.

11. Allegro, *The End of a Road*.

12. J. C. King, *A Christian View of the Mushroom Myth*.

13. von Strahlenburg, *An Histori-Geographical Description of the North and Eastern Part of Europe and Asia*.

14. Krasheninnikov, *Description of the Land of Kamchatka*.

15. Krasheninnikov, *Description of the Land of Kamchatka*, 694–95.

16. Moser, *Keys to Agarics and Boleti;* Bresinsky and Besl, *A Colour Atlas of Poisonous Fungi;* Takashi et al., "Molecular Phylogeny of Japanese *Amanita* Species Based on Nucleotide Sequences of the Internal Transcribed Spacer Region of Nuclear Ribosomal DNA," 57–64; Néville and Poumarat, "Étude sur les Variations du Complexe d'*Amanita muscaria*," 277–381.

17. Liljefors et al., *Textbook of Drug Design and Discovery*.

18. Nielsen et al., "Excitatory Amino Acids," 725–31.

19. Snodgrass, "Use of 3H–Muscimol for GABA Receptors Studies," 392–94.

20. Kanasaki et al., "Gamma-Aminobutyric AcidA Receptor Agonist, Muscimol, Increases KiSS-1 Gene Expression in Hypothalamic Cell Models," 386–91.

21. Bowden et al., "Constituents of *Amanita muscaria*," 1359–60.

22. Frydenvang and Jensen, "Structures of Muscarine Picrate and Muscarine Tetraphenylborate," 985–90.

23. H. King, "The Isolation of Muscarine, the Potent Principle of *Amanita muscaria*," 1743–53.

24. Good et al., "Isolation and Characterization of Premuscimol and Muscazone from *Amanita muscaria*," 927–30.

25. Fritz et al., "The Structure of Muscazone," 2075–76; Reiner and Eugster, "Zurkenntnis des Muscazons. 24. Mitteilung uber Inhaltsstoffe von Fliegenpilzen," 128–36.

26. Stadelmann et al., "Investigations on the Distribution of the Stereoisomeric Muscarines within the Order of Agaricales," 2432–36.

27. Kögl et al., "Über Muscaridin. *Recueil des Travaux Chimiques des*

Pays-Bas," 278–81; Matsumoto et al., "Isolierung von (–) -R-4-Hydroxy-pyrrolidon-(2) und einigen weiteren Verbindungen aus *Amanita muscaria,*" 716–20; Chilton and Ott, "Toxic Metabolites of *Amanita pantherina, A. cothurnata, A. muscaria* and Other *Amanita* Species," 150–57; Döpp and Musso, "Fliegenpilzfarbstoffe, II," 3473–82; Musso, "The Pigments of Fly Agaric," 2843–53; Faulstich and Cochet-Meilhac, "Amatoxins in Edible Mushrooms," 73–75; Larcan et al., "Phalloidian Toxins," 233–72.

28. Deja et al., "Do Differences in Chemical Composition of Stem and Cap of *Amanita muscaria* Fruiting Bodies Correlate with Topsoil Type?"

29. Austin, 2013.

30. Tsunoda et al., "Change in Ibotenic Acid and Muscimol Contents in *Amanita muscaria* during Drying, Storing or Cooking," 153–60.

31. Tsujikawa et al., "Analysis of Hallucinogenic Constituents in *Amanita* Mushrooms Circulated in Japan," 172–78.

32. Tsujikawa et al., "Determination of Muscimol and Ibotenic Acid in *Amanita* Mushrooms by High-Performance Liquid Chromatography and Liquid Chromatography-Tandem Mass Spectrometry," 430–35.

33. Falandysz et al., "Metallic and Metalloid Elements in Various Developmental Stages of *Amanita muscaria* (L.) Lam," 174–82.

34. Kneifel and Bayer, "Stereochemistry and Total Synthesis of Amavadin, the Naturally Occurring Vanadium Compound of *Amanita muscaria,*" 3075–77.

35. Berry et al., "The Structural Characterization of Amavadin," 795–97.

36. Watkinson, "A Selenium-Accumulating Plant of the Humid Regions," 1239–40.

37. Michelot et al., "Update on Metal Content Profiles in Mushrooms," 1997–2012; Siobud-Dorokant et al., "Multivariate Analysis of Metal Concentration Profiles in Mushrooms," 315–70.

38. Kuehnelt et al., "Arsenic Compounds in Terrestrial Organisms I."

39. Festi and Bianchi, *"Amanita muscaria,"* 79–89.

40. Michelot and Melendez-Howell, *"Amanita muscaria,"* 131–46.

41. Lescaudron et al., "GM1 Ganglioside Effects on Astroglial Response in

the Rat Nucleus Basalis Magnocellularis and Its Cortical Projection Areas after Electrolytic or Ibotenic Lesions," 85–95.

42. Satora et al., "Fly Agaric (*Amanita muscaria*) Poisoning, Case Report and Review," 941–43.

43. Warrell, "Poisonous Plants and Aquatic Animals."

44. Benjamin, "Mushroom Poisoning in Infants and Children," 13–22.

45. Afonso et al., "Drugs of Abuse and Cardiotoxicity," 356–82.

46. Pérez Silva and Herrera Suárez, *Iconografia de Macromicetos de Mexico*.

47. Festi, *Funghiallucinogeni* [Hallucinogenic mushrooms].

48. Ott, "Recreational Use of Hallucinogenic Mushrooms in the United States," 231–43.

49. Catalfomo and Eugster, "L'Amanita Muscaria," 35–43.

50. Pahapill et al., "Tremor Arrest with Thalamic Microinjections of Muscimol in Patients with Essential Tremor," 249–52; Levy et al., "Lidocaine and Muscimol Microinjections in Subthalamic Nucleus Reverse Parkinsonian Symptoms," 2105–18.

51. Kondeva-Burdina et al., "Effects of *Amanita muscaria* Extract on Different in Vitro Neurotoxicity Models at Sub-Cellular and Cellular Levels," 110687.

52. Tamminga et al., "Stimulation of Prolactin and Growth Hormone Secretion by Muscimol, a Gamma-Aminobutyric Acid Agonist," 1348–51.

53. Tamminga et al, "Improvement in Tardive Dyskinesia after Muscimoltherapy," 595–98.

54. Krogsgaard-Larsen, "Muscimol Analogues," 584–88; Krogsgaard-Larsen et al., "Design of Excitatory Amino Acid Receptor Agonists, Partial Agonists and Antagonists," 515–37; Krogsgaard-Larsen et al., "GABA(A) Agonists and Partial Agonists," 1573–80; Tamminga et al., "Stimulation of Prolactin and Growth Hormone Secretion by Muscimol," 1348–51.

55. Matsumoto et al., "Isolierung von (–) -R-4-Hydroxy-pyrrolidon-(2) und einigen weiteren Verbindungen aus *Amanita muscaria*," 716–20.

56. Mandell and Sande, "Antimicrobial Agents," 1199–218.

57. Johnston, "Muscimol as an Ionotropic GABA Receptor Agonist," 1942–47.

58. Krogsgaard-Larsen, "THIP/Gaboxadol, a Unique GABA Agonist."

59. Johnston et al., "Herbal Products and GABA Receptors," 1095–101.

60. Krogsgaard-Larsen et al., "GABA(A) Agonists and Partial Agonists," 1573–80.

61. Ludvig et al., "Transmeningeal Muscimol Can Prevent Focal EEG Seizures in the Rat Neocortex without Stopping Multineuronal Activity in the Treated Area," 182–91.

62. Biziulevicius and Vaitkuviene, "Taking Advantage of the Experience in Ethnomedicinal Use of Mushrooms," 946–47.

63. Kiho et al., "Structure and Antitumor Activity of a Branched (1→3)-β-d-glucan from the Alkaline Extract of *Amanita muscaria*," 237–43.

64. Michelot and Melendez-Howell, "*Amanita muscaria*," 131–46.

65. Ruthes et al., "Fucomannogalactan and Glucan from Mushroom *Amanita muscaria*," 761–69.

66. Wilensky et al., "Rethinking the Fear Circuit," 12387–96.

67. Chapman et al., "Relation of Cortical Cell Orientation Selectivity to Alignment of Receptive Fields of the Geniculocortical Afferents That Arborize within a Single Orientation Column in Ferret Visual Cortex," 1347–58.

68. Beach and Wade, "Masculinisation of the Zebra Finch Song System," 324–34.

Chapter 3. *Amanita muscaria*
Microdose General Information

1. Tsunoda et al., "Change in Ibotenic Acid and Muscimol Contents in *Amanita muscaria* during Drying, Storing or Cooking," 153–60.

2. Fadiman, *The Psychedelic Explorer's Guide.*

3. Fadiman, *The Psychedelic Explorer's Guide.*

Chapter 4. *Amanita muscaria*
Microdose Effects on Various Conditions

1. Smith, "Can You Microdose to Treat Depression?"

2. Andersson and Kjellgren, "Twenty Percent Better with 20 Micrograms?," 63.

3. Johnson et al., "Long-Term Follow-Up of Psilocybin-Facilitated Smoking Cessation," 55–60.

4. Sewell et al., "Response of Cluster Headache to Psilocybin and LSD," 1920–22.

5. Andersson and Kjellgren, "Twenty Percent Better with 20 Micrograms?," 63.

Chapter 6. *Amanita muscaria*
Microdose Effects on Various Addictions

1. Chastain, "Alcohol, Neurotransmitter Systems, and Behavior," 329–35.

2. Zaiko et al., *Pathological Physiology*.

3. Zaridze et al., "Alcohol and Cause-Specific Mortality in Russia," 2201–14.

4. Zupanetsi et al., "Pharmaceutical Guardianship," 4.

5. Neafsey and Collins, "Moderate Alcohol Consumption and Cognitive Risk," 465–84.

6. Kornilov et al., "Parental Alcoholism and Mental Retardation."

7. Baykova and Merinov, "Influence of Parents' Alcoholism on Suicidal and Personality-Psychological Characteristics of Offspring," 547–58.

Appendix. Similarities in Biosynthetic
Pathways in Humans and Fly Agaric

1. Zhang et al., "Recent Advance in Oxazole-Based Medicinal Chemistry," 444–92.

2. Giomi et al., "Isoxazoles," 365–486.

3. Zimecki et al., "Isoxazole Derivatives as Regulators of Immune Functions," 2724.

4. Panda and Chowdary, "Synthesis of Novel Indolyl-Pyrimidine Anti-inflammatory, Antioxidant and Antibacterial Agents," 208–15.

5. McEnery and Siegel, "Neurotransmitter Receptors," 552–64.

6. Suppiramaniam et al., "Neurotransmitter Receptors," 101–28.

7. Liljefors et al., *Textbook of Drug Design and Discovery*.

8. Suppiramaniam et al., "Neurotransmitter Receptors," 101–28.

9. Dutta et al., "Glutamic Acid Analogues Used as Potent Anticancer," 263–72.

10. Cruzat et al., "Glutamine," 1564.

11. Obermaier and Müller, "Ibotenic Acid Biosynthesis in the Fly Agaric Is Initiated by Glutamate Hydroxylation," 12432–35.

Bibliography

Afonso, L., T. Mohamad, and A. Badheka. "Drugs of Abuse and Cardiotoxicity." *Comprehensive Toxicology* 13 (2018): 356–82.

Allegro, J. M. *The End of a Road*. London: McGibbon & Kee, 1970.

Andersson, M., and A. Kjellgren. "Twenty Percent Better with 20 Micrograms? A Qualitative Study of Psychedelic Microdosing Self-Rapports and Discussions on YouTube." *Harm Reduction Journal* 16, no. 1 (2019): 63.

Austin, Trent. Method for Producing Muscimol and/or Reducing Ibotenic Acid from Amanita Tissue. US Patent 8.784,835 B2, filed 2013.

Baykova, M. A., and A. V Merinov. "Influence of Parents' Alcoholism on Suicidal and Personality-Psychological Characteristics of Offspring" [in Russian]. *Russian Medical Biological Herald* 26, no. 4 (2018): 547–58.

Beach, L. Q., and J. Wade. "Masculinisation of the Zebra Finch Song System: Roles of Oestradiol and the Z-Chromosome Gene Tubulin-Specific Chaperone Protein A." *Journal of Neuroendocrinology* 27, no. 5 (2015): 324–34.

Benjamin, D. R. "Mushroom Poisoning in Infants and Children: The *Amanita pantherina/muscaria* Group." *Journal of Toxicology: Clinical Toxicology* 30, no. 1 (1992): 13–22.

Berry, R. E, E. M. Armstrong, R. L. Beddoes, D. Collison, S. N. Ertok, M. Helliwell, and C. D. Garner. "The Structural Characterization of Amavadin." *Angewandte Chemie International Edition* 38, no. 6 (1999): 795–97.

Biziulevicius, G. A., and A. Vaitkuviene. "Taking Advantage of the Experience in Ethnomedicinal Use of Mushrooms: Anti-Inflammatory and Related Pharmacological Activities of Fly Agaric (*Amanita muscaria*) Ethanolic Extract Deserve a Modern Evaluation." *Medical Hypotheses* 69, no. 4 (2007): 946–47.

Bogoraz-Tan, V. G. *The Chukchee.* Vol. 11. New York: E. J. Brill, 1904.

Bowden, K., A. C. Drysdale, and G. A. Mogey. "Constituents of Amanita Muscaria." *Nature* 206 (1965): 1359–60.

Bresinsky, A., and H. Besl. *A Colour Atlas of Poisonous Fungi.* London: Wolfe Publishing, 1990.

Brown, Jerry, and Julie Brown. *The Psychedelic Gospels: The Secret History of Hallucinogens in Christianity.* Rochester, Vt.: Park Street Press, 2016.

Catalfomo, P., and C. H. Eugster. "L'Amanita Muscaria: Connaissance Actuelle de Ses Principes Actifs." *Bulletin des Stupefiants* 22 (1970): 35–43.

Chapman, B., K. R. Zahs, and M. P. Stryker. "Relation of Cortical Cell Orientation Selectivity to Alignment of Receptive Fields of the Geniculocortical Afferents That Arborize within a Single Orientation Column in Ferret Visual Cortex." *Journal of Neuroscience* 17, no. 5 (1991): 1347–58.

Chastain, G. "Alcohol, Neurotransmitter Systems, and Behavior." *Journal of General Psychology* 133, no. 4 (2006): 329–35.

Chilton, W. S., and J. Ott. "Toxic Metabolites of *Amanita pantherina, A. Cothurnata, A. muscaria* and Other *Amanita* Species." *Lloydia* 39, no. 2–3 (1975): 150–57.

Cruzat, V., M. M. Rogero, N. K. Keane, R. Curi, and P. Newsholme. "Glutamine: Metabolism and Immune Function, Supplementation and Clinical Translation." *Nutrients* 10, no. 11 (2018): 1564.

Deja, S., P. Wieczorek, M. Halama, I. Jasicka-Misiak, P. Kafarski, A. Poliwoda, and P. Młynarz. "Do Differences in Chemical Composition of Stem and Cap of *Amanita muscaria* Fruiting Bodies Correlate with Topsoil Type?" *PLoS ONE* 9, no. 12 (2014): e104084.

Döpp, H., and H. Musso. "Fliegenpilzfarbstoffe, II. Isolierung und Chromophore der Farbstoffeaus *Amanita muscaria.*" *Chemische Berichte* 106 (1973): 3473–82.

Dutta, S., S. Ray, and K. Nagarajan. "Glutamic Acid Analogues Used as Potent Anticancer: A Review." *Der Pharma Chemica* 2, no. 2 (2011): 263–72.

———. "Glutamic Acid as Anticancer Agent: An Overview." *Saudi Pharmaceutical Journal* 21, no. 4 (2013): 337–43.

Fadiman, J. *The Psychedelic Explorer's Guide: Safe, Therapeutic, and Sacred Journeys*. Rochester, Vt.: Park Street Press, 2011.

Falandysz, J., A. Hanc, D. Baralkiewicz, J. Zhang, and R. Treu. "Metallic and Metalloid Elements in Various Developmental Stages of *Amanita muscaria* (L.) Lam." *Fungal Biology* 124, no. 3–4 (2020): 174–82.

Faulstich, H., and M. Cochet-Meilhac. "Amatoxins in edible mushrooms." *FEBS Letters* 64, no. 1 (1976): 73–75.

Festi, F. *Funghiallucinogeni: Aspettipsicofisiologici e Storici* [Hallucinogenic mushrooms: Psychophysiological and historical aspects]. Rovereto: Museo Civico, 1985.

Festi, F., and A. Bianchi. "*Amanita muscaria*." *Integration Journal of Mind-Moving Plants and Culture*, no. 2–3 (1992): 79–89.

Fritz, H., A. R. Gagneux, R. Zbinden, and C. H. Eugster. "The Structure of Muscazone." *Tetrahedron Letters* (1965): 2075–76.

Frydenvang, K., and B. Jensen. "Structures of Muscarine Picrate and Muscarine Tetraphenylborate." *Acta Crystallographica* C49, no. 5 (1993): 985–90.

Geml, J., G. A. Laursen, K. O'Neill, H. Nusbaum, and D. L. Taylor. "Beringian Origins and Cryptic Speciation Events in the Fly Agaric (*Amanita muscaria*)." *Molecular Ecology* 15, no. 1 (2005): 225–39.

Geml, J., R. E. Tulloss, G. A. Laursen, N. A. Sazanova, and D. L. Taylor. "Evidence for Stronger Inter- and Intracontinental Phylogeographic Structure in *Amanita muscaria*, a Wind-Dispersed Ectomycorrhizal Basidiomycete." *Molecular Phylogenetics and Evolution* 48, no. 2 (2008): 694–701.

Giomi, D., F. Cordero, and F. Machetti. "Isoxazoles." In *Five-Membered Rings with Two Heteroatoms, Each with Their Fused Carbocyclic Derivatives*, edited by J. A. Joule, 365–486. Vol. 4 of *Comprehensive Heterocyclic Chemistry III*, ed. A. Katritzky, C. A. Ramsden, E. F. Scriven, and R. J. K. Taylor. Amsterdam: Elsevier Science, 2008.

Goldsmith, O. *The Citizen of the World*. Dublin: Printed for George and Alex Ewing, 1762.

Good, R., G. F. Müller, and C. H. Eugster. "Isolation and Characterization of

Premuscimol and Muscazone from *Amanita muscaria* (L. ex Fr.). Hooker." *Helvetica Chimica Acta* 48 (1965): 927–30.

Hajicek-Dobberstein, S. "Soma Siddhas and Alchemical Enlightment: Psychedelic Mushrooms in Buddhist Tradition." *Journal of Ethnopharmacology* 48, no. 2 (1995): 99–118.

Heim, R. *Les Champignons Toxiques et Hallucinogenes.* Paris: Boubée, 1964.

Hoffman, M. A. "Entheogens (Psychedelic Drugs) and the Ancient Mystery Religions." In *Toxicology in Antiquity,* 2nd ed., edited by P. Wexler. Cambridge, Mass.: Academic Press, 2019.

Iohelson, V. I. *Samples of Folk Literature Yukaghir* [in Russian]. St. Petersburg, 1900.

Johnson, M. W., A. Garcia-Romeu, and R. R. Griffiths. "Long-Term Follow-Up of Psilocybin-Facilitated Smoking Cessation." *American Journal of Drug Alcohol Abuse* 43, no. 1 (2017): 55–60.

Johnstad, P. G. "Powerful Substances in Tiny Amounts: An Interview Study of Psychedelic Microdosing." *Nordic Studies on Alcohol and Drugs* 35 (2018): 39–51.

Johnston, G. A. "Muscimol as an Ionotropic GABA Receptor Agonist. *Neurochemical Research* 39, no. 10 (2014): 1942–47.

Johnston, G. A., M. Chebib, R. K. Duke, S. P. Fernandez, J. R. Hanrahan, T. Hinton, and K. N. Mewett. "Herbal Products and GABA Receptors." *Encyclopedia of Neuroscience* 4 (2009): 1095–101.

Kanasaki, H., T. Tumurbaatar, A. Oride, T. Hara, H. Okada, and S. Kyo. "Gamma-Aminobutyric AcidA Receptor Agonist, Muscimol, Increases KiSS-1 Gene Expression in Hypothalamic Cell Models." *Reproductive Medicine and Biology* 16, no. 4 (2017): 386–91.

Kiho, T., M. Katsurawaga, K. Nagai, S. Ukai, and M. Haga. "Structure and Antitumor Activity of a Branched $(1{\rightarrow}3)$-β-d-glucan from the Alkaline Extract of *Amanita muscaria.*" *Carbohydrate Research* 224, no. 7 (1992): 237–43.

King, H. "The Isolation of Muscarine, the Potent Principle of *Amanita muscaria.*" *Journal of the American Chemical Society, Transactions* 121 (1922): 1743–53.

King, J. C. *A Christian View of the Mushroom Myth*. London: Hodder & Stoughton, 1970.

Kneifel, H., and R. Bayer. "Stereochemistry and Total Synthesis of Amavadin, the Naturally Occurring Vanadium Compound of *Amanita muscaria*." *Journal of the American Chemical Society* 108, no. 11 (1986): 3075–77.

Kögl, F., C. A. Salemink, and P. L. Schuller. "Über Muscaridin." *Recueil des Travaux Chimiques des Pays-Bas* 79, no. 3 (1960): 278–81.

Kondeva-Burdina, M., M. Voynova, A. Shkondrov, D. Aluani, V. Tzanova, and I. Krasteva. "Effects of *Amanita muscaria* Extract on Different in Vitro Neurotoxicity Models at Sub-Cellular and Cellular Levels." *Food and Chemical Toxicology* 132 (2019): 110687.

Kornilov, A. A., A. M. Seledtsov, A. V. Maksimenko, V. S. Letunova, M. V. Krysyuk, and A. L. Novoseltsev. "Parental Alcoholism and Mental Retardation" [in Russian]. *Health Sciences* no. 1 (20) (2005):4.

Krasheninnikov, S. P. *Description of the Land of Kamchatka* [in Russian]. Vol. 2. St. Petersburg, Russia: Russian Imperial Academy of Science, 1755.

Krogsgaard-Larsen, P. "Muscimol Analogues. II. Synthesis of Some Bicyclic 3-Isoxazolol Zwitterions." *Acta Chemica Scandinavica* 31b (1977): 584–88.

———. "THIP/Gaboxadol, a Unique GABA Agonist." Elsevier Reference Module in Biomedical Sciences (online). Available online February 10, 2018. https://doi.org/10.1016/B978-0-12-801238-3.97290-8.

Krogsgaard-Larsen, P., B. Ebert, T. M. Lund, H. Bräuner-Osborn, F. A. Sløk, T. N. Johansen, L. Brehm, and U. Madsen. "Design of Excitatory Amino Acid Receptor Agonists, Partial Agonists and Antagonists: Ibotenic Acid as a Key Lead Structure." *European Journal of Medicinal Chemistry* 31, no. 7–8 (1996): 515–37.

Krogsgaard-Larsen, P., B. Frølund, T. Liljefors, and B. Ebert. "GABA(A) Agonists and Partial Agonists: THIP (Gaboxadol) as Non-Opioid Analgesic and Novel Type of Hypnotic." *Biochemical Pharmacology* 68, no. 8 (2004): 1573–80.

Kuehnelt, D., W. Goessler, and K. J. Irgolic. "Arsenic Compounds in Terrestrial Organisms I: *Collybiamaculata, collybiabutyracea* and *Amanita muscaria* from Arsenic Smelter Sites in Austria." *Applied Organometallic Chemistry* 11, no. 4 (1998): 289–96.

Larcan, A., M. Lamarche, and H. Lambert. "Phalloidian Toxins." [In French.] *Agressologie* 20 (1979): 233–72.

Lescaudron, L., B. S. Bitran, and D. G. Stein. "GM1 Ganglioside Effects on Astroglial Response in the Rat Nucleus Basalis Magnocellularis and Its Cortical Projection Areas after Electrolytic or Ibotenic Lesions." *Experimental Neurology* 116, no. 1 (1992): 85–95.

Levy, R., A. E. Lang, J. O. Dostrovsky, P. Pahapill, J. Romas, J. Saint-Cyr, and A. M. Lozano. "Lidocaine and Muscimol Microinjections in Subthalamic Nucleus Reverse Parkinsonian Symptoms." *Brain* 124, no. 10 (2001): 2105–18.

Liljefors, N., P. Krogsgaard-Larsen, and U. Madsen. *Textbook of Drug Design and Discovery.* 3rd ed. Boca Raton, Fla.: CRC Press, 2002.

Lindenau, Y. *Description of the Peoples of Siberia* [in Russian]. Moscow: Magadan Publishing House, first published in 1983.

Ludvig, N., H. M. Tang, N. S. Artan, P. Mirowski, G. Medveczky, S. L. Baptiste, S. Darisi, R. I. Kuzniecky, O. Devinsky, and J. A. French. "Transmeningeal Muscimol Can Prevent Focal EEG Seizures in the Rat Neocortex without Stopping Multineuronal Activity in the Treated Area." *Brain Research* 1385 (2011): 182–91.

Mandell, G. L., and M. A. Sande. "Antimicrobial Agents: Drugs Used in the Chemotherapy of Tuberculosis and Leprosy." In *Goodman & Gilman's the Pharmacological Basis of Therapeutics,* 8th ed., edited by A. G. Gilman, L. S. Goodman, T. W. Rail, and F. Murad, 1199–218. New York: MacMillan Publishing, 1992.

Matsumoto, T., W. Trueb, R. Gwinner, and C. H. Eugster. "Isolierung von (–) -R-4-Hydroxy-pyrrolidon-(2) und einigen weiteren Verbindungen aus *Amanita muscaria.*" *Helvetica Chimica Acta* 52 (1969): 716–20.

McEnery, M. W., and R. E. Siegel. "Neurotransmitter Receptors." In *Encyclopedia of the Neurological Sciences,* 2nd ed., edited by M. J. Aminoff and R. B. Daroff, 552–64. London: Elsevier, 2014.

Merck, K. *Ethnographic Materials of the Northeastern Geographic Expedition of 1785–1795* [in Russian]. Magadan, Russia: Kniznoe Izdatelstvo, 1978.

Michelot, D., and L. M. Melendez-Howell. *"Amanita muscaria:* Chemistry, Biology, Toxicology, and Ethnomycology." *Mycological Research* 107, no. 3 (2003): 131–46.

Michelot, D., E. Siobud, J. C. Doré, C. Viel, and F. Poirier. "Update on Metal Content Profiles in Mushrooms—Toxicological Implications and Tentative Approach to the Mechanisms of Bioaccumulation." *Toxicon* 36, no. 12 (1998): 1997–2012.

Moser, M. *Keys to Agarics and Boleti: Polyporales, Boletales, Agaricales, Russulales.* London: Roger Phillips Publishers, 1983.

Musso, H. "The Pigments of Fly Agaric, *Amanita muscaria." Tetrahedron* 35, no. 24 (1979): 2843–53.

Neafsey, E. J., and M. A. Collins. "Moderate Alcohol Consumption and Cognitive Risk." *Neuropsychiatric Disease and Treatment* 7 (2011): 465–84.

Néville, P., and S. Poumarat. "Étude sur les Variations du Complexe d'Amanita Muscaria." *Bulletin de la Société Mycologique de France* 117 (2001): 277–381.

Nielsen, E. Ø., A. Schousboe, S. H. Hansen, and P. Krogsgaard-Larsen. "Excitatory Amino Acids: Studies on the Biochemical and Chemical Stability of Ibotenic Acid and Related Compounds." *Journal of Neurochemistry* 45, no. 3 (1985): 725–31.

Obermaier, S., and M. Müller. "Ibotenic Acid Biosynthesis in the Fly Agaric Is Initiated by Glutamate Hydroxylation." *Angewandte Chemie International Edition* 59, no. 30 (2020): 12432–35.

Ott, J. "Recreational Use of Hallucinogenic Mushrooms in the United States." In *Handbook of Mushroom Poisoning: Diagnosis and Treatment,* edited by H. Rumack and E. Salzman, 231–43. West Palm Beach, Fla.: CRC, 1978.

Pahapill, P. A., R. Levy, J. O. Dostrovsky, K. D. Davis, A. R. Rezai, A. R. Tasker, and A. M. Lozano. "Tremor Arrest with Thalamic Microinjections of Muscimol in Patients with Essential Tremor." *Annals of Neurology* 46, no. 2 (1999): 249–52.

Panda, S. S., and P. V. R. Chowdary. "Synthesis of Novel Indolyl-Pyrimidine Anti-Inflammatory, Antioxidant and Antibacterial Agents." *Indian Journal of Pharmaceutical Sciences* 70, no. 2 (2008): 208–15.

Pérez Silva, E., and T. Herrera Suárez. *Iconografia de Macromicetos de Mexico: I Amanita*. Mexico: Instituto de Biologia, Universidad Nacional Autonoma de Mexico, 1991.

Reiner, R., and C. H. Eugster. "Zurkenntnis des Muscazons. 24. Mitteilung uber Inhaltsstoffe von Fliegenpilzen. *Helvetica Chimica Acta* 50, no. 1 (1967): 128–36.

Rose, David. "The Poisoning of Count Achilles de Vecchj and the Origins of American Amateur Mycology." *McIlvainea* 16, no. 1 (2006): 37–55.

Rubel, William, and David Arora. "A Study of Cultural Bias in Field Guide Determinations of Mushroom Edibility Using the Iconic Mushroom, *Amanita muscaria*, as an Example." *Economic Botany* 62, no. 3 (2008): 223–43.

Ruck, C., M. A. Hoffman, and J. Celdrán. *Mushrooms, Myth & Mithras: The Drug Cult That Civilized Europe*. San Francisco: City Lights Books, 2011.

Ruthes, A. C., E. R. Carbonero, M. M. Córdova, C. H. Baggio, G. L. Sassaki, P. A. J. Gorin, A. R. S. Santos, and M. Iacomini. "Fucomannogalactan and Glucan from Mushroom *Amanita muscaria*: Structure and Inflammatory Pain Inhibition." *Carbohydrate Polymers* 98, no. 1 (2013): 761–69.

Samorini, G. "The Oldest Representations of Hallucinogenic Mushrooms in the World (Sahara Desert, 9000–7000 B.P.)." *Integration Journal of Mind-Moving Plants and Culture,* no. 2/3 (1992): 69–78.

Satora, L., D. Pach, B. Butryn, P. Hydzik, and B. Balicka-Slusarczyk. "Fly Agaric (*Amanita muscaria*) Poisoning, Case Report and Review." *Toxicon* 45, no. 7 (2005): 941–43.

Sewell, R. A., J. H. Halpern, and H. G. Pope. "Response of Cluster Headache to Psilocybin and LSD." *Neurology* 66, no. 12 (2006): 1920–22.

Siobud-Dorokant, E., J. C. Dorée, D. Michelot, F. Poirier, and C. Viel. "Multivariate Analysis of Metal Concentration Profiles in Mushrooms." *Environmental Research* 10, no. 4 (1999): 315–70.

Smith, P. "Can You Microdose to Treat Depression?" The Third Wave (website), February 24, 2017.

Snodgrass, R. S. "Use of 3H–Muscimol for GABA Receptors Studies." *Nature* 273, no. 5661 (1978): 392–94.

Spencer, B., and F. J. Gillen. *The Native Tribes of Central Australia*. Cambridge, Mass.: Cambridge University Press, 2010.

Stadelmann, R. J., E. Müller, and C. H. Eugster. "Investigations on the Distribution of the Stereoisomeric Muscarines within the Order of Agaricales." *Helvetica Chimica Acta* 59, no. 7 (1976): 2432–36.

Steller, G. W. *Reise von Kamtschatkanach Amerika mit dem Commandeur-Capitän Bering: Ein Pendant Zudessen Beschreibung von Kamtschatka*. St. Petersburg: Johann Zacharias Logan, 1793.

Suppiramaniam, V., E. A. Abdel-Rahman, and K. Parameshwaran. "Neurotransmitter Receptors." In *Comprehensive Toxicology*, 2nd ed., edited by C. A. McQueen, 101–28. London: Elsevier, 2010.

Takashi, O., T. Chihiro, and M. Tsuda. "Molecular Phylogeny of Japanese *Amanita* Species Based on Nucleotide Sequences of the Internal Transcribed Spacer Region of Nuclear Ribosomal DNA." *Mycoscience* 40 (1999): 57–64.

Takemoto, T., T. Nakajima, and T. Yokobe. "Structure of Ibotenic Acid." *Yakugaku Zasshi* 84 (1964): 1232–33.

Tamminga, C. A., J. W. Crayton, and T. N. Chase. "Improvement in Tardive Dyskinesia after Muscimoltherapy." *Archives of General Psychiatry* 36, no. 5 (1979): 595–98.

———. "Muscimol: GABA Agonist Therapy in Schizophrenia." *American Journal of Psychiatry* 135, no. 6 (1978): 746–47.

Tamminga, C. A., A. Neophytides, T. N. Chase, and L. A. Frohman. "Stimulation of Prolactin and Growth Hormone Secretion by Muscimol, a Gamma-Aminobutyric Acid Agonist. *Journal of Clinical Endocrinology & Metabolism* 47, no. 6 (1978): 1348–51.

Tamminga, C. A., M. H. Schaffer, R. C. Smith, and J. M. Davis. "Schizophrenic Symptoms Improve with Apomorphine." *Science* 200, no. 4341 (1978): 567–68.

Tsujikawa, K., K. Kuwayama, H. Miyaguchi, T. Kanamori, Y. Iwata, H. Inoue, T. Yoshida, and T. Kishi. "Determination of Muscimol and Ibotenic Acid in *Amanita* Mushrooms by High-Performance Liquid Chromatography and Liquid Chromatography-Tandem Mass Spectrometry. *Journal of Chromatography B* 852 (2007): 430–35.

Tsujikawa, K., H. Mohri, K. Kuwayama, H. Miyaguchi, Y. Iwata, A. Gohda, S. Fukushima, H. Inoue, and T. Kishi. "Analysis of Hallucinogenic Constituents in *Amanita* Mushrooms Circulated in Japan." *Forensic Science International* 164 (2006): 172–78.

Tsunoda, K., N. Inoue, Y. Aoyagi, and T. Sugahara. "Change in Ibotenic Acid and Muscimol Contents in *Amanita muscaria* during Drying, Storing or Cooking." *Food Hygiene and Safety Science* 34, no. 2 (1993): 153–60.

———. "Simultaneous Analysis of Ibotenic Acid and Muscimol in Toxic Mushroom, *Amanita muscaria,* and Analytical Survey on Edible Mushrooms." *Food Hygiene and Safety Science* 34, no. 1 (1993): 12–17.

Viess, Debbie. "Further Reflections on *Amanita muscaria* as an Edible Species," *Mushroom, The Journal,* no. 110 (2011–2012): 42–50.

von Strahlenberg, P. J. *An Histori-Geographical Description of the North and Eastern Part of Europe and Asia; but More Particularly of Russia, Siberia, and Great Tartary.* London: W. Innys, R. Manby, and L. Gilliver, 1730.

Waldman, A. *A Really Good Day: How Microdosing Made a Mega Difference in My Mood, My Marriage, and My Life.* New York: Anchor Books, 2018.

Warrell, D. A. "Poisonous Plants and Aquatic Animals." In *Hunter's Tropical Medicine and Emerging Infectious Diseases,* 9th ed., edited by A. J. Magill, E. T. Ryan, D. Hill, and T. Solomon, 924. New York: Elsevier, 2013.

Wasson, R. G. *Soma: Divine Mushroom of Immortality.* New York: Harcourt, Brace & World, 1959.

Wasson, V. P., and R. G. Wasson. *Mushrooms, Russia, and History.* New York: Pantheon Books, 1957.

Watkinson, J. H. "A Selenium-Accumulating Plant of the Humid Regions: *Amanita muscaria.*" *Nature* 202, no. 4938 (1964): 1239–40.

Wilensky, A. E., G. E. Schafe, M. P. Kristensen, and J. E. LeDoux. "Rethinking the Fear Circuit: The Central Nucleus of the Amygdala Is Required for the Acquisition, Consolidation, and Expression of Pavlovian Fear Conditioning." *Journal of Neuroscience* 26, no. 48 (2006): 12387–96.

Wong, S. "Leading the High Life." *New Scientist* 234, no. 3130 (2017): 22–23.

World Health Organization. *Aminita [sic] muscaria, Amanita Pantherine and Others.* Group monograph available at Inchem (website), accessed November 29, 2021.

Zaiko, N. N., Y. V. Byts, and A. V. Ataman. *Pathological Physiology* [in Russian]. Kiev: Logos, 1996.

Zaridze, D., P. Brennan, J. Boreham, A. Boroda, R. Karpov, A. Lazarev, I. Konobeevskaya, V. Igitov, T. Terechova, P. Boffetta, and R. Peto. "Alcohol and Cause-Specific Mortality in Russia: A Retrospective Case-Control Study of 48,557 Adult Deaths." *Lancet* 373, no. 9682 (2009): 2201–14.

Zhang, H.-Z., Z.-L. Zhao, and C.-H. Zhou. "Recent Advance in Oxazole-Based Medicinal Chemistry." *European Journal of Medicinal Chemistry* 144 (2018): 444–92.

Zimecki, M., U. Bachor, and M. Maczynski. "Isoxazole Derivatives as Regulators of Immune Functions" [in Russian]. *Molecules* 23 (2018): 2724.

Zupanetsi, A., N. V. Bezdetko, and L. V. Derimedved. "Pharmaceutical Guardianship: Clinical and Pharmaceutical Aspects of the Use of Alcohol in Medicine" [in Russian]. National University of Pharmacy (Ukraine). *Provisor* 4 (2003).

Index